ETHICS & ISSUES
IN CONTEMPORARY NURSING

Margaret A. Burkhardt

PhD, RN, CS, FNP

Alvita K. Nathaniel

MSN, RN, CS, FNP

Dedication
To Joe and Tim

Delmar Publishers

an International Thomson Publishing company I(T)P®

Albany • Bonn • Boston • Cincinnati • Detroit • London • Madrid
Melbourne • Mexico City • New York • Pacific Grove • Paris • San Francisco
Singapore • Tokyo • Toronto • Washington

Cover design: Brucie Rosch
Cover photo courtesy of NYS Department of Economic Development

Delmar Staff

Publisher: William Brottmiller
Acquisitions Editor: Cathy Esperti
Assistant Editor: Hillary Everson-Schrauf

Project Editor: Pat Gillivan
Production Coordinator: Sandra Woods
Art and Design Coordinator: Carol D. Keohane

Printed in the United States of America
4 5 6 7 8 9 10 XXX 03 02 01 00

For more information, contact Delmar, 3 Columbia Circle, PO Box 15015, Albany, NY 12212-0515; or find us on the World Wide Web at http://www.delmar.com

International Division List

Japan:
Thomson Learning
Palaceside Building 5F
1-1-1 Hitotsubashi, Chiyoda-ku
Tokyo 100 0003 Japan
Tel: 813 5218 6544
Fax: 813 5218 6551

UK/Europe/Middle East:
Thomson Learning
Berkshire House
168-173 High Holborn
London
WC1V 7AA United Kingdom
Tel: 44 171 497 1422
Fax: 44 171 497 1426

Canada:
Nelson/Thomson Learning
1120 Birchmount Road
Scarborough, Ontario
Canada M1K 5G4
Tel: 416-752-9100
Fax: 416-752-8102

Australia/New Zealand
Nelson/Thomson Learning
102 Dodds Street
South Melbourne, Victoria 3205
Australia
Tel: 61 39 685 4111
Fax: 61 39 685 4199

Latin America:
Thomson Learning
Seneca, 53
Colonia Polanco
11560 Mexico D.F. Mexico
Tel: 525-281-2906
Fax: 525-281-2656

Asia:
Thomson Learning
60 Albert Street, #15-01
Albert Complex
Singapore 189969
Tel: 65 336 6411
Fax: 65 336 7411

Library of Congress Cataloging-in-Publication Data

Burkhardt, Margaret A.
  Ethics and issues in contemporary nursing / Margaret A. Burkhardt,
Alvita K. Nathaniel.
    p.   cm.
  Includes bibliographical references and index.
  ISBN 0-8273-7702-9
  1. Nursing ethics.   I. Nathaniel, Alvita K. II. Title.
  [DNLM: 1. Ethics, Nursing.   WY 85 B959e 1998]
RT85.B766   1998
174'.2—dc21
DNLM/DLC   97-38418
for Library of Congress   CIP

Contents

Preface   xiii
Acknowledgments   xvi

PART I   **Guides for Principled Behavior   1**

Chapter 1   **History of Nursing as an Ethical Science   2**
Objectives   2
Introduction   3
Influence of Social Need   3
Spiritual and Religious Influences   6
   Ancient Times   6
   Early Christian Era   7
   Middle Ages   8
   Renaissance and Reformation   10
Influence of the History of Women   11
   Ancient Times   12
   Early Christian Era   12
   Middle Ages   12
   Renaissance and Reformation   16
Summary   17
Chapter Highlights   17
Discussion Questions and Activities   18
References   18

Chapter 2   **Ethical Theory   20**
Objectives   20
Introduction   21
   Ethics and Nursing   22
Philosophy   23
Ethics   24
   Philosophical Basis for Ethical Theory   25
Theories of Ethics   26
   Utilitarianism   28
   Deontology   31
   Virtue Ethics   33
Summary   36

Chapter Highlights   36
Discussion Questions and Activities   37
References   37

Chapter 3   **Ethical Principles   39**
Objectives   39
Introduction   40
  Respect for Persons   40
Autonomy   40
  Recognizing Violations of Patient Autonomy   42
  Informed Consent   44
  Paternalism/Parentalism   45
  Noncompliance   46
Beneficence   47
Nonmaleficence   48
Veracity   50
Confidentiality   53
  Limits of Confidentiality   55
Justice   57
Fidelity   58
Summary   58
Chapter Highlights   58
Discussion Questions and Activities   59
References   61

Chapter 4   **Ethical Decision Making   63**
Objectives   63
Introduction   64
Ethical Dilemmas   64
  Practical Dilemmas   65
  Moral Distress   65
Making Decisions   66
  Nursing Process and Ethical Decision Making   67
  Scientific Process and Ethical Decision Making   67
Ethical Decision Making   68
  Emotions and Ethical Decisions   68
Process of Ethical Decision Making   69
  Gather Data and Identify Conflicting Moral Claims   70
  Identify Key Participants   70
  Determine Moral Perspective and Phase of Moral
    Development of Key Participants   70
  Determine Desired Outcomes   71
  Identify Options   71

Acting on the Choice   71
Evaluate Outcomes of Action   71
Applying the Decision Making Process   73
Gathering Data and Identifying Conflicting Moral Claims   73
Identifying Key Participants   74
Determining Moral Perspective and Phase of Moral
Development of Key Participants   74
Determining Desired Outcomes   74
Identifying Options   74
Acting on the Choice   75
Evaluating Outcomes of Action   75
Summary   75
Chapter Highlights   76
Discussion Questions and Activities   76
References   77

PART II   **Developing Principled Behavior   79**

Chapter 5   **Values Clarification   80**
Objectives   80
Introduction   81
What Are Values?   81
Moral Values   81
Acquiring Values   81
Self-Awareness   82
Enhancing Self-Awareness   83
Values in Professional Situations   85
Impact of Institutional Values   87
Clarifying Values with Patients   89
Summary   91
Chapter Highlights   91
Discussion Questions and Activities   92
References   92

Chapter 6   **Values Development   94**
Objectives   94
Introduction   95
Transcultural Considerations in Values Development   95
Theoretical Perspectives of Values Development   96
Piaget's Stages of Cognitive Development   96
Kohlberg's Theory of Moral Development   97
Gilligan's Study of the Psychological Development
of Women   98

Fowler's Stages of Faith Development   99
Some Nursing Considerations   101
Summary   103
Chapter Highlights   103
Discussion Questions and Activities   104
References   104

PART III   **Principled Behavior in the Professional Domain   107**

Chapter **7**   **Legal Issues   108**
Objectives   108
Introduction   109
Relationship Between Ethics and the Law   109
General Legal Concepts   111
    Sources of Law   111
    Types of Law   112
Recent Legal Trends   122
    Legal Trends Involving Managed Care Organizations   122
    Malpractice Claims Against Nurses   123
    Criminalization of Nurses' Professional Negligence   124
Risk Management   125
    Maintaining Communication with Patients   126
    Maintaining Conscientious Practice   126
    Maintaining Autonomy and Empowerment   127
    Liability Insurance   127
Nurses as Expert Witnesses   128
Summary   129
Chapter Highlights   130
Discussion Questions and Activities   130
References   131

Chapter **8**   **Professional Issues   133**
Objectives   133
Introduction   134
Professional Status   134
    Nurses as Professionals   136
Expertise   137
Autonomy   138
Accountability   141
    Mechanisms of Accountability   141
Authority   145
Unity   146
Summary   148

Chapter Highlights   148
Discussion Questions and Activities   149
References   149

Chapter 9   **Issues Involving Nurses and the System   151**
Objectives   151
Introduction   152
Problem Solving in the Professional Realm   152
    Attentiveness to Personal Values   153
    Obligation   153
    Determine Nature of the Problem   155
Nurses' Relationships with Institutions   157
Nurses' Relationships with Other Nurses   160
Nurses' Relationships with Physicians   162
Nurses' Relationships with Subordinates   164
Discrimination and Harassment   165
    Racial Discrimination   166
    Discrimination Against Persons with Disabilities   167
    Sexual Harassment and Discrimination   168
Summary   169
Chapter Highlights   169
Discussion Questions and Activities   170
References   170

Chapter 10   **Practice Issues Related to Technology   172**
Objectives   172
Introduction   173
Benefits and Challenges of Technology   173
    Quality of Life   174
    Principles of Beneficence and Nonmaleficence   175
Current Technology—Issues and Dilemmas   175
    Treating Patients: When to Intervene and to What End   175
    Issues of Life, Death, and Dying   176
    Medical Futility   179
    Do Not Resuscitate Orders   183
    Artificial Sources of Nutrition   185
    Legal Issues Related to Technology   186
    Examples of Potential Dilemmas with Other Technology   188
Nursing Practice in the Midst of Technology   190
    Attitudes and Values   191
    The Importance of Communication—Who Decides?   191
    Caring—The Human Focus   192
Summary   193

Chapter Highlights   193
Discussion Questions and Activities   194
References   194
Suggested Readings   195

Chapter 11   **Practice Issues Related to Patient Self-Determination   196**
Objectives   196
Introduction   197
Autonomy and Paternalism   197
   How Far Does Autonomy Go?   199
Informed Consent   200
   Decision Making Capacity   200
   Ethical and Legal Elements of Informed Consent   202
   Nursing Role and Responsibilities   204
   Advance Directives   205
Choices Concerning Life and Health   207
   Choices Regarding Recommended Treatment   208
   Controversial Choices   210
   Confidentiality   214
Summary   215
Chapter Highlights   215
Discussion Questions and Activities   216
References   217

Chapter 12   **Scholarship Issues   218**
Objectives   218
Introduction   219
Academic Honesty   219
Research Issues and Ethics   221
   Ethical Issues in Research   222
   Special Considerations: Vulnerable Populations   227
   More than Protection of Human Rights   227
Ethical Treatment of Data   229
Summary   230
Chapter Highlights   231
Discussion Questions and Activities   231
References   232

PART IV   **Global Issues That Impinge on Nursing Practice   233**

Chapter 13   **Health Care Changes and Challenges   234**
                 By Barbara Kupchak
                 Objectives   234
                 Introduction   235
                 A Brief History of Health Care Delivery
                   The Euro-American Experience   235
                     Early Eras of Health Care Delivery   236
                     Changes Through the Middle Ages and Reformation   237
                     Changes Influencing Development of Modern Health Care
                       in the United States   238
                 Health Care Perspectives—A Global Concern   243
                 Alternative Traditions of Health Care   246
                 Challenges for Rural and Urban Aggregates   247
                 Summary   248
                 Chapter Highlights   249
                 Discussion Questions and Activities   249
                 References   250
                 Suggested Readings   250

Chapter 14   **Political Issues   252**
                 Objectives   252
                 Introduction   253
                 Political Issues   253
                 Health Policy   257
                     The Health Policy Process   258
                     Ethics in Policy Making   260
                     Research Data in Policy Making   261
                 Nursing, Policy, and Politics   262
                     Policy Goals for Nursing   263
                 Lobbying   264
                     Methods of Lobbying   264
                     Political Campaigns   267
                 Summary   267
                 Chapter Highlights   267
                 Discussion Questions and Activities   268
                 References   268

Chapter 15   **Economic Issues   270**
                 Objectives   270
                 Introduction   271
                 Overview of Today's Health Care Economics   271

Distributive Justice   273
   Entitlement   273
   Fair Distribution   276
   Distribution of Resources   276
   Theories of Justice   277
Recent Trends and Health Economic Issues   278
   Health Care Reform   280
   The Move Toward Managed Care   280
Summary   282
Chapter Highlights   282
Discussion Questions and Activities   283
References   284

Chapter 16   **Social Issues   285**
By Mary Jo Butler
Objectives   285
Introduction   286
Social Issues   286
   Poverty   286
   Homelessness   288
   Domestic Violence   289
   Increasing Elder Population   291
   Racism   293
Ethical Principles Applied to Social Issues   294
   Justice   294
   Nonmaleficence   294
   Beneficence   294
   Autonomy   295
Personal Impediments to Intervening with Vulnerable Groups   295
   Victim Blaming   295
   Language of Violence   296
Social Issues and Scholarship   296
Summary   297
Chapter Highlights   298
Discussion Questions and Activities   298
References   298

Chapter 17   **Gender Issues   301**
By Sandra L. Cotton
Objectives   301
Introduction   302
Historical Perspectives and Overview of Gender Based Issues   302
   Societal Expectations   302

Gender and Race   303
Sex Discrimination in Nursing   304
  Gender Issues in Women's Health   305
  Expanding Numbers of Men in the Profession   305
  Gender and Caring   306
Sexual Harassment in Nursing   307
Communication Issues Related to Gender   308
  The Doctor-Nurse Game   308
  Communicating with Patients   309
  Gossip   310
Modern Sexism   310
Sexual Orientation   311
Summary   312
Chapter Highlights   312
Discussion Questions and Activities   313
References   313

Chapter 18   **Transcultural and Spiritual Issues   317**
Written in collaboration with Mary Gail Nagai-Jacobson

Objectives   317
Introduction   318
Transcultural Issues   318
  Understanding Culture   319
  Cultural Values and Beliefs   320
  Culture and the Health Care System   324
  Complementary Therapies   325
  Legal Considerations Related to Transcultural Issues   326
Issues Related to Spirituality and Religion   327
  Approaching Spirituality   327
  Spirituality and Religion   329
  Nurturing Spirit   331
Summary   331
Chapter Highlights   332
Discussion Questions and Activities   332
References   333

PART V   **The Power to Make a Difference   335**

Chapter 19   **Empowerment for Nurses   336**
Written in collaboration with Barbara C. Banonis

Objectives   336
Introduction   337
Influences on Nursing's Perceptions of Principled Practice   337

Influence of Mind Sets   337
Metaphors of Nursing   338
How Nursing Is Perceived by Others   339
Understanding Power and Empowerment   340
Personal Empowerment   341
Professional Empowerment   343
Unity in Diversity   344
Re-Visioning Nursing   344
Summary   346
Chapter Highlights   346
Discussion Questions and Activities   347
References   347

Chapter 20   **Enabling Patient Empowerment   349**
Objectives   349
Introduction   350
Patients and Empowerment   350
Nurses and Patient Empowerment   350
Attitudes of Nurses That Enable Empowerment   350
Nursing Knowledge and Skills Necessary
for Enabling Empowerment   351
Enhancing Patient Capacity for Decision Making   352
Barriers to Empowerment   353
Fostering Patient Empowerment   353
Summary   354
Chapter Highlights   355
Discussion Questions and Activities   355
References   356

APPENDIX A   **American Nurses Association: Code for Nurses with
Interpretive Statements   357**

APPENDIX B   **American Hospital Association: A Patient's Bill of Rights   370**

APPENDIX C   **Canadian Nurses Association: Code of Ethics for
Registered Nurses   374**

APPENDIX D   **International Council of Nurses: Code for Nurses—
Ethical Concepts Applied to Nursing   382**

Glossary   385
Index   396

Preface

We who lived in the concentration camps can remember the men who walked through the huts comforting others, giving away their last piece of bread. They may have been few in number, but they offer sufficient proof that everything can be taken from a man but one thing: The last of his freedoms—to choose one's attitude in any given set of circumstances, to choose one's own way.

(Frankl, 1984, p. 86)

As contemporary nurses, we must deal with the challenge of facing complex personal, interpersonal, professional, institutional, and social issues. Appropriate responses to these issues are seldom clear. Ethical dilemmas, in particular, involve choices with no clearly correct solutions. We believe that declaring that there is one correct approach to solving ethical problems risks imposing personal values on others. We must be sensitive to that possibility and recognize that our responses to dilemmas depend upon such variables as contextual factors, patient and family values, relationships, moral development, religious beliefs, spiritual perspective, cultural orientation, and legal constraints.

It is our intention in this book to (1) acknowledge that each person is a moral agent, (2) raise awareness of the myriad of factors that need to be considered when dealing with ethical decisions, (3) present a decision making model to help individuals learn to process information and move toward action, and (4) affirm nursing as an ethically responsible profession. We present ethical issues from the perspective of nursing, recognizing that relationships and the authority to make decisions are affected by contextual factors such as professional status; gender; the development of the profession; personal ethical stance; social, economic, institutional, and political climate; and personal and professional empowerment.

Dealing with ethical issues requires skill in the processes of values clarification, ethical decision making, self-awareness, empowerment, transcultural sensitivity, and challenging injustice. The text poses questions about contemporary issues and provides processes for the development of sensitivity and skill in resolving ethical problems. Highlighting nurses in a variety of settings and roles, exercises and activities are intended to facilitate self-reflection and awareness of personal approaches to issues and decision making. Our goal is that you will become engaged in active learning throughout the text through the use of *Case Presentations* based upon real-life situations, *Ask Yourself* and *Think About It* exercises derived from thought provoking material and case presentations, and *Discussion Questions and Activities.*

Though acknowledging the rich and divergent history of nursing in other cultures, we have chosen to write primarily from the Western perspective. The background that we give explains the many factors that lead to social systems which either encourage or prohibit certain people from critically examining issues and making authoritative decisions. The book begins with a chapter that explores the impact of historical factors, particularly religion and gender, on the profession of nursing in Western culture. We hope that this will help you to more fully understand the context of nursing and question arbitrary and artificial barriers to ethical decision making.

With a strong groundwork of ethical theories and principles in Part I, subsequent chapters deal with various issues as they pertain to ethics and ethical decision making. As you explore political, professional, legal, social, and gender issues, we encourage you to look at the related ethical questions and to continually move back and forth from the concrete to the abstract, from the general to the specific, from the global to the personal, and from issue to principle—recognizing the interrelatedness of many factors.

Principled behavior in personal and professional situations is the organizing theme of this text. Beginning with a brief descriptive history of nursing as it relates to ethics, Part I, *Guides for Principled Behavior,* presents ethical theories, models, and principles that serve as guides for principled behavior. Part II, *Developing Principled Behavior,* discusses personal issues including values clarification and moral development. Part III, *Principled Behavior in the Professional Domain,* presents professional and legal overviews and chapters related to specific issues important to contemporary nursing. This section includes discussion about autonomy, authority, accountability, codes of practice, scholarship issues, practice issues related to health care providers, systems within which nurses work, technology, and patient self-determination. Part IV, *Global Issues That Impinge on Nursing Practice,* addresses health care changes and challenges as a background for understanding issues that nurses encounter in the contemporary health care system. Considerations related to political, economic, social, gender, transcultural, and spirituality issues are discussed in light of nursing role, potential dilemmas, and professional practice. Part V, *The Power to Make a Difference,* focuses on developing skills to empower both nurses and patients to make principled choices and act with courage.

Throughout this book, we have chosen to refer to the recipient of nursing care as *patient* rather than *client.* Since nurses function as members of interdisciplinary health care teams and the term *patient* is commonly used by other health providers, using a common language fosters better communication, understanding, and collegiality. In addition, the American Nurses Association (1996) *Nursing's Social Policy Statement* notes that though the term *client* is preferred by some nurses, it implies that the recipient of care is able to choose one nurse from among many, a choice that typically does nor occur. We recognize that the term *client, person,* or *individual* may be the better choice in some circumstances and encourage the reader to make that distinction if needed.

Though we have written from the Western perspective, we recognize that our culture is a melding of traditions and people from many other cultures. We have attempted to be sensitive in reflecting transcultural situations and issues. In that vein, you will notice that when referring to the dates of historical events, we have used the designation *B.C.E.* (Before the Common Era) rather than the more familiar *B.C.*

This book is meant to be very personal. You should become engaged, examining and questioning your options and values as they relate to real-life situations. As learning is demonstrated by changed behavior, we hope that you will become a more sensitive, capable, courageous, and responsible decision maker and citizen. We believe with Phyllis Kritek (1994) that "the measure of [one's] character and worth is not whether [one has] avoided making poor choices, but how willing [one is] to learn from these errors in an effort to not repeat them, and how [one elects] to attend to their consequences. . . . Finding meaning, discovering that which is of worth, becomes a searching process where everyone's help is welcome." (pp. 21, 33). This book is offered as a guide to help in the process of learning to make sound choices and act in principled ways in both personal and professional realms. As you use this book, we echo the same sentiment voiced by Florence Nightingale in the preface to her *Notes on Nursing:* "I do not pretend to teach her how, I ask her to teach herself, and for this purpose I venture to give her some hints" (1859, preface).

REFERENCES

American Nurses Association. (1996). *Nursing's social policy statement.* Washington, DC: Author.

Frankl, V. E. (1984). *Man's search for meaning* (Rev. ed.). New York: Washington Square Press.

Kritek, P. B. (1994). *Negotiating at an uneven table: A practical approach to working with difference and diversity.* San Francisco: Jossey-Bass.

Nightingale, F. (1859). *Notes on nursing: What it is, and what it is not.* London: Harrison & Sons.

Delmar Publishers' Online Services
To access Delmar on the World Wide Web, point your browser to:
http://www.DelmarNursing.com
To access through Gopher: gopher://gopher.delmar.com
(Delmar Online is part of "thomson.com", an internet site with information
on more than 30 publishers of the International Thomson Publishing organization.)
For information on our products and services:
email: info@delmar.com
Or call 800–347–7707

Acknowledgments

The journey of writing a book requires solitude and the companionship and support of many people. We express gratitude to the many friends and colleagues who have encouraged us along the way. Special thanks are due to Mary Jo Butler who, in her role as director of the Charleston Division of WVU School of Nursing, has encouraged scholarship and principled behavior in the midst of challenges to both. We are grateful to Barbara C. Banonis, Mary Jo Butler, Sandra L. Cotton, Barbara Kupchak, and Mary Gail Nagai-Jacobson for their chapter contributions, and to Anna Nicoloudakis for secretarial assistance and general support in innumerable ways. Thanks go to all those who gave the time and care to review the manuscript at various stages in the writing process, providing us with helpful comments and guidance, particularly to our reviewers Dr. Luz Porter, Dr. Harriet Duncan, and Mary Gail Nagai-Jacobson; to Candy Stanley; and most especially to Hilary A. Schrauf, assistant editor at Delmar Publishers, through whose guidance we have been able to stay on track and reach our journey's destination.

Finally, we are eternally grateful to our families, Joe Golden and Tim, Josh, and Maggie Nathaniel, for their loving patience, humor, caretaking, and encouragement throughout this challenging and growthful journey.

Contributors

Barbara C. Banonis, MSN, RN
Well-Being Consultant
LifeQuest International
Charleston, WV

Mary Jo Butler, EdD, RN
Associate Professor and Director
West Virginia University
School of Nursing, Charleston Division
Charleston, WV

Sandra L. Cotton, MS, RN, C-ANP
Instructor
West Virginia University
School of Nursing
Morgantown, WV

Sr. Barbara Kupchak, PhD, RN-C
Associate Professor
West Virginia University
School of Nursing
Morgantown, WV

Mary Gail Nagai-Jacobson, MSN, RN
Community Health Consultant
San Marcos, TX

PART I

GUIDES FOR PRINCIPLED BEHAVIOR

Part I lays a foundation for nurses to begin critically examining issues and systematically participating in ethical decision making. Examining the history and context of nursing in Western cultures, Chapter 1 gives nurses insight into the profession of nursing as part of an overall social system—focusing specifically upon the influence of the practice of religion and the status of women in society upon the profession. Recognizing that knowledge of ethical theories and principles can help the nurse to develop a cohesive and logical system for making individual decisions, Chapters 2 and 3 describe philosophical stance, various classic ethical theories, and ethical principles. Utilizing the information from these chapters and recognizing differences among individuals, Chapter 4 describes a systematic decision making process for nurses to use when making ethical decisions.

CHAPTER 1

History of Nursing as an Ethical Science

> *You know that the beginning is the most important part of any work, especially in the case of a young and tender thing; for that is the time at which the character is being formed and the desired impression is more readily taken. . . .*
>
> **(Plato, *Republic*)**

OBJECTIVES

After completing this chapter, the reader should be able to:

1. Discuss the relationship between social need and the origin of the profession of nursing.
2. Briefly discuss the relationship between moral thinking and the origin of nursing.
3. Describe the mutually beneficial relationship between the broader society and its professions.
4. Explain the effect of a culture's prevailing belief system on the practice of nursing.
5. Identify how historic spiritual beliefs and religious practices influenced evolutionary changes in nursing.
6. Discuss how the historical background of the status of women in various cultures is related to the practice of nursing.
7. Make plausible inferences relating the evolution of the practice of nursing to the current state of the profession.

INTRODUCTION

Jameton (1984) calls nursing the "morally central health care profession" (p. xvi). Though the development of the profession is at times difficult to trace, moral action is the historical basis for the genesis, evolution, and practice of nursing. The spirit and substance of nursing are based upon social and individual moral codes. This chapter looks at three aspects of the history of nursing as a moral discipline. The moral foundations of nursing will be examined in light of the relationships of the historical influences of social need, spirituality, and women's standing in various western cultures.

Morals and ethics affect nursing in many ways. The motivation to care for others through nursing is generated by moral thinking. On another level, moral thinking produces rules of action, or ethics, which are an integral part of nursing. Expressions of ideals, discussions of moral issues, statements of moral principles, and codes of ethics can be found throughout the history of nursing. "Moreover, nursing is morally worthy work: Caring for and treating the sick, and comforting and protecting the suffering, are basic benefits of human culture" (Jameton, 1984, p. 1). As health care technology extends the boundary of what is possible, all of society is challenged to examine emerging ethical issues. Nurses are faced with ethical tension in a system that requires moral decision making, yet sometimes restricts nurses' legitimate roles in the process. An examination of the history of the profession is helpful in understanding the position of nurses within the health care system.

It is difficult to establish a clear picture of the development of the profession of nursing through history. The origins of medicine and nursing are intertwined in the history of healers. It is not possible to determine the exact origin of either profession, since the earliest stages of each are so closely interwoven (Donahue, 1996). The history of nursing is one of social need fulfilled by individuals with practical, moral, or spiritual motivation. It is also the story of a profession inescapably linked to the status of women. The history of healers, and subsequently that of nurses, has gone through many phases and has been a substantial part of social movements. It is the narrative of a professional group whose status has always been affected by the prevalent standards of society (Donahue, 1996).

INFLUENCE OF SOCIAL NEED

Helping professions find their origin, purpose, and meaning within the context of culturally accepted moral norms, individual values, and perceived social need. By serving others, those who respond to human need explicitly express moral belief.

The term **moral thought** relates to an individual's cognitive examination of right and wrong, good and bad. The term *moral thought* describes any level of this type of thinking: it may be complex and well developed or it may be rudimentary. The origin of moral thought is explained in different ways. Some moral and ethical philosophy describes the motive for moral thinking and ethical action in terms related to the concept of empathy. As one visualizes the circumstance of another person, one can begin to imagine oneself in the same condition. The desire to help others is described by many as a natural outcome of social consciousness and motivation similar to that ascribed in the golden rule of "Do unto others as you would have them do unto you." The golden rule is such a universal notion that it designates a guide to conduct thought fundamental in most major moral traditions including those of Jesus, Confucius, or Hillel (Honderich, 1995). The object of the action is both to help someone in need and, to some degree, assure oneself similar consideration. Ethics based upon pure religious belief, on the other hand, often motivates people to act with the objective of obeying a commandment, fulfilling a perceived duty to God, or serving others as a means to attain spiritual rewards. Whether the original motivation of ethical action is based upon a desire to help others or is a religious duty, the outcome of the action is the same: meeting the needs of others. As the morally central health care profession, nursing has historically responded to human suffering.

Ask Yourself

What Is the Motivation for Helping?

Imagine a "Utopian" world in which all people are happy and healthy and have satisfying relationships. There is neither illness nor death. Each person's needs are entirely met without the help of other people. Within this model society, because everyone is satisfied, healthy, and happy, there is no social disorder and no need for any helping profession: no police, doctors, nurses, lawyers, or social workers. Neither is there need for moral discernment. Now, imagine the social disorder that would follow the introduction of serious disease. Individuals who become ill are unable to care for themselves and to meet their own basic needs.

- How does society deal with this problem?
- Are the ill entirely responsible for themselves?
- Do unaffected members of society continue to live the "Utopian" existence, ignoring the suffering of others, or is the whole of society responsible for helping those in need?
- Does society allow the diseased members to suffer, or do healthy members act to help those afflicted, thus altering their own "perfect" lives—and in turn the prevailing social order?

It is likely that at least some members of the hypothetical community described in the Ask Yourself example will recognize the importance of helping those in need. These people will begin to exercise moral thinking as they examine their beliefs. Ethics will emerge in the form of rules of action that are specifically related to solving the moral problem. Those committed to helping the ill will devise methods to utilize individual abilities to the best advantage and fairly distribute the burden of providing services and resources. As this example implies, nursing can be described as a profession that exists to meet certain needs of individuals and groups and, thus, is a product of the moral thinking of people in society.

Think About It

What Makes People Service Oriented?

- Why do you think people are motivated to help those who are in need?

- The actions of those who choose to help others in specific situations might be described as based upon self-interest, altruism, or a combination of other motives. How would you describe the motivation to care for others within the healing professions today?

The needs of society, combined with the technological capabilities and knowledge base of the time, determine the existence and parameters of any profession. Dynamic boundaries of the profession are established by the society, based primarily upon the criteria of need and the perceived knowledge base and abilities of members of the profession. Nursing is a part of the society from which it evolved and can be said to be owned by the society "in the sense that nursing's professional interest must be and must be perceived as serving the interests of the larger whole of which it is a part" (American Nurses Association [ANA], 1980, p. 3). The landmark document *Nursing: A Social Policy Statement* (ANA, 1980) was the profession's first description of its social responsibility. Both this document and a subsequent revision entitled *Nursing's Social Policy Statement* (ANA, 1996) can be used as the framework for understanding the profession's relationship with society and its obligation to those who receive nursing care (1996, p. 1). These documents express the mutually beneficial relationship between the broader society and its professions as follows:

> A profession acquires recognition, relevance, and even meaning in terms of its relationship to that society, its culture and institutions, and its other members. Professions acquire recognition and relevance primarily in terms of needs, conditions, and traditions of particular societies and their members. It is societies (and often vested interests within them) that determine, in accord with their different technological and economic levels of development and their socioeconomic, political and cultural conditions, and values, what professional skills and knowledge they most need and desire. By various financial means, institutions will then emerge to train interested individuals to supply those needs. Logically, then, the professions open to individuals in any particular society are the property not of the individual but of society. (ANA, 1980, p. 3)

Nursing is a profession that was created by society for the purpose of meeting specific perceived health needs. In response, the profession has made an implicit promise to ensure, by various means, that members are competent to provide the service and, further, that they are the *only* members of society that can qualify to provide the service.

The relationship of social need and individual motivation to care for others is complementary. It is fortunate that human nature is such that there are individuals who, for whatever reason, are interested in serving others. There were periods in history, however, when capable and caring nurses were not available. At those times society compelled slaves, servants, inmates, prostitutes, and others to care for the ill. Collectively, if not individually, during those dark periods in history, social institutions devised means of caring for the less fortunate.

SPIRITUAL AND RELIGIOUS INFLUENCES

The spiritual and religious foundation of past and present cultures determines many facets of health care. Spiritual belief and religious practices have made major contributions to the moral foundation of nursing and other healing professions; they have also influenced both the gender and, to some degree, much of the activity of healers. Spirituality and religious doctrine also give rise to beliefs related to the value of individuals, life, death, and health. Historically, many of the dominant religious institutions made determinations about the origin and essence of healing and described (and sometimes certified) those who would hold positions as legitimate healers. The path that nursing has taken since ancient times is not linear. There have been advances and setbacks: libraries have been destroyed, widely diverse groups have held the title of nurse, and those who were the nurses in some early cultures left few records. Nevertheless, nursing of some sort has existed in every culture and has been influenced by spiritual beliefs, religious practices, and related cultural values.

Ancient Times

According to Jeanne Achterberg (1990), the **cosmology** of a culture indirectly determines specific beliefs about the origin of disease and healing. Cosmology is a branch of philosophy that describes the structure, origin, and processes of the universe and includes beliefs about the gods of the culture. The nature of the gods worshiped in any culture directly affects prevailing healing beliefs. Regarding ancient cultures, Achterberg says,

> When gods lived in the earth, the whole planet was worshiped as the manifestation of the divine. The rivers, the rocks, and especially humans were the inhabitants of a sacred place. All—what we call living and nonliving alike—was alive and related. All humans breathed the breath of the spirit and drank the waters of the spirit. (p. 188)

Thus, in ancient cultures, the healer was involved with the sacred elements of the earth and the spirit in healing practices.

The vocation of healer was viewed by early cultures in terms associated with the sacred. In ancient times the position of healer was practiced by those thought to have special spiritual gifts. Through the study of relics, it has been determined that the healing arts in the ancient cultures of Sumer, Denmark, Greece, and others were performed in sacred ceremonies by priests, priestesses, or shamans. These ancient healers represented the embodiment of the cultures' gods on earth (Achterberg, 1990). In ancient Persia there are indications that there were three types of healers: those who healed with the knife, those who healed with herbs, and those who healed with sacred words. Practitioners who used sacred words were considered to have the greatest prestige (Dolan, 1973). Archeological evidence suggests that in all early cultures the position of the healer was associated with the sacred.

Having a great influence on Western thought, early Hebrew teaching codified health practices as an integral part of the religion. The Mosaic health code applied to every aspect of individual, family, and community life. It included principles related to rest, sleep, cleanliness, hygiene, and childbearing (Dolan, Fitzpatrick, & Herrmann, 1983). The code required inspection of food, detection and reporting of disease, methods of disposal of excreta, feminine hygiene, and isolation of those with communicable illness. It specified particular methods of hand washing and care of food. The Hebrew high priest served in the capacity of priest-physician, and the people were admonished to honor him. Thus, for the early Hebrews, that which was "right" to do in regard to health was mandated by religious doctrine.

Early Christian Era

Arguably the most profound religious influence on healing beliefs and practices in Western civilization occurred with the advent of the Christian era. The effect of Christian belief and organized Christian religion upon the history of health and healing is multifaceted. It is interesting to closely examine textbooks on nursing history and recognize divergent opinions that exist among authors. The pendulum swings from authors' bias that presents only the positive aspects of the Christian influence upon the history of nursing to those that condemn Christianity as a destructive, misogynistic force that hindered nursing progress.

In a text on nursing history that has been popular since its original edition in 1916, Dolan writes, "Man and the universe were made to exist in the profound execution of the plan of Creation" (1973, p. 3). She utilizes the New Testament of the Bible in describing Jesus's message about caring for others in the following way: (1) caring for others represents caring for Jesus; (2) there is spiritual reward to be gained by caring for others; (3) even in a world of selfishness and hatred one should love God and one's neighbor; (4) every person, even the "poorest and most miserable," is an important member of the Kingdom of God; and (5) every person has worth and dignity. As this example shows, nursing texts, in the United States, often reflect the prevailing influence of the early Christian church and Christian teaching upon healing practices and the nursing profession.

Early Christian nurses were frequently women of high social status and often became independent practitioners. Many set aside special places in their homes for hospitality and care of the sick. These places were called Christrooms (Dolan, 1973; Dolan, Fitzpatrick, & Herrmann, 1983). Early Christians exhibited caring and respect for the intrinsic value of each human.

As centuries passed, the path of healing practices assumed a tortuous course. Jeanne Achterberg describes the first five hundred years after the birth of Christ as the "calm before the storm." She says, "These were fluid times, when religion was a satisfying and exotic blend of ingredients taken from pre-Christian, pagan, and folk traditions" (1990, p. 39). As time progressed, war, pestilence, and the inculcation of Catholic dogma effectively altered the course of the healing traditions.

Middle Ages

As the early Middle Ages began, many believed that the world was falling into ruins. During this time, pestilence, famine, and war interacted to produce a predictable sequence: war drove the farmer from his fields and destroyed his crops, destruction of the crops led to famine, and the starved and weakened populace fell easy victim to the onslaught of pestilence and plague (Cartwright, 1972). The established social structure was deteriorating, and disorganized communities turned to feudalism, monasticism, and, in certain regions, to Islam as solutions to the chaos they were experiencing. During this time, monasticism and other religious groups offered the only opportunities for men and women to pursue careers in nursing and other healing professions. Much of the hospital nursing was carried out by repentant women and widows called sisters and by male nurses called brothers. Deaconesses, matrons, and secular nursing orders were among the organized groups that had religious foundations and offered nursing services. According to Dolan, these early nurses believed they were following the command of God to imitate Jesus who spent his life ministering to those in need. For many, this service was viewed as a means of securing salvation. Dolan quotes the Sisters of Charity founder Saint Louise De Marillac, who wrote in a letter dated 1633, "We do not want those who have no desire to work at their spiritual perfection in the service of God. They should have no motive in coming except the one of serving God and their neighbor" (1973, p. 100). Women who entered nursing orders donated their property and wealth to the Church and devoted their lives to service. Believing that "charity" was synonymous with "love," many early Christians sold their possessions and gave everything to the Church or the poor. Though in many cases "nursing" care was given by slaves or servants, religious orders offered the only route through which respectable women and men could serve as nurses.

The overall belief system of a culture influences the extent to which members accept various healing methods and health care practices. An example of this can be seen in historical accounts of the healing arts in the Middle Ages. The term **empirical** relates to knowledge gained through the processes of observation and experience. Many people, especially those involved with the Church, had deeply antiempirical beliefs. This antiempiricism caused a profound distrust of the senses. People believed there was no reason to look for natural laws governing physical phenomena because the world is created anew by God in every instant. Consequently, people were more likely to seek healing through religious intervention, touching of religious relics, visiting of sacred places, incantations, and other methods sanctioned by the Church. Because of religious fervor during this time, empirical treatment (particularly if provided by anyone not explicitly sanctioned by the Church), even if it was successful, was thought to be generated by the devil, since the position of the Church was that only God and the devil had the power to cause either illness or healing.

Because of increasingly influential Christian doctrine, there was a constant war waged against the flesh. Achterberg (1990) relates that people during the Middle Ages believed that they should "mortify the flesh" in the name of exalting the spirit. There was little attention to physical needs. People were dirty and covered with rashes and "foul eruptions." These problems were made worse by rough, dirty, woolen clothing and the constant presence of ticks and fleas. Thus, as a direct result of Christian dogma, health care practices during the Middle Ages actually caused the spread of disease, accentuated health problems, and curtailed effective empirical healing practices.

The Crusades, which began in 1096 and lasted nearly two hundred years, marked many changes in the health of the population. These holy wars led to deplorable sanitary conditions, fatigue, poor nutrition, diarrhea, and the spread of communicable disease. These problems subsequently led to a need for more hospitals and greater numbers of health care providers. In response to the compelling need, military nursing orders were formed. These orders drew large numbers of men into the field of nursing (Dolan, 1973).

Another direct result of the Crusades was the collection of relics by the Catholic Church. These spoils of war included body parts and exudations of the martyrs of the Crusades and were believed to offer the potential of healing miracles. Through their sale the Church obtained significant wealth and power. Achterberg (1990) compares this time to an earlier Roman mythology in which large numbers of deities or sainted mortals, their relics, and pilgrimages to their sacred sites were believed to hold the key to health.

For most of the Middle Ages, the Roman Catholic Church held tremendous influence over the people and governments of all European countries. Powerful leaders within the Church determined the appropriateness of various healing practices. Official credentialing of physicians, nurses, and midwives was left in the hands of the Church. Even after civic legislation became common, the Roman Catholic Church continued to enforce the law and monitor practitioners (Achterberg, 1990). As will be seen in the following section, this power was also used to enforce religious doctrine related to the status of women in society.

Accounts of the actual treatment of patients in early times vary. In some hospitals operated by religious orders, patients were treated as welcome guests and were sometimes known to feign illness to be admitted. In contrast, there are reports indicating that some groups of patients were treated inhumanely, even by members of nursing orders. If these nurses believed their duty was to God and to the spiritual rather than physical needs of the patients, they were undoubtedly less attentive to physical, emotional, and comfort needs.

For centuries the treatment of the mentally ill was based upon the fixed idea that they were possessed by devils or that they were being punished for their sins (Dolan, 1973). Chained and manacled, they were often starved and kept under filthy conditions. There was even a time when it was thought that torture was useful in driving out madness. Because the public perception of mental illness was based upon religious beliefs related to demon possession and punishment for sin, the mentally ill were treated inhumanely.

Renaissance and Reformation

The sixteenth century heralded the beginning of two great movements—the Renaissance and the Reformation. Resulting from a revolutionary spirit and quest for knowledge, the Renaissance produced an intellectual rebirth that began the scientific era. The Reformation was a religious movement precipitated by the widespread abuses that had become a part of Church life and doctrinal disagreement among religious leaders (Donahue, 1996).

The Renaissance gave birth to the Scientific Revolution and a new era in the healing arts. Beginning its gradual escape from the control of the Church, the scientific community made advances in mathematics and the sciences. Rene Descartes is credited with proposing a theory that quickly altered philosophic beliefs about the separation of mind and body. Descartes proposed that the universe is a physical thing and all therein is analogous to machines that can be analyzed and understood. Descartes further theorized that the mind and body are separate entities (Durant, 1926). Based upon Descartes's work, **Cartesian philosophy** began to replace religious beliefs related to the physical and spiritual realms of humankind. As a direct result, a separation was created between the acts of caring and curing in the healing arts. The advent of this philosophy, while elevating the sciences and making scientific inquiry possible, did not improve the status of nursing. Achterberg identifies this time as an important turning point. Regarding Cartesian philosophy, she says,

> When spirit no longer is seen to abide in matter, the reverence for what is physical departs. Hence medicine no longer regarded itself as working in the sacred spaces where fellow humans find themselves in pain and peril, and where transcendence is most highly desired. (1990, p. 103)

As Cartesian philosophy became popular, nurses' place in the health care system assumed the "caring" realm. Caring was given lower priority than curing within the hierarchy of the healing arts. Some would argue that this legacy is one that remains with nursing today.

The Reformation produced a split in the Church. Engendered by widespread abuses and differences in belief among Church leaders, a struggle between Catholic and Protestant groups spread across Europe. As a result, Catholicism lost its power in many countries. According to Donahue (1996), laws and customs in Protestant countries discouraged the humane care of the "downtrodden and the weak" (p. 193). Religious nursing orders were driven out of hospitals, many of which were ultimately closed. It was during this era that hospitals became places of horror. There was no qualified group to take the place of the religious nursing orders. Unqualified and undesirable women were assigned nursing duties. Known as the "Dark Period of Nursing," conditions were at their very worst between 1550 and 1850 when convalescent patients, prostitutes, prisoners, and drunkards provided hospital nursing care (Donahue, 1996).

The influence of many of these events is seen in the life and writing of Florence Nightingale (1820–1910). Known as the founder of modern nursing, Nightingale, though devoutly religious, worked to free nursing from the bonds of the Church, which she called "an over busy mother" (Roberts & Group, 1995). As a person, Nightingale remains an enigma. Though she saw nursing as a profession separate from the Church, she began her career as the result of a mystic experience. Showalter reports that, according to Nightingale, God spoke to her four times, calling her into his service. Her experience in the Crimean was the direct result of her second revelation which was "a call from God to be a savior" (1981, p. 400). Her religious beliefs were evident in her dealings with students, admonishing them to work, work, work because "if there is no cross, there is no crown" (Achterberg, 1990). In addition, Nightingale's description of nursing as "caring for the mind and the body" implies a rejection of Descartes's philosophy on the separation of these two human spheres.

Thus entering the twentieth century, nursing in Western culture had been shaped by religious and spiritual influences of the past. As a tapestry woven of one piece over time, nursing owns the heritage of those early times. Recently there has been a resurgence of interest in spirituality and its relationship to health and healing. There is also a growing movement of religious zeal that will certainly affect how people view health care practices. Nurses must be sensitive to the relationship of health and spirituality and recognize that patients' beliefs affect both their attitude and response to treatment.

INFLUENCE OF THE HISTORY OF WOMEN

One of the most crucial factors that influences nursing practice is the role of women in society. Because nursing has generally been a profession of women, the status accorded women in society is pivotal in determining the measure of freedom and respect accorded to nurses. It is the society that allows or fails to allow women to assume roles of authority, roles that allow independent decision making or participation in the decision making process.

In every culture women have been healers. Because nursing has always consisted primarily of women (from the beginning ninety-five to ninety-eight percent of nurses have been women), the profession has been molded by social forces that ascribe gender roles in society. As a result of the perception that women are more humane and more caring by nature, they have been viewed as naturally endowed with nursing talents. Florence Nightingale said, "Every woman . . . has, at one time or another of her life, charge of the personal health of somebody, whether child or invalid—in other words, every woman is a nurse" (Nightingale, 1859, preface). This kind of stereotyping has been both the bane and blessing of nursing. There are periods in history in which women were the honored sole practitioners of the healing arts, and there are periods in which women were forced into submissive and subservient healing roles. The authority to practice has been granted to women based upon prevailing social beliefs.

The overall belief system of any culture describes the population's views related to the nature of God and the universe. This prevailing system of beliefs is referred to as the culture's cosmology. Achterberg (1990) proposes that the cosmology of any culture determines, among other things, which members of society assume positions of leadership and honor. Healers who exercise freedom and power in any culture are those members of the society who reflect the predominant beliefs about the nature of the god(s).

Ancient Times

In ancient times when the reigning deity had a feminine, bisexual, or androgynous nature, women were leaders in the healing arts. Achterberg (1990) reports that many diverse and widely placed cultures have left evidence that there was a very early time when women served in the esteemed roles of healer and priestess. As the world became a harsher place and the gods assumed a masculine nature, women's role as independent, primary healer was taken away.

Early Christian Era

As religious belief moved toward a single male god, women's healing role changed from that of sacred healer to subservient caregiver. By the time Jesus lived, women's place in the healing arts was minimal. Jesus called this into question with an assault on patriarchy. According to Achterberg, Jesus challenged tradition by associating freely with women. He selected the most "compassionate, maternal images from the Jewish tradition, creating a Christian god as androgynous . . . as any male god in history. In some of the early sects, God was even seen as a dyadic being (mother-father), rather than the trinity (father-son-holy spirit)" (1990, p. 38). As a result, women enjoyed a renewal as honored healers. Their intellect and contribution to the religious movement were respected by the early Christians. Women enjoyed this resurgence of power and respectability for only a few centuries after the birth of Christ.

Middle Ages

During the Middle Ages, the status of women plummeted. In many ways this was directly related to Church doctrine. St. Thomas Aquinas, ironically known within the Church as the "angelic doctor" (Donahue, 1996), wrote that one should "only make use of a necessary object, woman, who is needed to preserve the species or to provide food and drink. . . . Woman was created to be man's [helper], but her unique role is in conception . . . since for all other purposes men would be better assisted by other men" (Achterberg, 1990, p. 68). Centuries earlier, another Church leader, St. Jerome, frequently recognized for his support of matrons in their calling as nurses, remarked, "woman is the gate of the devil, the path of wickedness, the sting of the serpent, in a word a perilous object" (Heer, 1961, p. 322). These religious leaders were setting the stage for the persecution of women that would last for hundreds of years and leave a persistent legacy of misogyny.

The Church was the only organized institution that provided an outlet for those wishing to practice nursing in the Middle Ages. Religious and Church sanctioned secular nursing orders afforded the only legitimate avenue for women wishing to care for those in need. The Church popularized the ideals of virginity, poverty, and a life of service. By the end of the thirteenth century, an estimated two hundred thousand women served as nurses within these orders (Achterberg, 1990). Caring for pilgrims in improvised infirmaries and clinics, women's nursing orders were particularly welcome during the Crusades. As was often the case, these orders were subordinate to the men's communities (Donahue, 1996). Nevertheless, some speculate that within the structure of the Church, these women exercised a degree of independence and autonomy. There is no doubt that they made a great contribution to the health care of the times.

During the Middle Ages, the Church and the newly formed medical profession were actively engaged in the elimination of lay female healers. Women were excluded from universities. Except for those devoting their lives to serving in nursing orders, they were not allowed by the Church to practice the healing arts. During a revival of learning in the thirteenth century, the Church imposed strict controls on the new profession of medicine and "allowed it to develop only within the terms set by Catholic doctrine" which officially prohibited practice by women (Achterberg, 1990, p. 15). Nevertheless, some women continued to covertly practice the healing arts, both within and outside the home. They used knowledge handed down for generations, intuitive knowledge, and empirical knowledge. Since the knowledge of illness and healing was thought to originate either from God or from the devil, those who practiced healing without the sanction of the Church were believed by the Church to be in collusion with the devil.

It was a popular ecclesiastical view that women are of an intrinsically evil nature. The pain of childbirth was believed to be punishment for Eve's transgression and to serve the purpose of reminding women of their original sinful nature. Those who dared provide pain relief to others during childbirth were severely punished (Achterberg, 1990). One can speculate about the role of empathy in caring for laboring women during these difficult times. Later, the Original Sin of Eve would be used to justify torturing and murdering thousands of women during the witch hunts.

Though the medical profession was officially sanctioned by the Church and male physicians were beginning to be trained in the university setting, there was scant scientific knowledge. When confronted with a sick person, the physician had only superstition upon which to rely (Ehrenreich & English, 1973). University trained physicians relied on such treatments as bloodletting, astrology, alchemy, and incantations. Their clientele consisted almost exclusively of the wealthy. Physicians' treatments were usually ineffective, often dangerous, and inaccessible to the majority of the poor.

Lacking access to doctors, poor villagers depended on female folk healers. Peasant women were often the only healers for people who had no doctors and suffered bitterly from poverty and disease (Ehrenreich & English, 1973). These wise women possessed extensive knowledge about cures that had been handed down by the oral tradition from generation to generation. They constantly improved their practice by the use of empirical methods of observation, trial, and evaluation. While physicians continued to rely on superstition, these women developed an extensive understanding of bones and muscles, herbs and drugs, and midwifery (Barstow, 1994; Ehrenreich & English, 1973). Some authorities believe these peasant folk healers were actually practicing some form of magic or witchcraft (Barstow). Others speculate that women were honoring the old pagan religions and worshiping the old gods who (to Church authorities) assumed the persona of the devil (Achterberg, 1990). It is likely that these women were simply assuming caring and curing roles in a manner that was consistent with prevailing folk belief—almost everyone in medieval Europe believed in the reality of magic (Barstow). This atmosphere set the stage for Church sanctioned crimes against women in the form of the witch hunts.

In its sweep across Europe, the witch hunts lasted from the fourteenth to the seventeenth century. The atmosphere that led to the witch hunts was a critical mixture of war, pestilence, and poverty combined with religious fervor, superstition, and political unrest. The witch trials were accomplished through an organized partnership between Church, state, and the emerging medical profession. Women, particularly women healers, represented a political, religious, and sexual threat to both Church and state. An atmosphere of superstition and widespread belief in magic set the stage that would allow the people to witness these heinous crimes against women (Achterberg, 1990; Barstow, 1994; Ehrenreich & English, 1973).

The witch hunts were indeed aimed at women. Armed with papal authorization to purge Germany of witches, Dominican inquisitors Kramer and Sprenger wrote *Malleus Maleficarum* (Barstow, 1994). In this witch hunters' manual, Kramer and Sprenger expressed virulent antifeminine and antisexual opinions. They claimed that women are "liars, more superstitious than men, more impressionable, wicked minded, and in need of constant male supervision" (Barstow, p. 172). They wrote that, "'If a woman dare to cure without having studied she is a witch and must die'" (Ehrenreich & English, 1973, p. 19) and that, "'No one does more harm to the Catholic Church than midwives'" (p. 13). They also wrote, "'When a woman thinks alone, she thinks evil. . . . Women are intellectually like children'" (Barstow, p. 172). Kramer and Sprenger defined witchcraft as treason against God and described it as female rebellion. According to Barstow, "the document reeks with fear and hatred of women, concluding with thanks to God 'who has so far preserved the male sex from so great a crime'" (1994, p. 62). The most authoritative document used by witch hunters, the *Malleus Maleficarum* was printed in four languages and at least twenty-nine editions between the years of 1486 and 1669 A.D.

What were the crimes of which the women were accused? Any woman who treated an illness, even if she applied a soothing salve to the diseased skin of her child, was likely to be accused of witchcraft. If the treatment failed, she was thought to have cursed the patient; if the treatment succeeded, she was believed to be in consort with the devil. Though women were permitted to practice midwifery (no one else wanted to do it), these women were in danger of being accused of witchcraft if anything went wrong with either mother or baby.

Ask Yourself

Healing or Witchcraft?

Imagine yourself the parent of a small child in the sixteenth century. You believe the Church doctrine about the origin of the knowledge of healing. Your family and neighbors are aware of the growing problem of witchcraft in the region. Your child becomes ill and you recall a remedy that your mother used successfully with the same ailment.

- Will you openly attempt to alleviate your child's suffering and risk being accused of witchcraft?
- How would you feel having to make this decision?

No one knows how many women were killed during the witch trials. When records were kept, they were abysmal. Often names were not used, and occasionally the verdict and sentence were not recorded. The most authoritative estimate of the number of executions is two hundred thousand, though some estimates are as high as ten million. Women constituted eighty-five to ninety-five percent of those killed (Barstow, 1994). During the twelfth century in Russia, when looking for witches, authorities simply rounded up all the women in an area. Some small European towns were left with one woman or no woman at all (Achterberg, 1990; Barstow, 1994; Ehrenreich & English, 1973).

It is difficult to comprehend the effect of the witch hunts on European society. Women had silently watched the public humiliation, torture, disfigurement, and death of other women. Often the accused women's breasts were publicly amputated prior to execution—symbolically eliminating the evil by removing the most obvious feature of her sex. Barstow believes that this public acknowledgment of the evil nature of the female sex left all women humiliated and frightened. Because both the accused and those viewing the proceedings were powerless to prevent the torture and executions, the witchcraze served to undermine women's belief in the ability and power of all women. Indeed, this was likely the inference made by all of society. Achterberg states that "women were never again given full citizenship in any country, nor was their role in the healing professions reinstated" (1990, p. 98). Even after the end of this terrible time, women were prohibited from independent healing professions by law in every country in Europe. This created a climate by which, under the protection and patronage of the ruling classes, males became the authoritative medical professionals (Ehrenreich & English, 1973). Though accounts of the witch hunts are absent in most popular nursing history texts, these events probably influenced the future of the profession more than any other single factor. As Ehrenreich and English write, "It was to become a theme of our history" (1973, p. 6).

 Think About It

Who Has the Right to Make Ethical Decisions?

Ethical decision making is not the sole domain of the physician. Nurses may be better prepared and have more opportunity to discuss ethical dilemmas with patients and families.

- Can you describe an instance in which the physician assumed the authority to make an ethical decision, denying nurses (and perhaps the patient and family) participation in the decision making process?

- If you feel you have an important contribution to make in a particular circumstance and your opinion is not considered, how do you react?

- How do you think nurses can overcome the strong heritage of subjugation?

Renaissance and Reformation

Though the world was beginning to change, the witch hunts lasted well into the Reformation. Following the end of the witch trials, the day-to-day life of women changed little. Though released from the grip of fear engendered by the witch hunts, women continued to live in subordination to men. For the most part, they were not allowed to be legitimate members of any profession. Nursing entered its "Dark Period" when much hospital nursing was performed by unqualified women. In the nineteenth century, nursing leaders began to emerge who would contribute to improving the status of nurses.

Florence Nightingale became a model for all nurses. She was a nurse, statistician, sanitarian, social reformer, and scholar. She was politically astute, intelligent, and single-minded. Unlike most women of her time, she addressed moral issues with courage and conviction and was not hesitant to challenge the established male hierarchy. Though much of her own life portrays a feminist viewpoint, it has been argued that Nightingale was not a feminist. Her writings instructed nurses to "do the thing that is good, whether it is 'suitable for a woman' or not" (Nightingale, 1859, p. 76). In any case, it is certain that she did not ascribe to the popular Cartesian notion that women do not have minds and souls and are put on the earth solely for man's purpose and pleasure (Roberts & Group, 1995).

Another of nursing's greatest leaders was Lavinia Lloyd Dock (1858–1956). Considered a radical feminist, Dock was actively engaged in social protest, picketing and parading for women's rights (Roberts & Group, 1995). She was concerned with the many problems plaguing nursing, warning that male dominance in the health field was the major problem confronting the nursing profession. Her concerns were unheeded by her contemporaries, and nurses found themselves fighting the same battles in the twentieth century.

Recurrent themes of paternalism and subjugation continued to affect the nursing profession well past the turn of the century. Following the examples set by nurse leaders like Florence Nightingale and Lavinia Dock, twentieth century women became more politically active. By the 1970s, many nurses were speaking out about sex discrimination. The women's movement encouraged political, social, and economic action to correct the wrongs suffered by women. Roberts and Group (1995) wrote, "Nurses' consciousness of their subordinated and oppressed group status became heightened, propelling some nurses to advocate radical role-breaking, risk-taking behaviors" (p. 187). Encouraged by society because of a critical need for primary caregivers, nurse practitioners, nurse midwives, and other advanced practice nurses began to assert themselves as independent professionals.

In the 1980s and 1990s nursing took a great leap forward. During these decades nurses moved into spheres of professional, social, and political responsibility. No longer forced into roles of subjugation, many nurses claimed legitimate authority to provide independent health care services and assume institutional and political leadership positions. Perceiving a health care crisis of growing proportions and recognizing a need for comprehensive, accessible, and affordable health care, society challenged established institutions to foster greater use of nurses in expanded roles.

Though many nurses have overcome social and institutional barriers to practice as full members of the healing professions, others continue to struggle within patriarchal, institutional hierarchy. Recognizing the legitimate need for both the caring and curing aspects of healing, nurses are charged with working together to improve the status of nurses and assure that the problems of the past are not repeated. Today's health care system is one that is experiencing rapid change. Managed care and other health care reform programs offer nurses both opportunities and challenges. The position of the professional nurse within these systems is far from assured. Recalling lessons from the past, nurses remain acutely aware of threats to newly won professional recognition.

SUMMARY

Nursing is a profession that was created by society for the purpose of meeting specific perceived health needs. The profession belongs to society and therefore is bound by the duty to competently meet the needs for which it was created. Individual nurses, therefore, have a duty to fulfill the promise the profession has made to society.

In all cultures, the profession has been profoundly influenced by various aspects of spirituality and the practice of religion. Both the nature of the healer and the healing act have been influenced by the prevailing cosmology. Until the last two centuries, healing was strongly associated with the sacred. Religious institutions have influenced the parameters and membership of the profession—by either including or excluding particular groups.

In every culture women have been healers. Because nursing is primarily a profession of women, the status of women in society has been an important factor in determining the role of nurses in the health care system. Women's status in society directly determines the freedom given to women to become educated, to think and act independently, and to participate fully in the healing arts. There are periods in history in which women were allowed freedom and responsibility, and there are dark periods in which women lived in subjugation. Nursing today is at a crossroads, free of many of the restrictions of the past, yet not fully franchised as a profession with power and authority.

CHAPTER HIGHLIGHTS

- Throughout history, spiritual beliefs, religious practice, cultural norms, and political factors have influenced evolutionary changes in nursing. These factors continue to influence the practice of nursing today.
- Social need is the criterion for the existence of all professions.
- Moral thinking originates as individuals or groups desire to meet the needs of others.
- The practice of nursing is focused upon meeting the health care needs of others; therefore, the practice of nursing originates in moral thinking.
- Professions exist to meet the needs of society.

- Society grants professionals the exclusive right to practice within defined parameters.
- Professionals have a reciprocal duty to society to practice competently.
- Because nursing is primarily a profession of women, the social status of women affects the status of the profession.
- The status of the nursing profession determines members' ability to practice with freedom and responsibility.

DISCUSSION QUESTIONS AND ACTIVITIES

1. Talk with nurses, physicians, and ministers. Ask them their opinions about why some people choose to help others in need. In class, analyze and compare the responses.

2. Discuss the historical developments that caused the separation of the professions of medicine and nursing. How were the distinctions drawn in regard to the boundaries of the professions? How would you change the boundaries today?

3. What is the relationship between the role of women in history and the status of nurses?

4. What is the relationship between the role of women today and the status of nurses?

5. Search out a few retired nurses. Ask them to describe the relationship between nurses and physicians in the mid-1900s. How was this related to the role of women in society during the same time period?

6. Discuss the relationship between the role of nurses in the health care system today and their role in ethical decision making in the clinical setting.

7. Discuss the challenges that the profession of nursing faces related to attaining or maintaining an authoritative role in the health care system of the future.

REFERENCES

Achterberg, J. (1990). *Woman as healer*. Boston: Shambhala.

American Nurses Association. (1980). *Nursing: A social policy statement*. Kansas City, MO: Author.

American Nurses Association. (1996). *Nursing's social policy statement*. Washington, DC: Author.

Barstow, A. L. (1994). *Witchcraze: A new history of the European witch hunts*. San Francisco: HarperCollins.

Cartwright, F. F. (1972). *Disease and history*. New York: Dorset Press.

Dolan, J. A. (1973). *Nursing in society: A historical perspective* (13th ed.). Philadelphia: Saunders.

Dolan, J. A., Fitzpatrick, M. L., & Herrmann, E. K. (1983). *Nursing in society: A historical perspective* (15th ed.). Philadelphia: Saunders.

Donahue, M. P. (1996). *Nursing: The finest art*. St. Louis, MO: Mosby.

Durant, W. (1926). *The story of philosophy*. New York: Washington Square Press.

Ehrenreich, B., & English, D. (1973). *Witches, midwives, and nurses: A history of women healers.* New York: The Feminist Press.

Heer, F. (1961). *The medieval world.* New York: New American Library.

Honderich, T. (Ed.). (1995). *The Oxford companion to philosophy.* New York: Oxford University Press.

Jameton, A. (1984). *Nursing practice: The ethical issues.* Englewood Cliffs, NJ: Prentice-Hall.

Nightingale, F. (1859). *Notes on nursing: What it is, and what it is not.* London: Harrison & Sons.

Plato. *Republic.*

Roberts, J. I., & Group, T. M. (1995). *Feminism and nursing: An historical perspective on power, status, and political activism in the nursing profession.* Westport, CT: Praeger.

Showalter, E. (1981). Florence Nightingale's feminist complaint: Women, religion, and suggestions for thought. *Journal of Women in Culture and Society, 6,* 395–412.

CHAPTER 2

Ethical Theory

Within Siddhartha there slowly grew and ripened the knowledge of what wisdom really was and the goal of his long seeking. It was nothing but a preparation of the soul, a capacity, a secret art of thinking, feeling and breathing thoughts of unity at every moment of life. This thought matured in him slowly, and it was reflected in Vasudeva's old childlike face: harmony, knowledge of the eternal perfection of the world, and unity.

(Hesse, 1971, p. 131)

OBJECTIVES

After completing this chapter, the reader should be able to:

1. Discuss the purpose of philosophy.
2. Define the terms *moral philosophy* and *ethics*.
3. Discuss the importance of a systematic study of ethics to nursing.
4. Discuss the importance of ethical theory.
5. Describe utilitarianism.
6. Describe deontological ethics, defining the terms *categorical imperative* and *practical imperative*.
7. Define the terms *virtue* and *virtue ethics*.

INTRODUCTION

At its core, nursing is a profession that deals with issues and situations that have elements of ethical or moral uncertainty. A spiraling dependence on technology and the resulting longer lifespans and higher health care costs coupled with increasing professional autonomy creates an atmosphere in which members of the profession are faced with problems of ever-increasing complexity. Nurses need to be able to recognize situations with ethical and moral implications and make coherent and logical ethical decisions based upon recognized ethical principles and theory. This text will prepare the student to examine issues and come to logical, consistent, and thoughtful ethical decisions. The study of ethics will make the student more rational, responsible, self-reliant, and effective.

Students and experienced nurses alike need to be able to recognize ethical components of practice and engage in a structured ethical decision making process. This requires four basic elements. First, nurses must have willingness and courage to participate in work that is emotionally painful. Ethical problems deal with issues of great significance to those involved and, by their very nature, have no easy or obvious solutions. Second, nurses must have a solid knowledge base that prepares them to identify circumstances that involve ethical components. Knowledge and insight of personal values, cultural norms, moral development, and ethical theory are necessary for the practicing nurse. Third, nurses must be sensitive, patient, and insightful. Recognition of subtle clues that may indicate when a situation is laden with ethical components demands that the nurse be attentive to all facets of the predicament. This requires time, focused attention, and sensitivity. Fourth, nurses need to be knowledgeable and adept in making logical, fair, and consistent decisions. Ethical decision making models offer a variety of methods for coming to rational conclusions. Each of these four components must be present for nurses to effectively participate in ethical decision making.

 CASE PRESENTATION

Nursing Students Face an Ethical Dilemma

Tonya and Lydia are two senior nursing students assigned to work in the intensive care unit with a critically ill patient. The patient, Mr. Dunn, is an eighty-seven-year-old retired ironworker. He lives alone in an old two-story frame house. Mr. Dunn is diabetic. He is nearly blind and has moderately advanced prostate cancer and Alzheimer's disease. Mr. Dunn was admitted to the intensive care unit after he was discovered unconscious in his home by a neighbor. At that time he was ketoacidotic and had a very severe necrotic wound on his left leg. The surgeon attending Mr. Dunn is planning amputation of his left leg but has been unable to get consent from either Mr. Dunn or his next of kin—a niece who lives out of town.

Tonya is proud of her efficiency as a nursing student. She makes rapid decisions. Tonya insists that Mr. Dunn must have the amputation. She boldly suggests to the physician that he have a surrogate appointed for Mr. Dunn so that the surgery can proceed. The course is clear to her. Lydia, on the other hand, is not certain of the correct course of action. She talks to Mr. Dunn and his niece about his condition. She wonders if the amputation is the best solution to his problem. She thinks about what his quality of life will be after the surgery. She worries about his ability to care for himself and about his state of mind should he be forced to live in a nursing home. She thinks about what she would want for her father if he were in the same situation. Lydia falls asleep at night pondering these thoughts. She does not know how to go about solving the problem. Tonya is impatient with Lydia. She sees no benefit to the time and energy spent worrying about this problem when the solution is apparent to her. She dislikes wasting her time talking to Lydia about these concerns.

In this example, we see nurses at both extremes. Tonya makes quick decisions. In all likelihood she recognizes neither the ethical nature of the problem, the bearing the outcome may have on the people involved, nor the conflicting possible solutions. She has great pride in her ability to make decisions and has confidence in the correctness of those decisions. Lydia, being more insightful and sensitive, recognizes intuitively that the problem presents no clear solution. She is troubled by the situation but has no tools with which to deal with the predicament. Each of these nurses will benefit from a study of nursing ethics.

 Think About It

Facing Ethical Dilemmas

- What alerts you to the presence of an ethical dilemma?
- How do you feel when confronted with difficult ethical decisions?
- To what degree do you think nurses should become involved in making decisions such as the one described in the situation above?
- With which qualities of each nurse do you identify?

Ethics and Nursing

Nursing is a profession that deals with the most personal and private aspects of humans' lives. From the beginning of time, and by definition, nurses, whether called healers, caretakers, nurturers, or nurses, have cared for those in need in a very personal and intimate way. Nurses are attentive to patients' needs over long periods of time. They may have made home visits and may know patients' families. They may care for patients at the bedside for hours and days on end. It is through the intimacy and trust inherent in the nurse-patient relationship that nurses become critical participants in the process of ethical decision making.

As participants in a dynamic profession, nurses are faced with ethical choices that affect the profession itself. For example, as the needs and demands of society change, boundaries of the domain of nursing contract and expand. This forces nurses to make decisions about such issues as the delegation of traditional nursing functions to non-nurse caregivers and the expanding boundaries of nursing. Because nursing is self-regulated, nurses are called on to review and discipline peers. This holds many ethical implications as nurses attempt to balance desires to advance the profession, protect the public, and maintain professional cohesiveness.

Nurses may also be called to take part in decision making on a broader scale. More than ever before, nurses are participating as members of policy making bodies. Community, state, and national task forces, committees, and boards of advisors are among those health care decision making groups in which nurses have become integral and respected legitimate members. It is imperative that nurses participating in decision making at this level be aware of the ethical implications of the decisions that are made, particularly those dealing with distribution of goods and services. These decisions are at the very heart of our society's beliefs about the value of the individual and, as such, compel those involved to cautiously deliberate every decision. A working knowledge of ethical theory will help nurses make clear and consistent decisions.

PHILOSOPHY

Philosophy is the intense and critical examination of beliefs and assumptions and, as such, is both natural and necessary to humanity. Philosophy gives coherence to the whole realm of thought and experience. It offers principles for deciding what actions and qualities are most worthwhile. Philosophy may also show inconsistency in meaning and context (Kneller, 1971). There are many philosophical schools of thought. Because of the nature of philosophy, it is impossible to verify philosophic beliefs or theories. Nevertheless, the study of philosophy helps give order and coherence to beliefs and assumptions. It gives shape to what would otherwise be a random chaos of thoughts, beliefs, assumptions, values, and superstition.

Philosophers examine questions dealing with life's most important aspects. Typical questions asked by philosophers include the following: What is the meaning of life? Is there a God? What is reality? What is the essence of knowledge? How can something be known? How can one describe the relationships among persons or between humans and the Divine? What is happiness? What is the ideal or virtuous human character? How can one understand human beliefs, values, and morals? Questions such as these have been asked by the most widely studied philosophers. Buddha asked, "How can one find the path that leads to the end of suffering?" Confucius asked, "What is the remedy for social disorder?" Socrates asked, "How should one live?" Through the centuries philosophy has concerned itself with topics that define the essence of human life. Martin Buber (1965) said, "With soaring power [man] reaches out beyond what is given him, flies beyond the horizon and the familiar stars, and grasps a totality" (p. 61).

Ayn Rand (1982), author and social philosopher, expressed her thoughts eloquently when she wrote the following:

> A philosophic system is an integrated view of existence. As a human being, you have no choice about the fact that you need a philosophy. Your only choice is whether you define your philosophy by a conscious, rational, disciplined process of thought and scrupulously logical deliberation—or let your subconscious accumulate a junk heap of unwarranted conclusions, false generalizations, . . . undefined wishes, doubts and fears, thrown together by chance, but integrated by your subconscious into a kind of mongrel philosophy and fused into a single weight: *self doubt,* like a ball and chain in the place where your mind's wings should have grown. (p. 5)

D. D. Raphael (1994) describes philosophy as essentially divided into two branches: the philosophy of knowledge and the philosophy of practice. He describes the philosophy of knowledge as attentive to critical examination of assumptions about matters of fact and argument. Included in this branch are epistemology (the study of knowledge), metaphysics (the study of ultimate reality), the philosophy of science, philosophy of the mind, and philosophical logic. Philosophy of practice, on the other hand, focuses on the critical examination of assumptions about norms or values and includes ethics, social and political philosophy, and the philosophy of the law. It is the philosophy of practice, particularly moral philosophy, that provides a groundwork for discussion of many of the troubling issues facing nurses.

Ethical theory provides the cement to produce cohesive and consistent ethical thinking and decision making. This chapter is devoted to an examination of the two ethical theories that have had the greatest influence on contemporary bioethics: utilitarianism and deontology. A description of virtue or character ethics is also included. There are many ethical theories, some more sound than others, and some consisting of combinations of other theories. Theories related specifically to resource allocation, such as libertarianism, are described in Chapter 15. Nurses who are interested in a more detailed examination of specific theories should read works by the original theorists as well as analysis by contemporary writers.

ETHICS

Moral philosophy is the philosophical discussion of what is considered to be good or bad, right or wrong. **Ethics,** on the other hand, answers the question, "What ought one do in a given situation?" Ethics offers a formal process for putting moral philosophy into practice. The study of ethics gives the nurse a groundwork for making logical and consistent decisions. These decisions may be based upon conventional moral principles or formal moral theory from which principles are derived. In the end, though, ethics does not tell us what we ought to do. We must decide that for ourselves.

Philosophical Basis for Ethical Theory

Unlike mathematics or other empirical sciences, there are no apparent absolute rules governing ethics. Scientists can say for certain that two plus two always equals four—regardless of the time factors, circumstances, feelings, or beliefs of those involved in the calculations. Ethical rules are less clear, and difficult or impossible to prove. For example, while some would declare that killing for any reason is always wrong, others might argue that euthanasia can be beneficial either for the individual or the society, that abortion to save the life of the mother is permissible, or that killing during war is justified. There are reasonable arguments, based upon opposing viewpoints, that support any of these beliefs. How can rational people come to such different conclusions? The answer to this question may lie in the particular perspective of the persons involved.

Ethical theories are derived from either of two basic schools of thought: naturalism or rationalism. An examination of these perspectives will help the reader to understand the various theories.

Ask Yourself

What Is Your Code of Ethics?

- Do you believe that there are some actions that are absolutely wrong in all circumstances? Give examples.
- Do you believe that you have an innate knowledge of right and wrong?
- How did you learn right and wrong? What was the influence of your parents? Society? Other forces?
- What are your thoughts about how beliefs concerning right and wrong originate? To what degree do you believe that rules about right and wrong originate from a universal source? From within oneself?

Naturalism. **Naturalism** is a view of moral judgment that regards ethics as dependent upon human nature and psychology. Naturalism attributes divergence in moral codes to differing social conditions, while suggesting that there is a basic congruence related to the possession, by nearly all people, of similar underlying psychological tendencies (Raphael, 1994). These similarities suggest, to the student of naturalism, that there is universality (or near-universality) in moral judgment. This viewpoint allows each group or person to make judgments, based upon feelings, about particular actions in particular situations. It further suggests that most people's judgments in similar circumstances will be much alike. Naturalism does not explain aberrant, selfish, or cruel choices that are made by apparently rational individuals.

Naturalism holds that, collectively, all people have a tendency to make similar ethical decisions. Though there are many value differences among cultures, the variations are not as great as they may seem. Most people desire to be happy, to experience pleasure, and to avoid pain. There seems to be a natural tendency to sympathize with wishes and feelings of other people and, as a consequence, to approve of helping people in need. Raphael (1994) outlines similarities among cultures:

> All societies think that it is wrong to hurt members of their own group at least (or to kill them unless there are morally compelling reasons); that it is right to keep faith; that the needy should be helped; that people who deliberately flout the accepted rules should be punished. (p. 16)

Raphael points to **sympathy** as a motivating factor in moral decision making. Sympathy is sharing, in imagination, of others' feelings. This entails imagining one-self in the shoes of the other and consequently sharing feelings. Sympathy involves such feelings as pleasure, the tendency to warm toward one who has pleased an-other, pain, and the tendency to feel hostile toward one who has caused pain to an-other. Sympathy, according to some, is a natural tendency and is the basis for moral reasoning.

Rationalism.   The opposing school of thought is that of **rationalism.** Rationalists argue that feelings or perceptions, though they may seem similar in many people, may not actually be similar. Rationalists believe there are absolute truths that are not depen-dent upon human nature. They argue that ethical values have an independent origin in the nature of the universe or in the nature of God and can be known to humans through the process of reasoning. Rationalists believe there are truths about the world that are necessary and universal and that these truths are superior to the information that we receive from our senses (Raphael, 1994).

To rationalists, moral rules are necessarily true. Rationalists see the knowledge gained through the senses as only contingently true (Raphael, 1994). For example, the grass is perceived as green, but the color may be different—or may be seen as differ-ent by some. One who feels bad when hearing of the misfortune of another may not feel the same way about all others. On the other hand, moral or ethical rules, originat-ing from a higher source and being free of the variances in human nature, are always true. For example, rationalists argue that it is good to help those in need and that the truth of this maxim will not change based upon different circumstances or perceptions.

The differences in the two schools of thought revolve around the question of the origin of ethics. Is ethics a matter of feeling or of reason? Are individuals free to make ethical choices based upon predictable human nature, or is the foundation of ethics based upon universal or theologic truth? The comparison between naturalism and ra-tionalism is seen clearly in the study of ethical theories. Students are challenged to con-sider these two viewpoints when reading ethical theory.

THEORIES OF ETHICS

Moral philosophy is the branch of philosophy that examines beliefs and assumptions about the nature of certain human values. Ethics is the practical application of moral philosophy; that is, given the moral context of good or bad, right or wrong, "What ought one to do in a given situation?" The philosopher reveals an integrated global vision in which elements, like pieces of a puzzle, have a logical fit. By developing theories of ethics, the philosopher hopes to explain values and behavior related to cultural and moral norms. Each theory is based upon the particular viewpoint of the individual philosopher, and maintains, within itself, philosophical consistency. The discussion related to naturalism and rationalism explains, in part, one basic difference among moral philosophers. Utilitarianism and deontology were chosen for inclusion in this chapter because they are complete and integrated and are the major theories central to bioethics.

 CASE PRESENTATION

Conflicting Duties

Ms. Washington is director of a local hospice service. Unrelated to her work with hospice, she serves on a statewide advisory board that makes recommendations about allocation of Medicaid services. In response to a dramatic decrease in federal appropriation, the board is mandated to recommend funding cuts to specific programs. Ms. Washington and other board members are asked to choose between eliminating funding for adolescent well-child screening programs that serve tens of thousands of youth or eliminating a single costly program that provides catastrophic assistance to only a few individuals. Because of her experience with hospice care, Ms. Washington recognizes the importance of programs to help with catastrophic illness; however, she is hesitant to advise eliminating a program that is proven to help large numbers of children.

 Think About It

Resolving Conflicting Duties

- To what degree does Ms. Washington have a primary duty to see that catastrophic programs benefiting her hospice patients continue to be funded?
- As an advisory board member, what is Ms. Washington's responsibility to the large number of adolescents who would be denied health care if the well-child program for adolescents were no longer funded?
- What basis should Ms. Washington use for making her decision?
- How would you decide what to do in this situation?

The preceding case presentation implies the differences among various ethical theories. Remember, there are no clear answers in ethical dilemmas. The reader's basic viewpoint is reflected in responses to the questions. In many instances answers are inconsistent, perhaps illustrating a need to identify and strengthen a cohesive ethical basis for practice.

Utilitarianism

Utilitarianism, sometimes called **consequentialism,** is a form of teleological theory. *Telos* comes from the Greek and literally means *end*. Utilitarianism is the moral theory that holds that an action is judged as good or bad in relation to the consequence, outcome, or end result that is derived from it. Utilitarianism is an important ethical philosophy that has its basis in naturalism. According to the utilitarian school of thought, right action is that which has greatest **utility** or usefulness, and no action is, in itself, either good or bad. Utilitarians hold that the only factors that make actions good or bad are the outcomes, or end results, that are derived from them (Quinn & Smith, 1987).

Utilitarianism is a broad term that relates to a number of important theories. One of the first utilitarians was the Roman philosopher Epicurus. The teachings of Epicurus date back to about 200–300 B.C.E. This philosopher believed that both good and evil lie in sensation, pleasure being good and pain being evil. He taught that pleasure can be gained by living a life of moderation, courage, and justice and by cultivating friendship. Epicurus also believed that deities dwell apart from humans and are not concerned with the state of human existence; therefore, humans control their own destiny (Honderich, 1995).

There was a rebirth of interest in utilitarian philosophy in the late eighteenth and early nineteenth centuries. Jeremy Bentham (1748–1832), a leading political philosopher, is considered to be the father of modern utilitarianism. According to Bentham's theory, actions can be considered to be right when they increase happiness and diminish misery, and can be considered to be wrong when they have the opposite effect. Following is Bentham's definition of the "principle of utility":

> By utility is meant that property in any object, whereby it tends to produce benefit, advantage, pleasure, good, or happiness . . . or . . . to prevent the happening of mischief, pain, evil, or unhappiness to the party whose interest is considered: if that party be the community in general, then the happiness of the community: if a particular individual, then the happiness of that individual. (Bentham, 1948, p. 2)

Bentham attempted to create a science derived from the principle of utility. He proposed that a person should measure the product of an act in terms of the value of a proposed pleasure. Seven criteria to measure the pleasure included intensity, duration, certainty, propinquity (nearness in place or time), fecundity (the chance of it being followed by sensations of the same kind), and purity (the chance of it not being followed by sensations of the opposite kind). Bentham proposed that each criterion be given a value and that the sum of the values related to the pleasure be weighed against a similar sum of values related to the pain that might result from any given act. The person should act in accordance with a mathematical formula resolving ethical decisions based upon the sum total of the value of a given act.

Though many critics describe Bentham as having a hedonistic tendency (his theory is often referred to as hedonistic utilitarianism), it is clear from his writings that his interest extended far beyond physical pleasure. He wrote that *pleasure* is synonymous with many other terms such as *good, profit, advantage, benefit,* and so forth. In fact, his interest in the common good of the community refutes those who charge that his theory is hedonistic. He describes a type of justice in which action should have a tendency to augment the happiness of the community as a whole, rather than diminish it.

John Stuart Mill (1806–1873) was a leading British moral philosopher of the nineteenth century. Like Bentham, Mill was a utilitarian. He described utilitarianism in terms of measuring acts according to the end result. He wrote, "All action is for the sake of some end; and rules of action, it seems natural to suppose, must take their whole character and color from the end to which they are subservient" (Mill, 1910, p. 2). The phrase *the end justifies the means* relates to Mill's theory. According to Mill, the only right actions are those that produce the greatest happiness. His "greatest happiness principle" holds that the right action in conduct is not the agent's own happiness, but the happiness of all concerned. He further believed that sacrifice is good only when it increases the total sum of happiness. For Mill, the object of virtue is the multiplication of happiness. He cautioned, however, that one must carefully attempt to avoid violating the rights of some in the process of maximizing the happiness of others.

Mill defined his concepts in ways that make the meaning of this theory clearer. He described happiness as a state of pleasure that is not restricted to physical pleasure alone. In fact, Mill made a strong argument in favor of prioritizing pleasure—with intellectual pleasure having greater priority than physical or hedonistic pleasure. Further, Mill condemned those who choose sensual indulgences to the injury of health. He described the greatest sources of physical and mental suffering as such things as "indigence, disease, and the unkindness, worthlessness, or premature loss, of objects of affection" (Mill, 1910, p. 14).

Mill, though disagreeing with the notion that rules of ethics are edicts from God, related utilitarianism to Judeo-Christian doctrine. He believed utilitarianism to be in the spirit of the golden rule, "do unto others as you would have them do unto you" (Random House et al., 1987). Thus, to do as you would be done by, and to love your neighbor as yourself, constitutes the ideal perfection of the utilitarian morality. He further wrote that the happiness of humankind is certainly within the interest of a benevolent God and that people are given the opportunity to make ethical choices according to these precepts. Interestingly, similar formulations of the golden rule designate guides to conduct fundamental to most major religions and moral traditions (Honderich, 1995).

Though the works of Bentham and Mill are the most frequently quoted, there are many other utilitarian theories. There are two basic types of utilitarianism. **Act-utilitarianism** suggests that people choose actions that will, in any given circumstance, increase the overall good. **Rule-utilitarianism,** on the other hand, suggests that people choose rules that, when followed consistently, will maximize the overall good.

Act-utilitarianism.   Act-utilitarianism allows for different, sometimes opposing, action in different situations. For example, while act-utilitarians probably believe that it is best to tell the truth (or keep promises, or avoid killing, and so on), they recognize that there are times when the overall consequences will be better for everyone concerned if this guideline is not followed, even if the rights of some individuals are violated (Beauchamp & Childress, 1994; Smart, 1993). Act-utilitarians recognize that there are tenets that are good to follow but which should be used as rough guidelines rather than strict rules.

Rule-utilitarianism.   Rule-utilitarianism, on the other hand, suggests that people should act according to rules that tend to maximize happiness and diminish unhappiness. Rule-utilitarianism requires that people tell the truth (keep promises, avoid killing, and so on) in all circumstances because the overall good is maximized by consistent following of such rules. An example of rule-utilitarian thinking regarding truth telling comes from the writing of Dr. Worthington Hooker, a prominent nineteenth century figure in medical ethics:

> The good, which may be done by deception in a few cases, is almost as nothing, compared with the evil which it does in many, when the prospect of its doing good was just as promising as it was in those in which it succeeded. And when we add to this the evil which would result from a general adoption of a system of deception, the importance of a strict adherence to the truth in our intercourse with the sick, even on the ground of expediency, becomes incalculably great. (Beauchamp & Childress, 1994, p. 51)

The argument of this rule-utilitarian was that even though the patient's health is sometimes maximized through the use of deception, a widespread use of deception will eventually cause more harm than good. Thus, though rule-utilitarians recognize that in some instances good might result from a particular act, in the end, the overall good is maximized by the following of strict rules in all situations.

Though utilitarianism is a widely accepted ethical theory, there are a few problems inherent in its use. Utilitarianism does not give sufficient thought to respect of persons. In fact, it is possible that harm can be done to minority groups or individuals in the name of overall good. It gives little recognition to the principle of autonomy, particularly when one considers utilitarian decision making relative to distributive justice. Critics argue that utilitarianism sacrifices rights of individuals in favor of the overall good.

Notwithstanding acknowledged problems inherent in utilitarianism, this ethical theory captures the imagination as an attractive moral philosophy. Its appeal lies in the simple precept of promoting happiness for as many people as possible. It is particularly useful as a method of deciding issues of distributive justice.

Ask Yourself

Is Utilitarianism Useful?

- What useful guidelines does utilitarianism provide in terms of distributing resources?
- To what degree is it permissible to sacrifice the rights of one to provide for the welfare of many?
- To what degree is it permissible to sacrifice the rights of many to provide for the welfare of one?

Deontology

Deontological theories of ethics are based upon the rationalist view that the rightness or wrongness of an act depends upon the nature of the act, rather than the consequences that occur as a result of it. The term *deontology* is taken from the Greek word for duty. Occasionally, deontology is called **formalism;** some writers refer to this type of ethical theory as **Kantian.** Kantianism is based upon the writings of the philosopher, Immanuel Kant, who shaped many deontological formulations. For the purpose of this chapter, the terms *deontology* and *Kantian ethics* are used interchangeably.

Kant was born at Konigsberg, Prussia, in 1724. After an uninspiring academic career, he surprised the world with his groundbreaking ethical theory. Late in his life, Kant published volumes of philosophical writings that shook the religious and political systems of his day and continue to have strong influence on contemporary ethical philosophy. Kant contended that ethical rules are universal and that humans can derive certain consistent principles to guide action. The awareness of these moral rules is the product of pure reason, and not of experience as the naturalists would maintain. Kant asserted that moral rules are absolute and apply to all people, for all times, in all situations. He believed that ethical rules could be known by rational humans. Knowledge of the right course of action in any given situation could be obtained by following a maxim that he called the **categorical imperative.** *Categorical* refers to moral rules that do not admit exceptions; *imperative* denotes a command that is derived from principle. Kant said there is only one categorical imperative:

> Act only according to that maxim by which you can at the same time
> will that it should become a universal law. (Kant, 1959, p. 39)

In other words, no action can be judged as right which cannot reasonably become a law by which every person should always abide. As an example, Kant related a moral problem in which a man needs money to feed his family. He knows that he will not be able to repay it, but sees that nothing will be lent to him if he does not promise to repay it at a certain time. In order to satisfy himself that the act of breaking the promise to repay the money is morally correct, the man asks himself the question, "Should every person always make promises which they know will not be fulfilled?" Through reasoning the man can see that this could not become a universal law because no one would ever believe what has been promised. As a consequence, promise making would hold no meaning. Kant gave similar examples of situations related to suicide, squandering of talent, and helping others. Rather than compile a list of specific ethical rules, Kant proposed that each rational person should use the test of the categorical imperative to guide actions.

Following the categorical imperative, Kant also described his formulation of the **practical imperative:**

> Act so that you treat humanity, whether in your own person or that of
> another, always as an end and never as a means only. (Kant, 1959,
> p. 47)

To treat another person as an end, according to Kant, is to make his or her ends your own and to act toward his or her purposes as you naturally do toward your own. Raphael (1994) makes the point that Kant's practical imperative automatically shows that domination of one person over another is morally wrong. Domination makes no allowance for the dominated person's power of decision making. He also notes that acting toward another as you would toward yourself mandates that, whenever possible, one must help people who need help. The practical imperative requires that one must fulfill certain duties owed to others.

When the categorical imperative and the practical imperative are merged, there is a strong implication that each person is a member of a *realm of ends*—a politically organized society. Kant calls this "a systematic union of rational beings through common objective laws" (1959, p. 51). This requires that one should act as a member of a community of equal and autonomous individuals and that each member treat all others as moral beings. Each person should have regard for the desires of others and allow them freedom of decision. In Kantian theory, there is an inherent recognition that all people are equal and equally competent to make universally legislative decisions. According to Raphael (1994), "Kantian ethics is in fact an ethics of democracy. It requires liberty, equality, and fraternity" (p. 57) within a politically organized society.

Deontology also implies that ethics are derived from one's fulfilling of duties. One must act for the sake of obligation. Kant believed that all *imperatives of duty* can be deduced from his categorical imperative (one should act as if one's actions could become universal law for all people) and must also comply with his practical imperative (treat all people as ends, none as means to an end). He also believed that an action done from duty has its moral worth, not in the results it attains, but from the principle of acting out of reverence for the law and doing one's duty—whatever that might be (Paton, 1961). Most professional codes of ethics are based upon Kantian principles. Nurses' codes of ethics stress the importance of fulfilling duties that are inherently owed to patients and the importance of preserving the dignity and autonomy of each individual patient.

There are some acknowledged problems with the practical application of Kantian or deontological ethics. Kantianism is exceptionless and rigid. It does not assist one in choosing among conflicting alternatives or principles and, in fact, may actually present a conflict between two equally compelling duties. In addition, it seems reasonable to speculate that the automatic disregard of the consequences of any given action can occasionally lead to disastrous results.

Like utilitarianism, deontology is an attractive ethical theory. It is, in fact, a most popular foundation for many contemporary beliefs. It provides clear guidelines for judging the rightness or wrongness of action. It recognizes the dignity and autonomy of individuals and allows all people equal consideration. It serves as a basis for much of the contemporary ethical thinking that guides health care delivery.

 CASE PRESENTATION

Weighing Rights and Duties in Questions of Justice

Sumiko is the home health nurse for Mrs. B. Her patient is an eighty-nine-year-old widow who lives in the home that she and her husband shared until his death five years previously. She suffers from severe rheumatoid arthritis and has a new colostomy. The colostomy was performed as a last resort for severe ulcerative colitis. Mrs. B. is unable to care for herself because of the advanced state of her arthritis. Her daughter, son-in-law, and two teenage grandchildren moved into her home to take care of her daily needs. After many months, the family feels that caring for the elderly woman has become an unbearable burden. They ask Sumiko to help arrange long-term care in a local nursing home. Mrs. B. wants to continue to live in her home.

Think About It

Whose Rights Are More Important?

- Does Mrs. B. have the right to stay in her home even if the entire family is made unhappy by her presence?
- According to Kantian ethics, what factors must the family consider in deciding?
- Kantian ethics is duty oriented. Assuming that a Kantian basis for ethical decision making is used, to whom does Sumiko owe a duty?
- To what degree should the rights of the other family members bear on the decision that Sumiko makes?
- How does the ANA *Code for Nurses with Interpretive Statements* offer Sumiko guidance as she responds to this situation?
- Apply the categorical imperative to Sumiko's decision.
- Whose decision is this to make? Why?
- What would you do if you were Sumiko? On what basis would you make your decision?
- How might cultural factors influence decisions in this situation?

Virtue Ethics

Virtue ethics, sometimes called **character ethics,** represents the idea that individuals' actions are based upon a certain degree of innate moral virtue. First noted in the writings of Homer, and subsequently in the works of Plato, Aristotle, and early Christian thinkers, Western moralism emerged with the idea of cardinal virtues: wisdom, courage, temperance, justice, generosity, faith, hope, and charity (Kitwood, 1990). Modern and contemporary writers also include such virtues as honesty, compassion, caring, responsibility, integrity, discernment, trustworthiness, and prudence. Though nearly absent in nursing ethics texts in the past twenty years, virtue ethics is reemerging as an important framework for examining moral behavior.

Aristotle (384–332 B.C.E.) considered goodness of character to be produced by the practice of virtuous behavior, rather than virtuous acts being the end result of a good character. According to Aristotle, virtues are tendencies to act, feel, and judge that are developed from a natural capacity by proper training and exercise. He believed that practice creates a habit of acting in a virtuous way and that virtue can be learned and improved. Virtue, according to Aristotle, depends on "clear judgment, self-control, symmetry of desire, and artistry of means" (Durant, 1926, p. 75). He considered virtue to be the fruit of intelligent pursuit. "It is not the possession of the simple [person], nor the gift of innocent intent, but the achievement of experience in the fully developed [person]" (Durant, p. 75). He considered excellence to be won by training and habituation, and believed that virtuous character is created by repeatedly acting in a virtuous manner. Aristotle's traits of a virtuous character provided three criteria:

1. Virtuous acts must be chosen for their own sake.

2. Choice must proceed from a firm and unchangeable character.

3. Virtue is a disposition to choose the mean. (Edge & Groves, 1994, p. 22)

The *golden mean* of virtuous behavior, for Aristotle, meant practicing moderation: avoiding both excess and deficiency. Aristotle did not list a number of moral principles. For him, the basic moral question is not "what should one do" but rather "what should one be" (Mayo, 1958).

Phillipa Foot (1993) adds another perspective to Aristotle's concept of a virtuous person. Foot proposes that virtue lies not only in engaging in virtuous acts, but also in will. She defines will as "that which is wished for as well as what is sought." According to Foot, a positive or moral will is sometimes the necessary ingredient in success. She says,

> sometimes one man succeeds where another fails not because there is some specific difference in their previous conduct but rather because his heart lies in a different place; and the disposition of the heart is part of virtue. What this suggests is that a man's virtue may be judged by his innermost desires as well as by his intentions and this fits with our idea that a virtue such as generosity lies as much in someone's attitudes as in his actions. (p. 252)

According to Foot, virtue is not like a skill or an art. It cannot merely be a practiced and perfected act: it must actually engage the will. In other words, an act, though apparently kind or generous, for example, cannot be considered to be virtuous if the agent's intention is not good. Though Aristotle's idea of virtue is one of hope (everyone has the capacity to learn virtuous action), Foot makes the road to virtuous character less easily accessed.

Focal Virtues. In the discussion of virtue as related to biomedical ethics, Beauchamp and Childress (1994) define character as being "comprised of a set of stable traits that affect a person's judgment and action" (p. 463). Like Aristotle, these authors suggest that although people have different character traits, all have the capacity to learn or cultivate those that are important to morality. Beauchamp and Childress propose that there are four focal virtues that are more pivotal than others in characterizing a virtuous person: compassion, discernment, trustworthiness, and integrity.

Compassion. **Compassion** is the ability to imagine oneself in the situation of another. Beauchamp and Childress (1994) define the term in the following manner: "The virtue of compassion is a trait combining an attitude of active regard for another's welfare with an imaginative awareness and emotional response of deep sympathy, tenderness, and discomfort at the other person's misfortune or suffering" (p. 466). This virtue embodies internalizing of the golden rule. Compassion is so important that many times the patient's need for a compassionate and caring presence outweighs the need for technical care. Nurses must be careful, however, that compassion does not impede the ability to make objective decisions.

Discernment. The virtue of **discernment** is in some ways related to the classical meaning of wisdom. "The virtue of discernment rests on sensitive insight involving acute judgment and understanding, and it eventuates in decisive action" (Beauchamp & Childress, 1994, p. 468). Discernment enables the nurse to have insight into appropriate actions in given situations. It requires sensitivity and attention attuned to the demands of a particular context. For example, a discerning nurse will recognize when a patient needs comfort and reassurance rather than privacy. Discernment requires that nurses continually strive to recognize and understand important nuances in human behavior.

Trustworthiness. **Trustworthiness** is another focal virtue for nurses. "Trust is a confident belief in and reliance upon the ability and moral character of another person. Trust entails a confidence that another will act with the right motives in accord with moral norms" (Beauchamp & Childress, 1994, p. 469). Trustworthiness is measured by others' recognition of the nurse's consistency and predictability in following moral norms. In practical terms, trustworthiness is accounted for in the reputation one has among coworkers. This virtue is important for the nurse in relationships with patients, physicians, and other nurses.

Integrity. **Integrity** is perhaps the cardinal virtue. Moral integrity, according to Beauchamp and Childress (1994), means soundness, reliability, wholeness, and an integration of moral character. It also refers to fidelity in adherence to moral norms that is sustained over time. It is "the character trait of a coherent integration of reasonably stable, justifiable moral values, together with active fidelity to those values in judgment and action" (p. 473). A person with integrity has a consistency of convictions, actions, and emotions and is trustworthy. Integrity is compromised when the nurse acts inconsistently or in a way that is not supported by professed moral beliefs. Deficiencies in moral integrity may include such vices as hypocrisy, insincerity, and bad faith.

Virtue Ethics in Nursing. How does the concept of virtue or character ethics fit with nursing as a principled profession? It is likely that principled behavior, while not the sole domain of a good moral character, is more likely to occur in the presence of one. Certainly Florence Nightingale thought virtue was an important trait of the good nurse. Traditionally recited by graduating nurses, the Nightingale Pledge implies virtue of character as nurses promise purity, faith, loyalty, devotion, trustworthiness, and temperance. It is reasonable to say that good character is the cornerstone of good nursing, and that the nurse with virtue will act according to principle. If Aristotle was correct in his belief that virtue can be practiced and learned, then students and young nurses can learn, through practice, those acts which, by their doing, create a virtuous person.

SUMMARY

Ethical theory helps nurses understand the origin and process of ethical and moral thinking and behavior. Two important theories are particularly important to nursing ethics. The ethical theory of utilitarianism was developed in part by Jeremy Bentham and later refined by John Stuart Mill. Utilitarianism suggests that ethical decisions should be made in regard to the outcome or end result. Accordingly, no action in itself is inherently right or wrong. This theory also provides for the greatest good for the greatest number. Utilitarianism is particularly useful in situations of distributive justice but tends to ignore the rights of the minority or the individual. Deontology, or Kantian ethics, was initially developed by Immanuel Kant. This theory, through the use of the categorical imperative, assists one in making ethical decisions. The categorical imperative demands that the agent ask the question, can this action be a law for all people in all circumstances? Additionally, the theory presents the practical imperative which requires that the agent treat all individuals as if they were ends only, rather than means. Kantian ethics provides clear guidelines for making ethical decisions but does not provide for making decisions when there are conflicting duties or obligations. Virtue or character ethics, as described by Aristotle, describes each person as capable of practicing and learning virtue through repetition of virtuous acts. Thus, the virtuous person is one in whom virtue is habituated. Virtue ethics complements other ethical theory and can be used to nurture or predict character in individuals. Ethical theories can help the nurse understand ethical decision making models and assist in developing a cohesive and logical system for making individual decisions.

CHAPTER HIGHLIGHTS

- Philosophy is the intense and critical examination of beliefs and assumptions.
- Moral philosophy is the philosophical discussion of what is considered to be good or bad, right or wrong.
- Ethics is a formal process for making logical and consistent decisions based upon moral philosophy.
- As the morally central health care profession, nursing requires astuteness of moral and ethical issues.
- Ethical theories explain values and behavior related to cultural and moral norms.
- Utilitarianism holds that right action is that which has the greatest utility or usefulness, and no action is in itself either good or bad.
- Deontology is based upon the rationalist view that the rightness or wrongness of an act depends upon the nature of the act, rather than the consequences that occur as a result of it.

- Kantianism is a particular deontological theory developed by Immanuel Kant.
- Categorical imperative is the Kantian maxim requiring that no action can be judged as right which cannot reasonably become a law by which every person should always abide.
- Practical imperative is the Kantian maxim requiring that one treats others always as ends and never as a means.
- Virtue ethics, usually attributed to Aristotle, represents the idea that individuals' actions are based upon innate moral virtue.

DISCUSSION QUESTIONS AND ACTIVITIES

1. Describe the differences in beliefs about the origin of ethical rules.

2. Describe a hypothetical situation in which an ethical dilemma exists and discuss solutions to the dilemma in terms of act-utilitarianism and rule-utilitarianism.

3. Identify specific health care funding policies and discuss these in terms of utilitarian theory.

4. Identify different ethical codes (including professional codes) that are based upon Kantian or deontological ethics.

5. Describe a real or hypothetical situation in which there is an ethical dilemma. Relate a solution to the dilemma using the rule of the categorical imperative.

6. List and describe the virtues that you feel are important for nurses.

7. Consider the following situation: Two nursing students are discovered to have cheated on several assignments. After being questioned by the instructor, both students deny having cheated, even though the evidence is irrefutable. Discuss these students in terms of virtue ethics and Kantian ethics. Do these students have integrity? Do these students have the character to become good nurses? How would you apply the categorical imperative?

REFERENCES

Beauchamp, T., & Childress, J. (1994). *Principles of biomedical ethics* (4th ed.). New York: Oxford University Press.

Bentham, J. (1948). *An introduction to the principles of moral legislation.* New York: Hafner Press.

Buber, M. (1965). *The knowledge of man: A philosophy of the interhuman.* New York: Harper & Row.

Durant, W. (1926). *The story of philosophy.* New York: Washington Square Press.

Edge, R. S., & Groves, J. R. (1994). *The ethics of health care: A guide for practice.* Albany, NY: Delmar.

Foot, P. (1993). Virtues and vices. In C. Sommers & F. Sommers, *Vice and virtue in everyday life: Introductory readings in ethics* (pp. 250–265). Fort Worth, TX: Harcourt Brace College. (Reprinted from P. Foot, *Virtues and vices,* Berkeley, CA: University of California Press)

Hesse, H. (1971). *Siddhartha.* New York: Bantam.

Honderich, T. (Ed.). (1995). *The Oxford companion to philosophy*. New York: Oxford University Press.

Kant, I. (1959). *Foundations of the metaphysics of morals*. (L. W. Beck, Trans.). Indianapolis, IN: Bobbs-Merrill.

Kitwood, T. (1990). *Concern for others: A new psychology of conscience and morality*. London: Routledge.

Kneller, G. F. (1971). *Introduction to the philosophy of education*. (2nd ed.). New York: John Wiley & Sons.

Mayo, B. (1958). *Ethics and the moral life*. London: Macmillan.

Mill, J. S. (1910). *Utilitarianism*. London: Dent & Sons.

Paton, H. J. (Trans. & Ed.). (1961). *The moral law*. London: Hutchinson & Co.

Quinn, C. A., & Smith, M. D. (1987). *The professional commitment: Issues and ethics in nursing*. Philadelphia: Saunders.

Rand, A. (1982). *Philosophy: Who needs it?* New York: Bobbs-Merrill.

Random House et al. (1987). *The Random House Dictionary of the English Language* (2nd ed. unabridged). New York: Random House.

Raphael, D. D. (1994). *Moral philosophy* (2nd ed.). New York: Oxford University Press.

Smart, J. J. C. (1993). Utilitarianism. In C. Sommers & F. Sommers, *Vice and virtue in everyday life: Introductory readings in ethics* (pp. 109–123). Fort Worth, TX: Harcourt Brace College. (Reprinted from J. J. C. Smart & B. Williams (Eds.), *Utilitarianism: For and against,* New York: Oxford University Press)

CHAPTER 3

Ethical Principles

*The quality of mercy is not strain'd
It droppeth as the gentle rain from heaven
Upon the place beneath. It is twice blest:
It blesseth him that gives, and him that takes.*
(William Shakespeare, *The Merchant of Venice*)

OBJECTIVES

After completing this chapter, the reader should be able to:

1. Discuss the principle of autonomy in terms of patients' rights, informed consent, parentalism, and noncompliance.
2. Discuss the principle of beneficence as it relates to nursing practice.
3. Define the principle of nonmaleficence and weigh actions in terms of harm and benefit.
4. Relate the principle of veracity to nursing practice.
5. Critically examine the principle of confidentiality in nursing practice, recognizing legal implications and reasonable limits to confidentiality.
6. Discuss the principle of justice as it relates to the delivery of health care goods and services.
7. Relate the principle of fidelity to nursing's promise to society.
8. Discuss situations in which there is a conflict between two or more ethical principles.

INTRODUCTION

Ethical issues are commonly examined in terms of a number of **ethical principles.** Ethical principles are basic and obvious moral truths that guide deliberation and action. Major ethical theories utilize many of the same principles, though either the emphasis or meaning may be somewhat different in each. For example, autonomy is a dominant principle in deontological theory but is less important in utilitarian theory. It is vital for nurses to understand ethical principles and be adept at applying them in a meaningful and consistent manner. (See Figure 3–1.) It is the authors' contention that consistent adherence to principle is an important basis for ethical practice in nursing. This chapter examines the following ethical principles: autonomy, beneficence, nonmaleficence, veracity, confidentiality, justice, and fidelity.

Figure 3–1 **Principles of Ethics**

Autonomy
Beneficence
Nonmaleficence
Veracity
Confidentiality
Justice
Fidelity

Respect for Persons

All of the principles discussed in this chapter presuppose that nurses have respect for the value and uniqueness of persons. Occasionally viewed as an ethical principle in its own right, **respect for persons** implies that one considers others to be worthy of high regard. Certainly, genuine regard and respect for others serves as the cornerstone of any caring profession. Discussion of the ethical principles in this chapter is based upon the belief that respect for persons is a value held by nurses.

AUTONOMY

The word **autonomy** literally means self-governing. *Autonomy* is a word that is frequently used, yet poorly understood. Nurses are told to respect the autonomy of patients but are given little guidance in understanding the meaning of this abstract concept. The term is more frequently used as a contrast to undesirable states such as dependency, coercion, paternalism, thoughtlessness, and habit (Jameton, 1984). Nurses are expected to understand the concept and be advocates to ensure the maintenance of autonomy for all patients. This advocacy may be very difficult in today's health care system.

The term *autonomy* denotes having the freedom to make choices about issues that affect one's life. Autonomy is closely linked to the notion of respect for persons and is an important principle in cultures where all individuals are considered to be unique and valuable members of society. In cultures that do not regard all members as being of equal worth or that respect the total social structure above individual rights, the concept of autonomy holds less meaning. Autonomy implies that each person has the freedom to make decisions about personal goals. It is a state in which the "individual is free to choose and implement one's own decisions, free from deceit, duress, constraint, or coercion" (Edge & Groves, 1994, p. 31). In societies where slavery exists, where women are expected to be subservient to men, where minority races are not respected, or where children are exploited, the notion of autonomy is meaningless. Autonomy cannot thrive in a climate that does not allow for either the independent planning of personal goals or the privilege of examining and choosing options to meet goals.

Implied in the concept of autonomy are four basic elements. First, autonomy implies a respect for persons. It is logical that those choosing the nursing profession would inherently value and respect the unique humanness of others. This element is essential to assuring autonomy. Second, one must be able to determine personal goals. These goals may be explicit and of a global nature or may be less well defined. For example, the patient with an ankle injury may have a goal to return to athletic play within two weeks of the injury or may simply wish to be pain free. In each case the patient develops personally chosen goals that are consistent with a particular lifestyle. Third, the concept of autonomy implies that the person has the capacity to decide upon a plan of action. One must be able to understand the meaning of the choice to be made and must be able to deliberate on the various options, while understanding the implications of possible outcomes. Imagine, for example, ordering from a restaurant menu written in a language you do not understand. You have the freedom and responsibility to make a choice but cannot make a meaningful choice without an understanding of the various foods offered. When it is believed that a patient is not able to comprehend the meaning of choices, goals, or outcomes, it is said that the person is incompetent to make decisions or lacks decision making capacity. There are certain groups of patients that are generally thought of as unable to make informed choices. Children, fetuses, and the mentally impaired are among these groups. Fourth, the concept of autonomy implies that one has the freedom to act upon the choices that are made. In situations where persons are capable of formulating goals, understanding various options, and making decisions, yet are not free to implement their plans, autonomy is either limited or absent. This may be seen in cultures where groups of people are systematically denied the freedom to act, as with communist or totalitarian governments. Autonomy may also be limited in situations where the means to accomplish autonomously devised plans do not exist. An example of the latter is seen in the case of the indigent person who does not have access to health care insurance. This person may choose to have, for example, a pancreas transplant in lieu of insulin injections, but does not have the financial means to meet this goal. In order to assure autonomy, each of the four elements must be present to a reasonable degree.

There are a number of intrinsic factors that threaten patient autonomy. The patient role is a dependent one. The patient seeks health care assistance because of a real or perceived need and, as a result, can be thought of as being dependent upon the health care provider. The role of the health care professional, on the other hand, is one of power. This power is based upon knowledge and authority and is inherent in the role. This complementary relationship, while a necessary one, can lead to violations of patient autonomy.

Ask Yourself

Is the Patient Role a Dependent One?

- Describe a time when you or a family member experienced the role of hospitalized patient.
- How did you or your family member feel when interacting with members of the health care team who were dressed, while you or your family member were in pajamas or a hospital gown (or worse yet, naked)?
- Describe the degree to which you or your family member were able to maintain dignity and autonomy.

Health care professionals are often insensitive to the way in which the health care industry systematically dehumanizes and erodes the autonomy of consumers. Patients are forced to comply with rules that require them to be and act dependent. Immediately upon admission to a hospital, patients are disrobed, asked questions about personal and private matters, forced to relinquish money and belongings, and expected to remain in a bed, emphasizing the dependency of the patient role. Patients are placed in rooms with doors that are seldom closed and asked to wear pajamas. Workers, who are strangers to patients, freely enter and leave the patients' rooms, making privacy impossible. Regardless of patients' personal habits or knowledge of their own health care, they are forced to bathe at certain times, eat at certain times, take medications at certain times, and are often prohibited from practicing self-care measures that may have been their habits for many years. Patients are expected to follow each plan that is made. Otherwise, they will be labeled difficult or *noncompliant*. For all the lip service given the importance of autonomy, health care professionals are often guilty of creating a climate of dependency for patients—of coercing otherwise autonomous, intelligent, and independent adults essentially into a very dependent role.

Recognizing Violations of Patient Autonomy

Often nurses and other health care workers fail to recognize subtle violations of patient autonomy. This occurs especially when nurses perceive choices to be self-evident. At least four factors are related to this failure. First, nurses may falsely assume that patients have the same values and goals as themselves. This state of mind compels nurses to believe that the only reasonable course of action is the one that is consistent with their own values. This leads to faulty conclusions. For example, if an elderly person chooses to stay in her own home, even though to others she seems to be incapable of caring for herself, the choice might be viewed as unreasonable and might become grounds to believe the patient incompetent to make decisions. In other words, "If you don't make the choices that seem correct to me, you must be incompetent to make decisions." In truth, the elderly person may recognize that life is drawing to a close and may want to remain in familiar surroundings, maintain dignity, remain independent, and prevent needless depletion of her life savings. The decision is based upon her thoughtful consideration of the consequences of staying home versus the consequences of living in a long-term care facility. There are some who would insist that she should be allowed to stay at home even if she places herself at considerable danger—as long as she does not jeopardize the autonomy of others.

 CASE PRESENTATION

Noncompliance Versus Autonomy

Cora is a forty-five-year-old woman who looks years older than her stated age. She has very limited monthly income and no health insurance. Cora smokes two and one-half packs of cigarettes per day. She has severe COPD with constant dyspnea and frequent exacerbations. The nurse who sees her at a local free clinic is interested in at least preventing further problems and speaks to Cora often about the importance of quitting smoking. The situation becomes very frustrating for all involved when Cora returns repeatedly for increasingly severe problems—having failed to quit smoking. Cora, of course, becomes labeled as noncompliant. During a particularly severe exacerbation, the nurse says to Cora, "You know you are committing suicide by continuing to smoke." Cora's reply is, "You don't understand. I live alone. I have no money, no friends, no family and will never be able to work. I know the damage I'm doing, but smoking is the only pleasure I have in life."

 Think About It

Do Nurses Coerce Patients?

- In attempting to persuade Cora to stop smoking, to what degree is the nurse disallowing Cora's right to autonomy?
- Does Cora have the right to choose to continue smoking?
- If rights and responsibilities are correlative, how should the clinic respond to Cora's continuing to smoke? Would you suggest that the clinic continue to serve Cora even though she is not following the plan of care?
- To what degree is coercion employed in situations such as Cora's? Is coercion an appropriate strategy?
- What would you do?

The second cause of failure to recognize subtle violations of patient autonomy lies in nurses failing to recognize that individuals' thought processes are different. Discounting a particular decision as incorrect may not take into consideration the fact that people process information in different ways. For example, there are those whose thought processes are very logical and methodical; others think in ways that are creative and free-flowing. It is particularly important to recognize these types of differences when several people are working together to come to a common decision. What is obvious to one will not be obvious to all—not necessarily because of a difference in values, knowledge base, or intellect, but because of different backgrounds and styles of thinking (Harrison & Bramson, 1982). This is an important consideration when collaborating with patients, families, and other professionals.

The third cause of failure to recognize subtle violations of patient autonomy lies in nurses' assumptions about patients' knowledge base. It is easy for nurses to forget that they have gained a specialized body of knowledge through their program of basic nursing education and extensive work experience. Knowledge about basic anatomy and physiology, disease process, the mechanism of action of drugs, and so forth is so ingrained in nurses' minds that it is easy to presume everyone has at least some of the same type of knowledge. Nurses often assume patients have more knowledge than is reasonable for them to have. Consequently, nurses may discount or criticize patients' decisions, even though flaws lie in the patients' level of knowledge rather than the appropriateness of decisions. Recall that an understanding of the choices, outcomes, and implications are inherently necessary for autonomous decision making. The nurse must accurately assess the patient's level of understanding in order to assure autonomy.

The fourth cause of the nurses' failure to recognize subtle violations of patient autonomy lies in the unfortunate fact that the "work" of nursing in some instances becomes the major focus. This produces a climate of industrious habit. As nurses go about their work—doing procedures, giving medications, writing care plans, and trying to keep up a frantic pace—attentiveness to assuring patient autonomy is sometimes neglected. In today's climate of advanced technology, fiscal uncertainty, staffing reductions, and bottom-line management, nurses should guard against focusing on industry rather than caring.

Autonomy for patients is more frequently discussed in terms of larger issues such as informed consent, paternalism, compliance, and self-determination. Let us review this principle as related to these and other recurrent themes.

Informed Consent

Informed consent relates to a process by which patients are informed of the possible outcomes, alternatives, and risks of treatments and required to freely give their consent. It assures the legal protection of a patient's right to personal autonomy in regard to specific treatments and procedures. The concept of informed consent is one that has come to mean that patients are given the opportunity to autonomously choose a course of action in regard to plans for medical care. This is usually discussed in relation to surgery and complex medical procedures. Informed consent will be discussed in more depth in Chapter 11.

Paternalism/Parentalism

Paternalism is a gender-biased term that literally means acting in a *fatherly* manner. The traditional view of paternal actions includes such role behaviors as leadership, benevolent decision making, protection, and discipline. As commonly used in nursing, the term *paternalism* carries negative connotations, particularly related to implied dominant male versus submissive female roles. The term *parentalism,* a nongender term that parallels the meaning of paternalism while avoiding gender-bias, is used in the subsequent discussion.

In the health care arena, the concept of parentalism translates to professionals who restrict others' autonomy, usually to protect that person from perceived or anticipated harm. Parentalism is appropriate when a patient is judged to be incompetent or to have diminished decision making capacity. As advocate, the nurse chooses to do for the patient that which it is reasonable to believe the patient would choose for self, if that were possible. For example, one would assume that a person would choose to be protected from injury. Within that context, and believing a patient to be incompetent, the nurse is justified in restraining an elderly person who is likely to fall or wander off if left unrestrained. Parentalism can be considered a form of advocacy when genuine concern for the patient is coupled with a well-founded belief that the patient is unable to make autonomous decisions.

The risk of harm is not enough by itself to judge a person incompetent. Virginia Henderson, the well-known nursing leader and author, recounts her experience as a hospitalized patient:

> I was in the room with another patient, and I couldn't stand being in bed any longer, and I would sit in a chair. This nurse came in and saw me sitting in the chair, and she said "Ms. Henderson if you keep doing that, we are going to have to tie you down" . . . I thought, You just try it. . . . (Goldsmith, 1992, p. 4)

Even though Ms. Henderson was ninety-four years old at the time of her hospitalization, she was certainly competent to make decisions for herself. Patients who are competent must be allowed to act autonomously—even if the choices can be predicted to cause them harm or render them incompetent (Quinn & Smith, 1987). The exception can be made that even competent persons cannot be allowed to act in a way that would cause harm to others.

The term *paternalism* generally evokes negative sentiments among nurses. This is due in part to a recognition that in the past patients' autonomy was frequently violated in the name of beneficence. Professionals sometimes make the dangerous assumption that they are uniquely qualified to make health care decisions by virtue of their professional knowledge and, further, that professional knowledge is the only knowledge needed to make decisions for patients. "Health care professionals often [believe they] understand better than patients do the full clinical implications of health risks, for they have seen the clinical results of its total actual results" (Quinn & Smith, 1987, p. 37). This kind of thinking allows the professional to ignore multiple factors that might be unrelated to physical outcomes, yet affect the whole person. These factors include, among others, economic considerations, lifestyle, values, role, culture, and spiritual beliefs. In making decisions, all possible factors must be taken into consideration. This dictates that the patient must be autonomously engaged in the decision making process.

It is interesting to compare discussion of the concept of paternalism in the nursing and medical literature. Nursing literature generally describes paternalism in a negative way. Nurses often think of paternalism as behavior that precludes autonomy. Medical literature, on the other hand, discusses paternalism as a benevolent quality. The following passage illustrates this point:

> In its strong version, the principle of paternalism justifies restricting someone's autonomy if by doing so we can benefit her. In such a case, our concern is not only with preventing the person from harming herself, but also with promoting her good in a positive way. The principle might be appealed to even in cases in which our actions go against the other's known wishes. (Munson, 1992, p. 43)

The differences between the nursing and medical community in relation to beliefs about paternalism probably relate to cultural and gender factors. Interdisciplinary discussion is needed in order to come to a consensus about the appropriateness of paternalism in health care decision making. Use of the term *parentalism* avoids negative gender reference and should be used in discussion.

Ask Yourself

Who Should Make Decisions?

- How do you feel when someone else makes a decision about you without your input?

- Since nurses and doctors know more about the science of health care, when, if ever, is it appropriate for them to make decisions about the health care regimen without participation of the patient?

Noncompliance

The term **noncompliance** is generally thought of as denoting an unwillingness on the part of the patient to participate in health care activities. This commonly entails lack of participation in a regimen that has been planned by the health care professional but must be carried out by the patient. Examples of such activities include taking medication as scheduled, maintaining a therapeutic or weight loss diet, exercising regularly, and quitting smoking. Use of the term *noncompliance* is just as likely to represent failure of the nurse as that of the patient. Discussion about noncompliance and care of the noncompliant patient centers around two basic factors. First, the autonomous participation of the patient in the health care plan is essential to success. When patients are fully aware of the choices in health care therapies and the consequences of nontreatment and are encouraged to make health care decisions, they are more likely to assume ownership of them and, as a result, to participate in care. Often nurses formulate plans of care that are consistent with a scientific base of knowledge but seem unreasonable to the patient. The nurse is amiss if the patient is not an autonomous participant in the formulation of the plan. Second, nurses and other health care professionals must assess patients' abilities to follow plans of care. Patients may be unable to comply with plans of care for a variety of reasons including lack of resources, lack of knowledge, lack of support from family members, psychological factors, and cultural beliefs that are not consistent with the proposed plan of care. An example of patients' inability to comply with a plan of care is seen every day in physicians' offices and emergency departments. Often patients are given prescriptions for medications that are prohibitively expensive. When they return with the same symptoms, not having taken the prescribed medication, they are invariably labeled as noncompliant. The problem is not one of compliance, but rather health care professionals' negligence in assessing patients' ability to follow a plan of care.

What are nurses to do when patients are well informed and apparently able to follow plans of care, yet do not? One hears stories of physicians who refuse to continue to care for patients who do not comply with instructions—smoking cessation, for example. In a climate of limited resources, this is a question worthy of contemplation. The American Nurses Association (ANA) *Code for Nurses with Interpretive Statements* (1985) states clearly that the nurse must "provide services with respect for human dignity and the uniqueness of the client unrestricted by considerations of social or economic status, personal attributes, or the nature of health problems" (p. 2). Further, the nurse must not be affected by patients' individual differences in background, customs, attitudes, and beliefs. Because health care practices are an integral part of patients' backgrounds, customs, and beliefs, refusal to participate in a plan of care, regardless of the outcome, is the prerogative of the patient and must not affect the care given by the nurse. Ultimately, choices about health care practices belong to patients. If allowed to choose, patients should not be labeled in a negative way for choices with which nurses do not agree. It is not appropriate for professionals who express the belief that all competent patients have the right to autonomous choice, to make value judgments about the choices made, and subsequently label patients as noncompliant.

BENEFICENCE

The principle of **beneficence** is one that requires nurses to act in ways that benefit patients. As with autonomy, beneficence, while appearing to be straightforward and simple, is a principle that is more complex than it first appears. The principle of beneficence lays the groundwork for the trust that society places in the nursing profession and the trust that individuals place in particular nurses or health care agencies. It requires that nurses act in ways that will help patients.

The ethical principle of beneficence has three major components. (See Figure 3–2.) It maintains, first, that one ought to do or promote good (Beauchamp & Childress, 1994). Even with the recognition that *good* might be defined in a number of ways, it seems safe to assume that the intention of nurses in general is to do good. Questions arise when, in particular situations, those involved cannot decide what is *good*. For example, consider the case of a patient who is in the process of a lingering, painful, terminal illness. There are those who believe that life is sacred and should be preserved at all costs. Others believe that death is preferable to a life of pain and dependence. The definition of *good* in any particular case will determine, at least in part, the action that is to be taken.

Figure 3–2 **Beneficence**

Do or Promote Good Prevent Harm Remove Evil or Harm

The principle of beneficence also maintains that one ought to prevent evil or harm (Beauchamp & Childress, 1994). The following statement from the ANA *Code for Nurses with Interpretive Statements* reflects this thought: "The nurse acts to safeguard the client and the public when health care and safety are affected by the incompetent, unethical, or illegal practice of any person" (1985, p. 6). Interpretive statements give specific guidance to the nurse in this situation:

> The nurse's primary commitment is to the health, welfare, and safety
> of the client. As an advocate for the client, the nurse must be alert to
> and take appropriate action regarding any instances of incompetent,
> unethical, or illegal practice by any member of the health care team
> or the health care system, or any action on the part of others that
> places the rights or best interests of the client in jeopardy. (1985, p. 6)

These steps are congruent with a third aspect of the principle of beneficence. Not only must nurses prevent, but they must also remove, evil or harm (Beauchamp & Childress, 1994). The *Code for Nurses with Interpretive Statements* (1985) very clearly delineates steps to be taken in the process of removing harm or evil. These steps include the following: expressing concern to the person carrying out the questionable practice, reporting the practice to the appropriate authority within the institution, and if not corrected, reporting the problem to other appropriate authorities such as practice committees of the pertinent professional organizations or licensing boards (pp. 5–6).

NONMALEFICENCE

The principle of **nonmaleficence** is related to beneficence. This principle requires nurses to act in such a manner as to avoid causing harm to patients. Included in this principle are deliberate harm, risk of harm, and harm that occurs during the performance of beneficial acts. It is obvious that nurses must not commit acts that cause deliberate harm. This principle prohibits, for example, experimental research that assumes negative outcomes for the participants and the performance of unnecessary procedures for economic gain or solely as a learning experience. Nonmaleficence may also be interpreted to mean avoiding harm as a consequence of doing good. In such cases, the harm must be weighed against the expected benefit. For example, sticking a child with a needle for the purpose of causing pain is always bad—there is no anticipated benefit to doing this. Giving an immunization, on the other hand, while causing similar pain, results in the benefit of protecting the child from serious disease. The harm caused by the pain of the injection is easily outweighed by the benefit of the vaccine. In day-to-day practice many situations are encountered by nurses in which the distinction is less clear, either because the harm caused may appear to be equal to the benefit gained, because the outcome of a particular therapy cannot be assured, or as a result of conflicting beliefs and values. For example, consider analgesia for patients with painful terminal illness. Narcotic analgesia may be the only type of medication that will relieve very severe pain. This medication, however, will result in dependence and can hasten death when given in amounts required to relieve pain. Each individual nurse must weigh the harm against the benefit within the context of personal values.

 ## CASE PRESENTATION

Beneficence Versus Nonmaleficence

A middle-aged nurse recounts an incident that she believes relates to the principle of nonmaleficence. As a senior nursing student she was responsible for the care of a man who had a shotgun wound to his abdomen. Surgery had been performed, and the surgeon was unable to adequately repair the damage. The man was not expected to survive the day. He was, however, awake and strong, though somewhat confused. He had a fever of 107° Fahrenheit. He was receiving intravenous fluids and had continuous nasogastric suction. The man begged for cold water to drink. The physician ordered nothing by mouth in the belief that electrolytes would be lost through the nasogastric suction if water were introduced into the stomach. The student had been taught to follow the physician's orders. She repeatedly denied the man water to drink. She worked diligently— giving iced alcohol baths, taking vital signs, monitoring the intravenous fluids, and being industrious. He begged for water. She followed orders perfectly. After six terrible hours she turned to find the man quickly drinking the water from one of his ice bags. She left the room, stood in the hallway, and cried. She felt she had failed to do her job. As a result of the gunshot wound, the man died the next morning. Today her view of the situation is different.

 ## Think About It

Weighing Harm Against Benefit

- Was this patient harmed? Discuss your answer.
- What was the benefit of the nothing by mouth order?
- Discuss whether the harm of thirst or the benefit of maintaining nothing by mouth should take precedence.

- What other ethical principles are relevant?
- Why did the student experience such extreme distress?

This case illustrates the difficulty encountered when attempting to honor the principles of beneficence and nonmaleficence.

VERACITY

The term **veracity** relates to the practice of telling the truth. Truthfulness is widely accepted as a universal virtue. Most were taught as children to always tell the truth. Philosophers, in general, favor openness and honesty. The philosophers most frequently cited in nursing literature, Immanuel Kant and John Stuart Mill, agree in favor of truth telling. Nursing literature promotes honesty as a virtue and truth telling as an important function of nurses. However, there are some differences in perspective among health care professionals. Bioethicists disagree on the absolute necessity of truth telling in all instances.

Ask Yourself

Is Truth Telling Always Beneficent?

- What situational variables influence how you feel about giving placebos?
- If your goal is to be beneficent and if the patient would benefit from a placebo, is deception justifiable if it will help the patient?
- What principles are in conflict when giving placebos?

Nurses' practice of telling the truth can be supported in many ways. Truth telling engenders respect, open communication, trust, and shared responsibility. It is promoted in all professional codes of nursing ethics.

A very general interpretation of the ideas of the contemporary philosopher Martin Buber (1965) suggests that true communication between people can take place only when there are no barriers between them. Lying or deception creates a barrier between people and prohibits both meaningful communication and the building of relationships. Recognizing that communication is the cornerstone of the nurse-patient relationship, an argument can be made that nurses must be truthful in order to effectively communicate with patients.

Nonadherence to the principle of veracity also shows lack of respect for others. Telling lies, or avoiding disclosure, implies that the specific function of the nurse or other person involved assumes prominence over the patient or, at the very least, the autonomy of the patient. Jameton (1984) suggests that manipulating information for the purpose of controlling others is like using coercion to control them. In essence this keeps them from participating in decisions on an equal basis. Used to benefit the patient, it is parentalism; used against the patient, it is fraud.

Jameton (1984) also suggests that deceiving others may constitute an unnecessary assumption of responsibility. When unfortunate consequences occur, the one responsible for the deception can also be assumed to be responsible for consequences. On the other hand, when bad consequences occur after one has reported the truth, one can attribute responsibility to the unfortunate nature of reality.

Truth telling engenders trust. The argument can be made that truth telling is imperative in assuring that patients continue to trust nurses and other health care professionals. It is by virtue of the trust that exists in these relationships that patients are willing to suspend some measure of autonomy and seek help in meeting health care needs. Without this trust the nurse-patient relationship would be destroyed, and it could be predicted that patients' needs would go unmet.

Veracity has been described as desirable by the American Hospital Association in the *Statement on a Patient's Bill of Rights* (1975). According to the second statement of this document, patients have the right to obtain complete, current information concerning diagnosis, treatment, and prognosis in terms they can be reasonably expected to understand. Though this position relates specifically to physicians' responsibility of disclosure, there are implications for nursing as well. As patient advocates, nurses are responsible for assuring that patients' rights are honored.

The ANA *Code for Nurses with Interpretive Statements* (1985) very specifically supports the principle of veracity. This document outlines nurses' responsibility in relation to truth telling:

> Truth telling and the process of reaching informed choice underlie the exercise of self-determination, which is basic to respect for persons.
>
> Clients should be as fully involved as possible in the planning and implementation of their own health care. Clients have the moral right to determine what will be done with their own person; to be given accurate information, and all the information necessary for making informed judgments. . . . (p. 2)

In subsequent statements, authors of the code support the principle of veracity but recognize that situations may warrant differences in approach. They conclude with the following statement, "The suspension of individual rights must always be considered a deviation to be tolerated as briefly as possible" (p. 3). Even though strongly promoting the practice of truth telling, the authors imply that there may be occasions when the patient's right to information may be suspended.

As with other principles, there is a dramatic discrepancy between nursing and medical literature in regard to veracity. Recognizing that nearly all health care is an interdisciplinary effort and that disclosure of information to patients involves both nurses and physicians, it is important for nurses to understand the medical perspective.

Physicians often make the claim that patients do not want bad news and that truthful information has the potential to harm patients. In the name of beneficence, some physicians proceed with either nondisclosure or outright lies. Lipkin (1991) argues that physicians should sometimes deceive their patients or withhold information from them. It is his view that patients do not have sufficient information about how their bodies function to interpret medical information accurately and sometimes do not want to know the truth about their illness. Joseph Ellin (1991) discusses special considerations that have been posed by the medical profession in relation to truth telling. He suggests that it does not seem beneficent to adopt an ethic of absolute veracity in which it is an obligation to cause avoidable anguish to someone who is already ill, especially when hope and positive outlook may promote healing and help prolong life. He writes, "One could hope to avoid this dilemma by holding that the duty of veracity, though not absolute, is to be given very great weight, and may be overridden only in the gravest cases . . ." (p. 82). Ellin draws a distinction between lying and deception: lying is the purposeful telling of untruths, whereas deception is usually accomplished through nondisclosure. He argues that there is an absolute duty to avoid lying to patients; however, there is no duty not to deceive. Examples he gives include withholding information about a poor prognosis or giving placebo medication. Consider the following situation: A mother of four is admitted to the emergency department after an automobile accident in which two of her children are killed. Recognizing that she is in very serious condition, according to Ellin, it would be appropriate to avoid telling her of the death of her children. If, however, she asks about their condition, she must be told the truth.

Ask Yourself

Is the Truth Sometimes Harmful?

- Do you think it is acceptable to deceive a patient in order to prevent unnecessary suffering?
- How would you feel if you were a patient and the health care team and your family conspired to deceive you—if, for example, you were ill and you had a bleak prognosis?

Bok (1991) examines the practice of physicians deceiving patients in the name of beneficence. She writes that lying to patients has historically been seen as an excusable act. "Some would argue that doctors, and only doctors, should be granted the right to manipulate the truth in ways so undesirable for politicians, lawyers, and others" (p. 75). In fact, truth telling has never been a principle that was given consideration in the medical literature. Veracity is absent from virtually all oaths, codes, and prayers. Even the Hippocratic Oath makes no mention of truthfulness. The 1847 version of the American Medical Association Code of Ethics endorses some forms of deception by stating that the physician has a sacred duty to avoid "all things which have a tendency to discourage the patient and to depress his spirits" (Bok, 1994, p. 683).

Nursing and medicine view veracity from two different perspectives. It is clear that physicians have traditionally seen disclosure or nondisclosure to be a facet of care within their control that can have implications for patient welfare. To withhold bad news is often considered a beneficent act if disclosure of the information is predicted to harm the patient. Nursing, on the other hand, upholds veracity as supporting individual rights, respect for persons, and the principle of autonomy. Recognition of the viewpoint of others is imperative for professionals who must collaborate. Chapter 4 discusses methods of making decisions about ethical problems when there are differences of perspective among those involved.

CONFIDENTIALITY

Confidentiality is the ethical principle that requires nondisclosure of private or secret information with which one is entrusted. Support for this principle is found in codes and oaths of nursing and medicine dating back many centuries. The ANA Committee on Ethics states a very clear position on confidentiality in point two of the *Code for Nurses with Interpretive Statements* (1985): "The nurse safeguards the client's right to privacy by judiciously protecting information of a confidential nature" (p. 4). Confidentiality is the only facet of patient care mentioned in the Nightingale Pledge. This oath has been recited for decades by graduating nurses: "I will do all in my power to elevate the standard of my profession and will hold in confidence all personal matters committed to my keeping and all family affairs coming to my knowledge in the practice of my profession." Physicians do not escape the promise of confidentiality. The Hippocratic Oath is very clear: "Whatever, in connection with my professional practice, or not in connection with it, I see or hear, in the life of men, which ought not to be spoken of abroad, I will not divulge, as reckoning that all such should be kept secret." Though there are compelling arguments in favor of maintaining confidentiality, there is disagreement about the absolute requirement of confidentiality in all situations.

The ability to maintain privacy in one's life is an expression of autonomy. The capacity to choose what others know about us, particularly intimate personal details, is important because it enables us to maintain dignity and preserve a measure of control over our own lives. Markus and Lockwood (1991) discuss the importance of privacy:

> Privacy is thus a value closely related to, and perhaps ultimately grounded on, the value of personal autonomy. To take this value of privacy seriously is to subscribe to a number of familiar precepts. It means that we should be reluctant to pry, that we should respect personal confidences, and that when we enter into relationships with others that render us privy to sensitive or intimate personal information, we should be [careful] about passing this information on, even in the absence of any specific request not to do so. (p. 349)

Thus, maintaining confidentiality of patients is an expression of respect of persons and, in many ways, is essential to the nurse-patient relationship. Consider the following case presentation.

CASE PRESENTATION

Making the Best Choice

Lora is a seventeen-year-old cheerleader. She comes to the local family planning clinic requesting birth control pills. Lora is a very attractive, neat, and pleasant patient. In the process of completing the initial physical examination, the nurse practitioner finds evidence of physical abuse including a recent traumatic perforated ear drum. Lora hesitantly and tearfully admits that her biological father slapped her across her left ear prior to her coming to the clinic. She reports that she recently moved into his home after living most of her life with her mother and stepfather. She tearfully reports that her stepfather was sexually abusive to her and that she wishes to remain with her biological father. She says that she can tolerate being slapped around occasionally, and she does not want to get her biological father in trouble or be forced to move back to her stepfather's home. State law requires that the nurse report any suspicion of child abuse. Both codes of ethics and federal law require that the nurse maintain confidentiality.

Think About It

To Tell or Not to Tell

- What are the principles involved?
- Does the nurse's obligation to report the incident of child abuse supersede the obligation to maintain confidentiality—particularly considering that the patient requested confidentiality? What if Lora was fourteen years old?
- What are the options for the nurse?
- What are the possible outcomes of the different options?
- Does Lora's autonomy outweigh the nurse's responsibility to report the abusive situation?

There are at least two basic ethical arguments in favor of maintaining confidentiality. The first of these is the individual's right to control personal information and protect privacy. The second argument is one of utility.

This right to privacy flows from autonomy and respect for persons. On one level, patients have the right to expect that personal and private information will not be shared unnecessarily among health care providers. Patient information is not an appropriate topic for elevator or dinner conversation. It is most likely that violations of this nature were what authors had in mind when writing early creeds and oaths that promise confidentiality. Nurses and other professionals often casually discuss private patient matters. On another level, nurses must keep in mind the number of people who have legitimate access to patient records. In a hospital situation, patient charts are accessible to many personnel. Nurses, physicians, dieticians, respiratory therapists, utilization review staff, financial officers, students, secretaries, physical therapists, and others have legitimate reason to view patient records. Information of a sensitive and private nature that the patient intends for the nurse alone can become widely known in a large health care facility. Care must be taken in choosing information to be recorded in patients' charts. It is important for nurses to be aware of the many threats to patient confidentiality.

Confidentiality is particularly important when revelation of intimate and sensitive information has the potential to harm the patient. Harm can take various forms such as embarrassment, ridicule, discrimination, deprivation of rights, physical or emotional harm, and loss of roles or relationships. Consider the plight of many AIDS victims whose diagnoses have become public knowledge. Confidentiality is particularly important when dealing with vulnerable populations (Winston, 1988).

The second argument is one of utility. If patients suspect that health care providers reveal sensitive and personal information indiscriminately, they are reluctant to seek care. Government policy makers recognize this problem. Because of the intimate and private nature of reproductive health issues, confidentiality of those seeking family planning services, for example, is mandated. Those caring for AIDS patients also recognize the need to maintain confidentiality. According to Winston (1988), many who work with AIDS patients find such arguments particularly compelling, believing that disclosure of patients' antibody status or a diagnosis of AIDS would have a "chilling effect," preventing those in high-risk groups from seeking care. There are other diagnoses such as mental illness, alcoholism, and drug addiction that, if revealed, could lead to public scorn, and subsequently discourage others from seeking care.

Limits of Confidentiality

Should the principle of confidentiality be honored in all instances? There are arguments that favor questioning the absolute obligation of confidentiality in certain situations. These arguments include theories related to the principles of harm and vulnerability (Winston, 1988). The harm principle can be applied when the nurse or other professional recognizes that maintaining confidentiality will result in preventable wrongful harm to innocent others. Mandatory premarital testing for syphilis, for example, is intended to prevent the spread of a serious communicable disease to innocent babies and spouses. In this instance, society chooses to override the privacy of the individual to protect the health of the innocent.

In rare instances, case law supports the harm principle. In July of 1976, the California Supreme Court ruled that a psychologist, Dr. Lawrence Moore, and his superior, Dr. Harvey Powelson, and the agency for which they worked were liable in the wrongful death of Tatiana Tarsoff. Prosenjit Poddar killed Tatiana Tarsoff in October of 1969. According to Tatiana's parents, two months earlier Poddar confided his intention to kill Tatiana to his psychologist, Dr. Moore. Though Dr. Moore initially tried to have his patient involuntarily committed, Dr. Powelson intervened and allowed Poddar to return home. Neither Tatiana nor her parents were informed of the patient's threats. The court found that the defendants were responsible for the wrongful death of

Tatiana because they knew in advance of the patient's intentions. The obligation to protect the innocent third party superseded the obligation to maintain confidentiality. According to the majority opinion in this case, the duty to warn arises from a special relation between the patient and the psychologist that imposes a duty to control the patient's conduct (Tobriner, 1991).

Foreseeability is an important consideration in situations in which confidentiality conflicts with the duty to warn. The nurse or other health care professional should be able to reasonably foresee harm or injury to an innocent other in order to violate the principle of confidentiality in favor of a duty to warn. This consideration precludes blanket disclosure of private information that might predict harm to others. The Tarasoff case exemplifies reasonable application of the harm principle. Subsequent court cases support the decision in the Tarasoff case. Courts have found that privacy is not absolute and is subordinate to the state's fundamental right to enact laws that promote public health.

The harm principle is strengthened when one considers the vulnerability of the innocent. The duty to protect others from harm is stronger when the third party is dependent on others or is in some way especially vulnerable. This duty is called the vulnerability principle. Vulnerability implies risk or susceptibility to harm when vulnerable individuals have a relative inability to protect themselves (Winston, 1988). For example, nurses have an absolute duty to report child abuse. Because children are dependent and vulnerable, they are at greater risk of harm. Coupling of the harm principle with the vulnerability principle produces a rather strong argument for abandoning the principle of confidentiality in certain instances.

Ask Yourself

Can Nurses Violate Confidentiality?

- How do you think confidentiality and the harm and vulnerability principles can be reconciled?
- How would you feel if a relative contracted HIV from a source who public health officials knew was infected, and had reason to believe would infect your relative, but neglected to warn?
- How would you feel if you were HIV infected and your health care provider violated your right to confidentiality?

Actions that are considered ethical are not always found to be legal. Though there is an ethical basis for subsuming the principle of confidentiality in special circumstances and there is some legal precedent for doing so, there is legal risk to disclosing sensitive information. There is dynamic tension between the patient's right to confidentiality and the duty to warn innocent others. Nurses need to recognize that careful consideration of the ethical implications of actions will not always be supported in bureaucratic and legal systems.

JUSTICE

Justice is the ethical principle that relates to fair, equitable, and appropriate treatment in light of what is due or owed to persons, recognizing that giving to some will deny receipt to others who might otherwise have received these things. Within the context of health care ethics, the relevant application of the principle focuses on distribution of goods and services. This application is called **distributive justice.** Unfortunately, there is a finite supply of goods and services, and it is impossible for all people to have everything they might want or need. One of the primary purposes of governing systems is to formulate and enforce policies that deal with fair and equitable distribution of scarce resources.

Decisions about distributive justice are made on a variety of levels. The government is responsible for deciding policy about broad public health access issues such as children's immunization and Medicare for the elderly. Hospitals and other organizations formulate policy on an institutional level and deal with issues such as how decisions will be made concerning who will occupy intensive care beds and which types of patients will be accepted in emergency rooms. Nurses and other health care providers frequently make decisions of distributive justice on an individual basis. For example, having assessed the needs of patients, nurses decide how best to allocate their time (a scarce resource).

There are three basic areas of health care that are relevant to questions of distributive justice. First, what percentage of our resources is it reasonable to spend on health care? Second, recognizing that health care resources are limited, which aspects of health care should receive the most resources? Third, which patients should have access to the limited health care staff, equipment, and so forth? (Jameton, 1984).

In making decisions of distributive justice, one must ask the question, "Who is entitled to these goods or services?" Philosophers have suggested a number of different ways to choose among people. Figure 3–3 lists some of the ways that people have historically made these types of decisions.

Figure 3–3 **Distributive Justice**

To each equally
To each according to need
To each according to merit
To each according to social contribution
To each according to the person's rights
To each according to individual effort
To each as you would be done by
To each according to the greatest good to the greatest number

There are those who believe that all should receive equally regardless of need. On the surface, nationalized health care systems would seem to meet this criterion, since all citizens are eligible for the same services. However, because some citizens would necessarily require more health care services than others, nationalized systems also meet the criterion of need. German philosopher, Friedrich Nietzsche, had a different perspective. He believed that there are superior individuals and that society's goal should be to enhance these "supermen." For Nietzsche, the choice of distribution was a clear one—to each according to his present or future social contribution (Durant, 1926). To each according to that person's rights indicates a libertarian viewpoint, and to each as you would be done by is a reflection of the golden rule. The idea that each should receive according to effort is a common belief in our culture and indicates the traditional "work ethic." Entitlement programs in the United States generally award benefits based upon a combination of need and the greatest good that can be accomplished for the greatest number of people. Chapter 15 discusses the application of the principle of distributive justice in greater detail.

FIDELITY

The ethical principle of **fidelity** is often related to the concept of faithfulness and the practice of keeping promises. Society has granted nurses the right to practice nursing through the processes of licensure and certification. "The authority for the practice of nursing is based on a social contract that acknowledges professional rights and responsibilities as well as mechanisms for public accountability" (ANA, 1995, p. 3). The process of licensure is one that ensures no other group can practice within the domain of nursing as defined by society and the profession. Thus, to accept licensure and become legitimate members of the profession mandates that nurses uphold the responsibilities inherent in the contract with society. Members are called to be faithful to the society that grants the right to practice—to keep the promise of upholding the profession's code of ethics, to practice within the established scope of practice and definition of nursing, to remain competent in practice, to abide by the policies of employing institutions, and to keep promises to individual patients. To *be* a nurse is to *make these promises*. In fulfilling this contract with society, nurses are responsible to faithfully and consistently adhere to these basic principles.

SUMMARY

As nurses participate in meeting the health care needs of society, they must be constantly aware of ethical implications inherent in many situations. Each nurse must develop a philosophically consistent framework from which to base contemplation, decision, and action. It is this framework that gives shape to the nurse's concept of various ethical principles. The principles discussed in this chapter presuppose nurses' innate respect of persons. Ethical principles include autonomy, beneficence, nonmaleficence, veracity, confidentiality, justice, and fidelity.

CHAPTER HIGHLIGHTS

- Ethical principles are basic and obvious moral truths that guide deliberation and action.

- All ethical principles presuppose a basic respect for persons.

- Autonomy denotes having the freedom to make choices about issues that affect one's life.

- Various intrinsic and extrinsic factors threaten patient autonomy.

- The principle of beneficence maintains that one ought to do or promote good, prevent evil or harm, and remove evil or harm.

- The principle of nonmaleficence requires one to avoid causing harm, including deliberate harm, risk of harm, and harm that occurs during the performance of beneficial acts.

- The principle of veracity relates to the universal virtue of truth telling.

- Confidentiality is the ethical principle that requires nondisclosure of private or secret information with which one is entrusted.

- Justice is the ethical principle that relates to fair, equitable, and appropriate treatment in light of what is due or owed to persons, recognizing that giving to some will deny receipt to others who might otherwise have received these things.

- Fidelity is the ethical principle that relates to faithfulness and promise keeping.

DISCUSSION QUESTIONS AND ACTIVITIES

1. Read the following hypothetical situation and answer the questions that follow:

An elderly gentleman presents himself to the emergency department of a small community hospital. The patient has contractures and paralysis of his left hand; he apparently has complete expressive and at least partial receptive aphasia. Upon questioning, the man takes off his right shoe and points to his right great toe and grimaces, apparently indicating a problem in that area. The nurse is unable to gather any further information from him because of his difficulty in communicating. In attempting to help him, she asks if he has a neighbor or friend accompanying him. He shakes his head, indicating that he is alone. Curious, the nurse asks him how he came to the hospital. The patient smiles and proudly produces a driver's license from his shirt pocket. Subsequently, the nurse leaves the room and returns a few minutes later to find that the patient left the hospital—having received no care. The nurse suspects that because of his current physical condition the man is unsafe to drive a motor vehicle.

- What are the ethical implications in this situation?
- What ethical principles are involved?
- Should the nurse pursue avenues to locate the patient and ensure that he is not endangering himself or others by driving? Would this be a breach of confidentiality? Autonomy?

- How does the nurse express fidelity in this situation?
- What is the beneficent action?

2. Describe situations you have witnessed in which decisions were made for patients in a *paternalistic* manner. Discuss your perception of the appropriateness of *parentalism* in given situations.

3. Read the following hypothetical case and answer the questions that follow:

Martha is a seventy-five-year-old woman who has terminal cancer of the bladder. During the course of her therapy, she sustains third-degree radiation burns to her lower abdomen and pelvic area. Her wounds are extensive and deep, involving her abdominal wall, bladder, and vagina. The physician orders frequent medicinal douches and wound irrigations. These treatments are very painful, and the patient wants the treatments discontinued but is too timid to actually refuse them. The physician will not change the order.

- Discuss the situation in terms of beneficence and nonmaleficence.
- How does this patient express her autonomy?
- What is the nurse's responsibility in assisting the patient to maintain autonomy?
- How does the nurse deal with conflicting loyalties and principles?

4. Do you think health care professionals should disclose information to patients related, for example, to a poor prognosis even though the information may cause distress? Discuss your views in depth.

5. Jameton (1984) says that for nurses to be less than competent is unethical. Discuss this statement in terms of fidelity.

6. Read the following hypothetical case and answer the questions that follow:

Nels Gruder is a forty-year-old disabled truck driver. He was injured several years ago in a trucking accident. He subsequently has had back surgery but continues to have severe pain. He has been seen by every local neurosurgeon and, for one reason or another, is not pleased with the care he has gotten. Because of the seriousness of his initial injuries, there is little doubt that Mr. Gruder has chronic back pain. Even though the local emergency room policy of not prescribing narcotic analgesics for chronic pain is clearly stated on signs in the waiting area, Mr. Gruder comes there frequently complaining of severe back pain. He reports a history of gastric ulcers and allergy to nonsteroidal anti-inflammatory drugs (NSAIDs). The nurse practitioner who sees Mr. Gruder is faced with a man who is in obvious pain. She wishes to help him relieve the pain he is experiencing. At the same time she realizes that narcotic analgesia is not appropriate for this type of problem and is unable to prescribe NSAIDs because of his reports of gastric ulcers and allergy. He says he has tried exercises and a local pain clinic, neither of which was effective. He is aware of the emergency room policy regarding narcotic analgesics for chronic pain, but he comes there in desperation. He insists that his pain is relieved only by narcotic analgesia.

- What ethical principles are involved?
- Does the benefit of pain relief outweigh the harm potentially caused by long-term narcotic analgesic use for this patient?
- Should Mr. Gruder's perceived need for narcotic pain medications be honored even though the nurse practitioner feels he has a problem with drug dependence?
- How does the nurse do what she thinks is right and yet respect Mr. Gruder's autonomy?
- Is it important whether or not the nurse's actions please the patient?

REFERENCES

American Hospital Association. (1975). *Statement on a patient's bill of rights*. Chicago: Author.

American Nurses Association. (1985). *Code for nurses with interpretive statements*. Washington: Author.

American Nurses Association. (1995). *Nursing's social policy statement*. Washington: Author.

Beauchamp, T., & Childress, J. (1994). *Principles of biomedical ethics* (4th ed.). New York: Oxford University Press.

Bok, S. (1991). Lies to the sick and dying. In T. A. Mappes & J. S. Zembaty, *Biomedical ethics* (pp. 74–81). New York: McGraw-Hill.

Bok, S. (1994). Truth telling. In W. Reich (Ed.), *Encyclopedia of bioethics* (pp. 1682–1686). New York: Macmillan.

Buber, M. (1965). *The knowledge of man: A philosophy of the interhuman*. New York: Harper & Row.

Durant, W. (1926). *The story of philosophy*. New York: Washington Square Press.

Edge, R. S., & Groves, J. R. (1994). *The ethics of health care: A guide for practice*. Albany, NY: Delmar.

Ellin, J. S. (1991). Lying and deception: The solution to a dilemma in medical ethics. In T. A. Mappes & J. S. Zembaty, *Biomedical ethics* (pp. 81–87). New York: McGraw-Hill.

Goldsmith, J. (Ed.). (1992). Virginia Henderson, RN: Humanitarian and scholar. *Reflections, 18*(1), 4–5.

Harrison, A. F., & Bramson, R. M. (1982). *Styles of thinking*. New York: Doubleday.

Jameton, A. (1984). *Nursing practice: The ethical issues*. Englewood Cliffs, NJ: Prentice-Hall.

Lipkin, M. (1991). On lying to patients. In T. A. Mappes & J. S. Zembaty, *Biomedical ethics* (pp. 72–73). New York: McGraw-Hill.

Markus, A., & Lockwood, M. (1991). Is it permissible to edit medical records? *British Medical Journal, 303*, 349–351.

Munson, R. (1992). Major moral principles. In *Intervention and reflection: Basic issues in medical ethics* (4th ed., pp. 31–45). Belmont, CA: Wadsworth.

Quinn, C. A., & Smith, M. D. (1987). *The professional commitment: Issues and ethics in nursing*. Philadelphia: Saunders.

Shakespeare, W. *The merchant of Venice*.

Tobriner, M. O. (1991). Majority opinion in Tarsoff v. Regents of the University of California. In T. A. Mappes & J. S. Zembaty, *Biomedical ethics*. (pp. 165–169). New York: McGraw-Hill.

Winston, M. E. (1988). AIDS, confidentiality, and the right to know. *Public Affairs Quarterly, 2,* 91–104.

CHAPTER 4

Ethical Decision Making

*Peace **requires that you do what in your heart you know—that your chosen values guide your actions.***
(Chinn, 1995)

OBJECTIVES

After completing this chapter, the reader should be able to:

1. Describe and differentiate ethical dilemmas, practical dilemmas, and moral distress.
2. Describe the process of making thoughtful decisions.
3. Discuss the nursing process as a decision making model.
4. Discuss similarities between scientific process and ethical decision making.
5. Describe the role of emotions in ethical decisions.
6. Examine the process of ethical decision making.
7. Apply the ethical decision making process to clinical case situations.

INTRODUCTION

Everyone makes decisions as part of everyday living. Some decisions seem routine, such as what to have for lunch or what to wear to work. Other decisions, like where to go to college, which job to accept, or whether to marry, call for more deliberation. Nurses constantly make decisions. They decide matters related to management of care, institutional policy, or when to collaborate or initiate referrals. Often nurses make decisions without conscious awareness of the process but have an innate sense of *knowing* what to do.

Ethical decision making may not seem as clear-cut as decisions made in other areas of one's life. How does one decide whether to remove life support measures for one's parent or whether to cut funding for childhood immunizations in lieu of other, equally important programs? What factors are involved in an ethical dilemma that makes "the right choice" either evident or obscure? This chapter defines the concept of ethical dilemma, relates ethical decision making to nursing process, and presents a guide for ethical decision making.

ETHICAL DILEMMAS

A dilemma exists when a difficult problem seems to have no satisfactory solution or when all solutions to a problem appear to be equally favorable (Davis, Aroskar, Liaschenko, & Drought, 1997). An **ethical dilemma** occurs when there are conflicting moral claims. Dilemmas present in at least two ways. According to Beauchamp and Childress (1994), a conflict can be experienced when there is evidence to indicate that a certain act is morally right and evidence to indicate that the act is morally wrong, but no evidence is conclusive. An example of this can be seen in the example of a terminally ill patient. While most would think it is morally right to preserve life, many would believe it is morally wrong to prolong suffering. A dilemma may also occur when the agent believes that one or more moral norms exist to support one course of action and one or more moral norms exist to support another course of action, and the two actions are mutually exclusive. Health care providers face this type of dilemma, for example, when they must decide who gets the critical care bed. Should they make the decision relative to who is most deserving, who arrives first, who can pay, or who has the best chance of survival? Different people perceive or conceptualize conflicts in different ways. Conflicting moral claims can be said to occur, for example, between obligations, principles, duties, rights, loyalties, and so forth.

Let us examine different perceptions of conflicting moral claims. The nurse might perceive a conflict between adherence to two different principles such as wishing to avoid the suffering a patient experiences as a result of hearing a bad prognosis while at the same time respecting the patient's right to know. In this instance, the nurse might perceive a direct conflict between the principles of nonmaleficence (the wish to do no harm) and autonomy (assuring that the patient is self-governing). In another instance, the nurse might perceive a conflict of duties. This type of conflict can occur, for example, when nurse managers must make decisions regarding staffing patterns. The nurse manager will recognize a duty to the institution but will also feel a duty to meet the needs of individual patients and nurses. This will often result in a conflict, when needs of the institution do not allow for meeting the needs of individuals.

There are instances in which the nurse might feel conflicting loyalties. For example, in caring for a promiscuous patient with AIDS, the nurse might experience a conflict between being loyal to the patient and being loyal to society. In this instance the nurse could experience a conflict between doing that which seems morally right and avoiding that which carries legal consequences. This situation can also be conceptualized as a conflict between the nurse's duty to maintain confidentiality and the duty to warn those at risk. All of these examples portray ethical dilemmas that nurses commonly experience. These moral problems offer conflicting moral claims, however conceptualized, and solutions that appear to be equally unfavorable.

Think About It

Facing Ethical Dilemmas

Put yourself in the position of the nurse in each of the examples noted in the discussion of ethical dilemmas above.

- How would the situation present a conflict for you?
- How do you think you would respond in each situation?
- Why would you respond in that manner?
- Think about a personal experience of a moral dilemma and describe why it was a dilemma for you.

Practical Dilemmas

One must be careful to differentiate between moral and **practical dilemmas.** Occasionally situations present themselves in which moral claims compete with nonmoral claims. Nonmoral claims can often be identified as claims of self-interest (Beauchamp & Childress, 1994). Consider, for example, the nurse who must to work overtime, caring for a gravely ill patient. The nurse might perceive a dilemma because she made a promise to take her children to the circus. Though the nurse might say that her duty to the children conflicts with her duty to care for the patient, it can be argued that the duties are not of equal moral weight. The duty to keep the promise to her children is a practical duty that is grounded in self-interest rather than having a moral claim. In decisions that involve practical dilemmas, moral claims have greater weight than nonmoral claims. Differentiating moral and practical dilemmas is an important facet of decision making.

Moral Distress

Occasionally nurses face situations that present moral problems which seem to have clear solutions, yet they are unable to follow their moral beliefs because of institutional or other restraints. Nurses in these predicaments are said to experience **moral distress**

(Jameton, 1984). These situations can be differentiated from those that present moral dilemmas. When moral distress occurs, there are no conflicting moral claims. The *right* action is clear, yet institutional or other restraints make it nearly impossible to pursue this course of action. For example, nurses in the hurried atmosphere of a particular hospital's same-day surgery report that they are expected to have sedated patients sign consent forms, recognizing that the physicians have often neglected to fully explain the scheduled procedures. The nurses know that this practice is one that does not respect patients' rights to informed consent, yet feel they have neither personal authority nor access to decision-making channels, and therefore believe themselves to be powerless to make the necessary changes. Jameton points out that in situations of this sort, it can be personally risky for staff to criticize a practice that helps the hospital make ends meet.

Situations in which nurses feel moral distress represent practical, rather than ethical, dilemmas. Nurses may face the choice of continuing to participate in a system that they feel is ethically flawed, resigning, or acting in a manner that they believe is correct but that could jeopardize employment. Moral distress will undermine integrity if it is easier for the nurse to comply with policies that are believed to be morally wrong than to pursue the ethically correct action.

Unrelieved moral distress over a period of time can erode the nurse's values and affect confidence and self-esteem. Unfortunately, there is no assurance that following the morally correct course of action will mean employer or legal support. Nurses should view these situations as practical dilemmas. Ethical decision making assures that moral claims hold greater weight than nonmoral claims. Thus, in the example offered above, the moral claim of respecting the right to informed consent constitutes greater weight than the nonmoral claim of system efficiency. The decision making guide described in this chapter is intended to be used with ethical dilemmas, but with some modification it can be used in helping individual nurses make practical decisions when facing moral distress.

Ask Yourself

Have You Experienced Moral Distress?

Moral distress occurs in situations that present moral problems which seem to have clear solutions, yet institutional or other restraints prohibit morally correct action. Consider a situation in which you experienced moral distress.

- What were the circumstances?
- How did you feel?
- How did you resolve the distress?

MAKING DECISIONS

The process of making thoughtful decisions follows a similar pattern in most circumstances. This pattern includes gathering data, comparing options, using some criteria for weighing the merit of each option, and making a choice. Evaluation of outcomes or circumstances surrounding the choice provides more data regarding the *rightness* of the choice. A simple example of this process is how you choose what clothes to wear today. The data you gather includes such things as where you are going, what you will be doing, the weather, what is clean or handy, your mood, the colors you prefer, and the style of clothing you anticipate others will be wearing. You may narrow choices down to one or several options that would be acceptable or appropriate, and you compare these based on some criteria. The criteria may be what is least wrinkled, or feels most comfortable, or makes you look or feel more confident, or is more appropriate for weather conditions, or a combination of such considerations. Using the criteria, you narrow down options and make a choice. As you move through the day, you gather more data about the *rightness* of your decision. For example, are you comfortable? Do you feel dressed appropriately for the meeting? Are you warm enough? Does the color seem to make you stand out? Your evaluation of whether you made the right decision provides information about the strength or validity of the criteria you used to guide your decision and whether to use these same criteria to guide similar decisions in the future.

Nursing Process and Ethical Decision Making

Nurses commonly use the **nursing process** as a model for decision making. Utilizing both logical thinking and intuitive knowing, the nursing process is a deliberate activity that provides a systematic methodology for nursing practice. The nursing process directs nursing practice, standardizes nursing care, and unifies nurses (Christensen & Kenney, 1990). Familiar to most nurses and endorsed by the American Nurses Association, the process generally includes the following interactive and sequential steps: problem identification based on assessment of subjective and objective data, development of a plan for care guided by desired outcomes, implementation of interventions, evaluation of the outcomes, and revision of the plan over time. Criteria used in making nursing care decisions derive from areas such as knowledge of normal anatomy, physiology, psychology, pathophysiology, therapeutic communication, family dynamics, pharmacology, microbiology, nursing and other theories, human energy fields, familiarity with standards of care and protocols, experience related to what has worked in similar situations, and intuitive knowing. The process is systematic and involves both logical thinking and intuitive knowing.

Scientific Process and Ethical Decision Making

The process of decision making in ethics follows a procedure that is similar to the process encountered in science. "A comparison between the giving of good reasons in science, which is called 'explanation,' and the giving of good reasons in ethics, which is called 'moral justification,' reveals striking procedural similarities bordering on identity" (Gibson, 1991, p. 3). Gibson notes similarities between the scientific process of explanation, which moves from *observation → hypothesis → law → theory*, and the moral justification process of ethics, which moves from *assessed ethical dilemma → rule → principle → theory*. A strong knowledge base regarding societal rules, ethical principles and theories, and professional codes and standards is as important to making ethical decisions as knowledge of principles related to physical, psychological, social, and human science is to other nursing judgments.

ETHICAL DECISION MAKING

Resolution of ethical dilemmas is often approached within a problem-solving frame of reference. Similar to both nursing process and scientific inquiry, the ethical problem solving process generally includes the following steps: (1) defining the problem, (2) identifying objectives to be achieved, (3) listing alternatives for meeting objectives, (4) evaluating each objective, and (5) choosing the best alternative.

Differences of culture or values among the various participants involved in ethical decision making often become an important issue. In this regard, defining the problem includes both determining the ethical issue at hand and identifying the value systems of those involved. Consider, for instance, parents who wish to terminate life support for a seriously injured child hospitalized with no hope of recovery. The parents believe that life support is causing harm by interfering with the natural process of death which they believe should be in God's hands, while the physician feels that removing life support constitutes murder. The problem includes both the issue of terminating life support and the conflicting values between physician and family. Although both parties might identify what is best for and least harmful to the child as the ultimate objective, the list of potential options would be different for the family and the physician. Determining which principles and theories guide the people involved enables the nurse to help clarify the issue and facilitate the process of coming to an ethical decision.

Emotions and Ethical Decisions

Many approaches to ethical decision making describe a primarily cognitive process in which emotions are subordinated to reason. In a holistic view of human persons, however, both thinking and feeling are credible ways of knowing, each having a legitimate role in ethical decision making. Callahan (1995) suggests that heart and mind should not be viewed as antagonistic in the moral arena; rather, both reason and emotion should be active and in accord as one comes to an ethical decision. Noting that emotions should tutor reason while reason is monitoring emotions, she describes emotions as personal signals providing information regarding both inner processes and interactions with the environment.

It is important to appreciate not only what one *thinks* about what is right or wrong in a situation but also what one *feels* in relation to the circumstances and decision to be made. If one is feeling discomfort, even though reason is pointing in a particular direction, it is wise to further explore both the arguments posed through reason and one's reactions to them. Callahan (1995) writes:

> In our technological culture perhaps the greatest moral danger arises not from sentimentality, but from devaluing feeling and not attending to or nurturing moral emotions. Numbness, apathy, isolated

disassociations between thinking and feeling are also moral warning signals . . . the absence of emotional responses of empathy and sympathy become critical bioethical issues. (pp. 30–31)

The goal is to have head and heart in harmony as the decision is made.

In the same way that people may approach an issue with differing moral reasoning, their emotional response might be quite different from one's own. In such situations one might see validity in the other's response and broaden one's own view. On the other hand, one may recognize that the chasm between the two is too deep to bridge. Callahan suggests that such social conflicts and challenges present new ethical dilemmas that may require dealing with the consequences of an ethical decision by repeating the decision making process.

Think About It

The Role of Emotions in Decision Making

Consider your emotional response to the following situations and how it would affect your dealing with and caring for the people involved.

• You work in a clinic serving primarily an indigent immigrant population and you hear one of your coworkers comment that "it's a waste of time trying to do health education because these people are all so stupid, and just a drain on the system."

• You just started working for a group of gynecologists and discover that the physician you are assigned to work with asks all his young patients about their sexual fantasies.

• You are working in an emergency department at the local hospital where a two-year-old child dies as a result of injuries sustained while being "disciplined" by the mother's boyfriend. The child had previously been placed in foster care due to neglect and had been returned to the mother's care only a week prior to this event.

PROCESS OF ETHICAL DECISION MAKING

The nature of the ethical dilemma requires a decision making process in which key facets are revisited from evolving perspectives even as one moves toward a decision or resolution. Many models for decision making describe step-by-step processes that are linear in nature, not reflecting the potential for an evolving perspective. The guidelines presented here provide a framework for entering a decision making process that requires an ongoing evaluation and assimilation of information. This decision making process is spiral in nature, with each step being revisited as often as is required and molded by the dynamics of changing facts, evolving beliefs, unexpected consequences, and participants who move in and out of the process. The following text describes the steps involved in the process of ethical decision making.

Gather Data and Identify Conflicting Moral Claims

When an ethical dilemma occurs, information or facts need to be gathered in order to clarify issues. Identification of the conflicting moral claims that constitute the ethical dilemma is the first part of the process. One should examine the situation for evidence of conflicting obligations, principles, duties, rights, loyalties, values, or beliefs. Additionally, data provide an understanding of the ethical components, principles of concern, and the various perceptions of issues and principles by those involved in the situation. Nurses must pay attention to societal, religious, and cultural values and beliefs. Often, a situation initially thought to constitute an ethical dilemma will be determined to actually be a practical dilemma. This recognition allows the participants to appropriately weigh choices and expedite decision making.

Identify Key Participants

It is important to identify the key persons involved in the decision making process and to delineate each person's role. Determining rights, duties, authority, context, and capabilities of decision makers is a critical component of the process (Curtin & Flaherty, 1982; Husted & Husted, 1995). The focal question is, "Whose decision is this to make?" Identification of the principal decision maker is sometimes all that is needed to facilitate the process. Recognition that one has the legitimate authority to make an important decision is an empowering event. Once the principle decision maker is identified, the roles of the other participants can be explicitly outlined. For example, nurses often feel the burden of difficult ethical decisions even though the responsibility for the decision making lies with the patient or the nearest relative. In these instances the nurse serves as a resource for information, a source of emotional support for those making the difficult decision, and a facilitator of the decision making process.

Determine Moral Perspective and Phase of Moral Development of Key Participants

Knowledge of developmental aspects and ethical theory may provide a helpful framework for understanding participants and their perspectives and responses in the process. An assessment of how those involved fit into paradigms of moral development provides useful information. It would be valuable to recognize, for instance, whether the principal decision maker is at a developmental level in which choices reflect a desire to please others, thus being rendered susceptible to choosing an alternative solely on the basis of seeking approval. (See Chapter 6 for an in-depth discussion of moral development.)

It is also crucial to identify the ethical perspective from which the participants make decisions. For example, if one of the major participants involved in discussions relative to discontinuing life support believes that it is always wrong to take a life (see discussion of deontology in Chapter 2), the process of negotiation with those who believe differently is likely to be frustrating. It would be more beneficial under those circumstances to begin the discussion by defining the point at which death actually occurs, thus finding common ground. When those involved present with diverse values, the nurse or others facilitate their coming to a consensus around goals and understanding of principles.

Determine Desired Outcomes

Identifying the desired outcomes and their potential consequences is a substantial step in the decision making process. At this point, participants will exclude those outcomes that are totally unacceptable. As with the nursing process, implementation of a plan of action cannot logically occur without explicit knowledge of the desired outcome. Likewise, evaluation of the success or failure of the plan is measured by the degree to which the outcome is met. Clarifying the outcomes and their anticipated consequences enhances the understanding of options and alternatives.

Identify Options

Having determined the desired outcomes, participants should identify possible options for action. Various options begin to emerge through the assessment process. Participants must consider consequences, and legal consideration of each alternative must be considered. Those involved in making the decision determine which alternatives best meet the identified outcomes and fit their basic beliefs, lifestyles, and values. This process helps to narrow the list of acceptable alternatives. It is critical to eliminate all unacceptable alternatives and begin the process of listing, weighing, ranking, and prioritizing those that are found to be acceptable. A choice among options is made with both head and heart; therefore, those involved should take time to dwell with remaining alternatives, recognizing that there is rarely a good solution. Once the selection is made, the decision makers must be willing to act upon the choice.

Act on the Choice

Taking action is a major goal of the process but can be one of the most difficult parts. It can stir numerous emotions laced with both certainty and doubt about the rightness of the decision. Participants must be empowered to make a difficult decision, setting aside less acceptable alternatives. Chapters 19 and 20 discuss empowerment in more depth. It is important to be attentive to the emotions involved at this point of the process.

Evaluate Outcomes of Action

After acting upon the decision, participants begin a process of response and evaluation. As in all decision making, reflective evaluation sheds light on the effectiveness and validity of the process. The action must be evaluated in terms of the effects upon those involved. Questions should be asked, such as "Has the original ethical dilemma been resolved?" and "Have other dilemmas emerged related to the action?" As the situation changes and new data emerge, participants must identify subsequent moral problems and adjust the course of action based upon both new information and responses to the previous decision.

Figure 4–1 presents a guide that may assist in the process of ethical decision making. The questions posed may need to be revisited several times and may emerge at various points as the process unfolds and new data is presented. For example, information about options may begin to emerge before all the parties involved are identified, and data regarding ethical perspectives of the various parties may be clarified only at the point when options are being discussed. No matter how much information the participants gather, they may make the decision with an awareness that they would like to have still more data, although having a long list of viable options may actually make it more difficult to come to a decision.

Figure 4–1 **A Guide for Decision Making**

Gather Data and Identify Conflicting Moral Claims

- What makes this situation an ethical dilemma? Are there conflicting obligations, duties, principles, rights, loyalties, values, or beliefs?
- What are the issues?
- What facts seem most important?
- What emotions have an impact?
- What are the gaps in information at this time?

Identify Key Participants

- Who is legitimately empowered to make this decision?
- Who is affected and how?
- What is the level of competence of the person most affected in relation to the decision to be made?
- What are the rights, duties, authority, context, and capabilities of participants?

Determine Moral Perspective and Phase of Moral Development of Key Participants

- Do participants think in terms of duties or rights?
- Do the parties involved exhibit similar or different moral perspectives?
- Where is the common ground? The differences?
- What principles are important to each person involved?
- What emotions are evident within the interaction and with each person involved?
- What is the level of moral development of the participants?

Determine Desired Outcomes

- How does each party describe the circumstances of the outcome?
- What are the consequences of the desired outcomes?
- What outcomes are unacceptable to one or all involved?

Identify Options

- What options emerge through the assessment process?
- How do the alternatives fit the lifestyle and values of the person(s) affected?
- What are legal considerations of the various options?
- What alternatives are unacceptable to one or all involved?
- How are alternatives weighed, ranked, and prioritized?

Act on the Choice

- Be empowered to make a difficult decision.
- Give oneself permission to set aside less acceptable alternatives.
- Be attentive to the emotions involved in this process.

Evaluate Outcomes of Action

- Has the ethical dilemma been resolved?
- Have other dilemmas emerged related to the action?
- How has the process affected those involved?
- Are further actions required?

APPLYING THE DECISION MAKING PROCESS

Application of the decision making guide in clinical situations is illustrated in the following case and discussion:

> A couple is pregnant with their second child after numerous unsuccessful attempts with artificial insemination. During a routine ultrasound at 28 weeks gestation, it is discovered that the fetus is anencephalic. This condition is such that there is a life expectancy of only a few days to weeks after birth. The couple is presented the option to terminate the pregnancy at this time or to carry the child to term.

Gathering Data and Identifying Conflicting Moral Claims

One conflict relates to the principle of nonmaleficence (the wish to do no harm). Terminating the pregnancy can be perceived as harmful to the baby, while carry- ing it to term may result in emotional or physical harm to the mother. Another conflict relates to the duty to preserve life, allowing the pregnancy, birth, and death of the baby to take its natural course versus the duty to alleviate the suffering that carrying the pregnancy to term might impose on the mother. Some of the important facts in this situation include knowing the life expectancy of a baby born with anencephaly, knowing the parents' attitudes toward abortion, appreciating the feelings that this news calls forth, and knowing the meaning of this pregnancy to the parents.

Identifying Key Participants

Notwithstanding the necessity of input from the physician and others, both parents have the moral and legal right and the responsibility to make the decision. They may want to consult religious ministers, family, or friends, and they may request a second opinion. Though mentally competent, the parents may have difficulty making a decision soon after receiving the painful news. Since this is not an emergency, the nurse and others should allow time and provide support while the parents process the information and deal with emotions. If, for example, one parent wants the pregnancy terminated and the other is strongly opposed, participants should further explore who has the right to make the ultimate decision.

Determining Moral Perspective and Phase of Moral Development of Key Participants

It is important to consider whether the stance of both parents is the same. Are they thinking about the rights of the infant versus the rights of the mother, or the duty to preserve the family integrity? If one parent thinks the pregnancy should be terminated and the other feels that the baby has a right to life, no matter how short it may be, can a common ground be reached? Do the parents seek guidance from those in authority or from beliefs regarding right and wrong in this situation? Do they talk of a relationship with the baby in utero and the impact of choosing to end its life—on the baby, its sibling, or their relationship?

Determining Desired Outcomes

Through discussion of outcomes, more insight into ethical theory may emerge. In this situation, participants could describe the desired outcome as prevention of unnecessary suffering for the mother and the baby. Further exploration might reveal the sense that carrying the baby to term would create such anguish for the mother that her emotional health, and even family integrity, would be threatened. In that instance, terminating the pregnancy would be viewed as more compassionate than prolonging the suffering of the mother and allowing the inevitable yet slow, natural death of the baby. Legal considerations would include laws related to abortion.

Identifying Options

In this case, the physician presented the options at the outset: the parents could terminate the pregnancy or allow it to go to term. One might well look at the risks for the mother involved in both choices. Participants need to clarify beliefs regarding life, abortion, family responsibility, duties, and the like. If carrying the pregnancy to term presents a health risk for the mother, an additional dilemma would arise regarding responsibility to the older sibling and family integrity versus responsibility to the baby.

If either carrying the pregnancy to term or terminating it now is acceptable, participants have the task of determining factors that may weigh one alternative more strongly than the other. They may decide that the grieving process of the baby's death has already begun and would only be intensified if the pregnancy were carried to term. With this in mind, they might decide to end the pregnancy.

Acting on the Choice

Deciding that terminating the pregnancy is the best alternative, the parents move toward action. As logistics of scheduling and preparing for the termination proceed, it is important to attend to the parents' emotional response and to ensure that they have other needed support.

Evaluating Outcomes of Action

The parents have resolved the dilemma of whether to terminate the pregnancy or carry it to term by choosing to proceed with termination. Reactions to the choice may emerge in the forms of guilt, depression, acceptance, or always wondering how things might have been different if the other path had been chosen. If the parents have long-term reactions, such as deep guilt or depression, they might come to a point of saying that, faced with such a situation again, they should decide to carry the pregnancy to term. On the other hand, they may examine issues surrounding the emotions with the awareness that the decision to terminate the pregnancy was the catalyst for dealing with these issues and that, in spite of the pain, they made the best decision at the time.

Various Responses to Terminating Pregnancy

Consider which areas of the "Guide for Decision Making" in Figure 4–1 may have to be revisited in the following variations of the case presented above.

- The mother indicates that she thinks she will "go crazy" if she carries the pregnancy to term, and the father says "no one is going to kill my child."
- This is a young single mother from another culture who believes she has been "witched" and that the baby will be normal if she has the proper ceremony.
- The local hospital has a religious affiliation that does not permit abortions. The parents feel that terminating the pregnancy is the better decision, but they have no transportation to the hospital, a two-hour drive away, where the procedure can be done.

SUMMARY

Ethical decision making requires knowledge and attention to many factors. Determining the existence of an ethical dilemma is a beginning step in the process which includes defining the problem, identifying desired objectives, listing and evaluating alternatives, choosing the best course of action based on one's knowledge and the current circumstances, and evaluating the outcomes of the action taken. One must consider both reason and emotion in making ethical decisions. Nurses are encouraged to utilize the decision making process described in this chapter as a guide in dealing with dilemmas encountered in clinical settings. As with every other nursing skill, comfort and competency with ethical decision making comes with repeated practice.

CHAPTER HIGHLIGHTS

- Dilemmas exist when difficult problems have no satisfactory solutions or when all the solutions appear equally favorable.
- In decisions involving practical dilemmas, moral claims hold greater weight than nonmoral claims.
- Making thoughtful decisions in any arena follows a pattern that includes gathering data, comparing options based on particular criteria, making and acting on a choice, and evaluating outcomes or circumstances surrounding the choice.
- One's value system affects how one defines and deals with an ethical issue; thus, resolution of ethical dilemmas requires determining the ethical issue at hand and identifying the value systems of those involved.
- Both emotion and reason have legitimate roles in ethical decision making.
- Ethical decision making requires ongoing evaluation and assimilation of information, with revisiting of various steps in the process as often as required by the dynamics of changing facts, evolving beliefs, unexpected consequences, and participants moving in and out of the process.
- Familiarity with and practice in applying ethical decision making enables the nurse to develop competence and confidence with the process.

DISCUSSION QUESTIONS AND ACTIVITIES

1. Working in small groups, discuss ethical and practical dilemmas that you have experienced, then choose an example of each type of dilemma to illustrate for the class.
2. Describe a situation in which you or someone you know experienced moral distress, noting moral and nonmoral claims in the situation.
3. Talk with practicing nurses about their experiences of ethical dilemmas. Identify their approaches to dealing with such dilemmas including their processes of ethical decision making.
4. With classmates, debate the role of reason and emotion in ethical decisions.
5. Use the ethical decision making process to revisit an ethical dilemma that you have encountered in the past or to guide you through a current dilemma. Examine your sense of comfort with each part of the process, noting areas of strength and areas needing more practice.
6. Discuss the interaction among moral development, moral perspective, and ethical decision making.

7. How would you approach an ethical dilemma in which the parties involved exhibit different moral perspectives?

8. How might legal considerations affect the process of making ethical decisions?

REFERENCES

Beauchamp, T. L., & Childress, J. F. (1994). *Principles of biomedical ethics* (4th ed.). New York: Oxford University Press.

Callahan, S. (1995). The role of emotions in ethical decision making. In J. H. Howell & W. F. Sale (Eds.), *Life choices: A Hastings Center introduction to bioethics*. Washington, DC: Georgetown University Press.

Chinn, P. L. (1995). *Peace and power: Building communities for the future* (4th ed.). New York: National League of Nursing Press.

Christensen, P. J., & Kenney, J. W. (1990). *Nursing process: Application of conceptual models* (3rd ed.). St. Louis, MO: Mosby.

Curtin, L., & Flaherty, M. J. (1982). *Nursing ethics: Theories and pragmatics*. Bowie, MD: Brady.

Davis, A. J., Aroskar, M. A., Liaschenko, J., & Drought, T. S. (1997). *Ethical dilemmas and nursing practice* (4th ed.). Norwalk, CT: Appleton & Lange.

Gibson, J. (1991). An introduction to the study of ethics and ethical theories. In B. R. Furrow, S. H. Johnson, T. S. Jost, & R. L. Schwartz (Eds.), *Bioethics: Health care, law, and ethics* (pp. 1–6). St. Paul, MN: West.

Husted, G. L., & Husted, J. H. (1995). *Ethical decision making in nursing*. St. Louis, MO: Mosby.

Jameton, A. (1984). *Nursing practice: The ethical issues*. Englewood Cliffs, NJ: Prentice-Hall.

PART II

DEVELOPING PRINCIPLED BEHAVIOR

Recognizing that values and beliefs are culturally relative, Part II describes theories related to moral development and values clarification. Because personal values and moral development influence perceptions and decisions, readers are encouraged to become aware of their own values and to examine personal levels of moral development in light of the different theories presented in Part I. Benefiting from this knowledge, readers can begin to be more sensitive to the perspectives, decision making abilities, and tendencies of other people and to acknowledge the influence of their own values and moral development on various decision making processes.

CHAPTER 5

Values Clarification

As your actions are informed by your awareness of values, your thinking and your ideas are shaped and changed by your experiences with those actions.

(Chinn, 1995, p. 3)

OBJECTIVES

After completing this chapter, the reader should be able to:

1. Define and differentiate personal values, societal values, professional values, organizational values, and moral values.

2. Discuss how values are acquired.

3. Discuss self-awareness as a tool for living an ethical life.

4. Explain the place of values clarification in nursing.

5. Explain the valuing process.

6. Describe values conflict and its implications for nursing care.

7. Describe the interaction between personal and institutional values.

8. Discuss the importance of attending to both personal values and patient values.

INTRODUCTION

Principled behavior flows from personal values that guide and inform one's responses, behaviors, and decisions in all areas of one's life. Ethical decision making requires self-awareness and knowledge of ethical theories and principles. Such awareness of self includes knowing what one values or considers important. The branch of philosophy that studies the nature and types of values is called **axiology,** a word that comes from the Greek for worth or worthy. Axiology includes the study of values in art, known as aesthetics, in human relations and conduct, known as ethics, and in relation to beliefs regarding relationship with the Divine, known as religion. This chapter discusses the importance of being aware of personal values and the impact of these values on the way one relates to self and others within personal and professional arenas.

WHAT ARE VALUES?

Values are ideals, beliefs, customs, modes of conduct, qualities, or goals that are highly prized or preferred by individuals, groups, or society. Omery (1989) notes that the fundamental nature of values includes a pattern of a "subjective, strongly motivational preference or disposition toward a person, object, or idea that is more likely to be manifest in an affective situation . . . and [is] more likely to be mobilized by the individual in a hierarchical order" (p. 500). Values, which are learned in both conscious and unconscious ways, become part of a person's makeup. When one is faced with choices, one's preferences and their hierarchy becomes evident. For example, if both comfort and appearance are valued in how one dresses, the hierarchy becomes evident when one chooses to wear the more restrictive suit rather than the more relaxed dress for a professional interview. One's values influence choices regardless of whether one is conscious that the values are guiding the choices. Values may be expressed overtly as espoused behaviors or verbalized standards, or they may manifest in an indirect way through verbal and nonverbal behavior.

Moral Values

As discussed in Chapter 2, individual cognitive evaluation of right and wrong, good, and bad, is reflective of **moral thought.** Flowing from this, preferences or dispositions reflective of right or wrong, should or should not, in human behavior are considered **moral values** (Omery, 1989). Moral values constitute a special case of values because the particular circumstances that call them forth deal with ethical issues or dilemmas. These values may be acquired within contexts such as the family, through one's religious or philosophical orientation, or through one's profession.

ACQUIRING VALUES

Personal ethical behavior flows from values held by an individual that develop over time. Cultural, ethnic, familial, environmental, educational, and other experiences of living help to shape one's values. We begin to learn and incorporate values into our beings at an early age and continue the process throughout our lives. As noted previously, values are acquired in both conscious and unconscious ways. Values may be learned in a conscious way through instruction by parents, teachers, religious ministers and educators, and professional and social group leaders. Many values are formally adopted by groups and are written in professional codes of ethics, religious doctrines, societal laws, and statements of an organization's philosophy. Socialization and role modeling, other ways values are acquired, lead to more subconscious learning. Some values stay with us for much of our lives, and others may change or be altered in response to our own development and experiences. "The most important step in values formation is one's freedom to choose those values that are most cherished and to relinquish those that have little meaning" (Seroka, 1994, p. 11).

Because values become a part of who we are, they often enter into decision making in less than conscious ways. We constantly make judgments that reflect our values, though not always realizing that we have a given set of values or that these values are affecting our decisions (Davis, Aroskar, Liaschenko, & Drought, 1997; Simon, Howe, & Kirschenbaum, 1995). Becoming more aware of one's values is an important step in being able to make clear and thoughtful decisions. Knowing one's own values in a conscious way and being able to help others to clearly name their values are particularly important in the area of ethical decision making.

Ask Yourself

How Have Your Values Developed?

Think of three ideals or beliefs that you prize in your personal life. Try to trace each belief or ideal back to the earliest time in your life when you were aware of its importance or presence.

- When and how did you learn to view each belief or ideal as important?
- How have they changed or evolved over time?
- Where do you find your support for them?
- How prevalent do you think these beliefs or ideals are among other people?
- What do you think of people who hold different beliefs or ideals?
- Think of a time in your life when one of these beliefs or ideals has been challenged. How did you feel? How did you react?

SELF-AWARENESS

Ethical relationships with others begin with self-knowledge and the willingness to honestly and appropriately express that awareness to others. Self-knowledge is an ongoing, evolving process that requires a person to make a commitment to know the truth about oneself. This is not an easy commitment to make. Although the truth can be painful at times, paradoxically, it can also set one free. It is important to keep in mind that what one believes to be the truth is always colored by one's perceptions and can change over time (Covey, 1990). Keep in mind that most situations are not black or white. All sides are present in each situation. Like the aperture of a camera, what one sees in any situation depends upon how close or far one is standing and the angle from which one is looking. From this perspective, there can be many views of a situation, depending upon how many people are picturing it. Understanding the truth of a situation is usually more accurate if people appreciate that there can be different views and openly share these perspectives (Banonis, 1997).

The term **values clarification** refers to the process of becoming more conscious of and naming what one values or considers worthy. It is a way of shedding light on one's personal perspective. Through developing insight into one's valuing, one's ability to make value decisions improves. Attentiveness to values enables one to consciously choose to be consistent in value decisions, thus enhancing personal integrity. As noted in Chapter 3, **integrity** refers to adherence to moral norms that is sustained over time. Implicit in integrity is trustworthiness and a consistency of convictions, actions, and emotions. It is only to the extent that one appreciates one's own values that there can be any true understanding of the values of another.

Since values include dimensions of knowing and of feeling, the process of becoming more clear about what one holds dear needs to address both the cognitive and the affective domains. Through behavior analysis and discovery of feelings one learns to discern which choices are rational and which are the result of preconditioning (Seroka, 1994). The process of assessing one's values requires a readiness and willingness to take an honest look within, at one's ideals and behaviors, at one's words, actions, and motivation, and at the congruencies and incongruencies among them. Moving toward the point of choosing one's own values rather than merely acting out prior programing is a goal of the process.

Enhancing Self-Awareness

Self-awareness is the ultimate tool for living a personally ethical life. Values clarification and **self-awareness** go hand in hand. The first and most important step in awareness of the self is an acknowledged intention to be aware. Consciousness of one's thoughts, feelings, physical and emotional responses, and insights in various situations can promote appreciation of one's values. Conversely, by identifying and analyzing personal values, one becomes more self-aware. Insight can be enhanced by developing the ability to step back and see what is going on in any situation, being aware of oneself and one's reactions in the present moment. Self-awareness can begin with as simple an act as tuning in to one's breathing, noting its rate, rhythm, depth, and other characteristics without any effort to change it. It is a way of becoming conscious of an act that usually occurs quite unconsciously. Another way to become more aware is to pay attention to how you are feeling physically and emotionally in any given situation—to name the feelings without judging them. You might ask, "What do I think I am reacting to here, and can I identify where that reaction comes from?" For example, when you see a beautiful sunset, you might note a feeling of peace, exhilaration, or relaxation and realize you are responding to beauty, with an ensuing memory that your mother was always one to be observant of beauty in her world. You thus recognize that you learned this value, at least in part, from your mother. Introspection, observation, reflection, meditation, journaling, art, writing, therapy, reading, discussion groups, and feedback assist people in expanding self-awareness.

Individual reflection and discussion with another or in small groups are approaches to self-awareness that can be useful in analyzing values. Group discussion enables one to react and hear the reactions of others. Such processes may lead to more clarity about values that have been accepted because of programming, modification of one's initial stance based on insights of others, and fuller articulation of values that have been personally chosen. Other tools that open one's perspective include: taking the other side of a debate, interviewing people with differing opinions, walking in another's shoes and defending their position, and asking for feedback on your positions. Another way to look at values is to ask general questions like "If I knew I would die in six weeks, what would I be doing today?" or "If I had to leave my house and could only take three things with me, what would they be?" or "Where would I like to be five/ten/twenty years from now?"

It has been suggested that the valuing process includes three areas:

Prizing and cherishing one's beliefs and behaviors, which includes knowing what one does and does not support and communicating this to others;

Choosing one's beliefs and behaviors by evaluating values received from others, which includes examining alternatives and their consequences then deciding what is one's own;

Acting on these beliefs with a consistent pattern that reinforces actions supportive of the values (Simon et al., 1995).

The intent of values clarification is to help people become more aware of their own values and the valuing process in their own lives; it does not aim to impose or instill particular values in their lives.

Journaling.   Kolkmeier (1995) describes **journals** as "records that are kept on a periodic or regular basis and contain factual material and subjective interpretations of events, thoughts, feelings, and plans" (p. 336). For many people, keeping a diary or journal of experiences and personal reactions to situations is a useful tool in developing awareness. A number of books such as those by Progoff (1992), Adams (1990), and Baldwin (1991) are available to guide someone new to journaling. Figure 5–1 offers guidelines that may help students utilize the journaling process to gain insight into personal values. The following are a few general considerations that may enhance the ability to gain insight through journaling. When writing in a journal, let your thoughts flow as freely as possible without censoring or judging what you are writing. Allow yourself time and privacy when you are journaling, and keep the journal in a place where you feel comfortable that you control who has access to it. Commit to journaling on a regular basis. Recognize that journaling is a personal process, so go with your style. If a format such as that suggested in Figure 5–1 helps you, go for it! If not, write as the thoughts flow from you.

Figure 5-1 **Journaling for Values Awareness**

- Describe a situation in your personal or professional experience in which you felt uncomfortable or felt that your beliefs or values were being challenged, or in which you felt your values were different from others involved.

- As you record the situation, include how you felt physically and emotionally at the time you experienced the situation.

- Write down your feelings as you remember the situation. Are your reactions now any different from when you were actually in this situation?

- What personal values do you identify in the situation? Try to remember where and from whom you learned these values. Do you totally agree with the values, or is there anything about them that you question or wonder about their validity?

- What values do you think were being expressed by others involved? Where are the similarities and differences relative to your values?

- What do you think you reacted to in the situation?

- Can you remember having similar reactions in other situations? If yes, how were the situations similar or different?

- How do you feel about your response to the situation? Is there anything you would change if you could repeat the scene? Rewrite the scene with the changes. What might be the consequences of these changes?

- How do you feel with the new scenario?

- What do you need to do to reinforce behaviors, ideals, beliefs, or qualities that you have identified as personal values in this situation? When and how can you do this?

Values in Professional Situations

Values clarification is important to nurses in several ways. To know and appreciate one's own value system provides a basis for understanding how and why one reacts and responds in decision making situations. Knowing one's own values enables one to acknowledge similarities and differences in values when interacting with others, enabling more effective communication and care. Attentiveness to analyzing personal values enables the nurse to be more effective in facilitating the process with others. In the professional realm, these others may be staff, patients, families, or institutions.

Values Conflict. When personal values are at odds with those of patients, colleagues, or the institution, internal or interpersonal conflict may result. This can subsequently affect patient care. Dealing in an effective way with **values conflict** requires conscious awareness of one's own values as well as the perceived values of the others involved. Such awareness enables the nurse to be more alert to situations in which the behaviors of others are judged according to one's own values, or in which personal values are being imposed upon another. When differences in values are identified, a choice can be made to respond to the other's viewpoint, seeking understanding and common ground, rather than reacting in a "knee-jerk" fashion. In this way the integrity of the caring relationship can be maintained.

The following case presentation provides an example of values conflict. As you read the case, think about the values that are evident in the situation. Put yourself in the position of each of the participants and ask yourself what you might do if you were in their shoes.

CASE PRESENTATION

A Conflict of Values

Nine-year-old Benton is a patient on the pediatric unit with a diagnosis of terminal stage Ewing's sarcoma. He has three sisters, aged seven, six, and three, who are presently being cared for by a grandmother. His father is self-employed and works long hours. His mother has never worked outside the home. Both parents have high school educations, and their primary activities outside of family are church-related. They belong to a small nondenominational rural church and state that they hold fast to what is taught in the Bible and put their faith in the word of God.

Prior to his illness, Benton, a healthy child, had been brought to the clinic only for acute health concerns. The family does not have health insurance. Shortly after entering second grade two years ago, he began limping. The family attributed the limp to a playground injury. When he continued to complain of pain and the limp persisted after three months, his mother took him to a local health clinic. Above-the-knee amputation followed diagnosis, but metastasis was evident in nine months. Chemotherapy has only been palliative.

The physician has discussed Benton's poor prognosis with the parents, recommending comfort care. The parents say they want everything possible to be done for him, and the father conducts nightly prayer sessions at Benton's bedside, affirming that God is healing Benton. Although Benton has asked whether he is going to die, his father refuses to allow staff to speak with him regarding fears or concerns about his condition. When asked what Benton has been told, the father responds, "He knows God is trying us and we must have faith." The mother, who appears less confident of a healing, is there twenty-four hours a day. She supervises Benton's care relentlessly, at times irritating staff with questions and demands. She keeps a notebook record of her son's care, including medication, times of care, intake and output, and personal assessments. Although Benton used to talk to staff, he now appears frightened and remains quiet, sleeping off and on.

Dealing with Values Conflict

Respond to these questions from the vantage point of the nurse in the situation:

- What is your first personal reaction to this situation? Identify your values relative to the situation.

- What do you perceive to be the values of the others involved?
- Identify value incongruencies that might lead to conflict. Give specific examples of how such a conflict can potentially affect patient care.
- Describe specific nursing interventions aimed at managing the conflict in a professional manner, and give examples of how nursing codes would guide such actions.
- Describe your own strengths and limitations as you consider dealing with this situation.

Impact of Institutional Values

Being conscious of values within the work setting is an important consideration for nurses. Values of individual institutions and organized health care systems that are explicitly communicated through philosophy and policy statements are called **overt values.** Values may also be implicit in expectations that are not in writing. Implicit or **covert values** are often identified only through participation in or controversies within the setting (Omery, 1989). Identifying congruencies or incongruencies between personal values and those of the institution is an important consideration for a nurse seeking employment in that institution, since accepting employment implies committing to the value system of the organization. Consider, for example, a nurse, Anton, who accepts a position at a health center because the center publicizes a commitment to providing quality care to all patients. Within two months he notices that patients with Medicaid cards are kept waiting longer than those with private insurance and are treated rudely by many of the staff. When he initiates teaching with the Medicaid patients, he is told not to waste his time because "those people won't change their ways." Overtly the health center is committed to quality care for all patients; however, the covert values reflect different attitudes toward and levels of care for those on public assistance. Anton's values of providing quality care for all may prompt a variety of responses in this situation. He may compromise his values if he wants to get along with other staff and do well in the job, he may expend much energy challenging the covert value system, or he may decide that he cannot continue to work in this system.

Ask Yourself

How Should Values Influence Job Selection?

Maria, a recently divorced mother of three, desperately needs to return to work, but nursing jobs in her area are scarce. There is one opening at a women's health clinic that performs abortions. The job, which has excellent salary and benefits, including on-site child care, looks great to Maria, except that abortions are against her religious and personal beliefs. A friend who works at the clinic said that, unless they are short staffed, Maria would not have to assist with abortions if she had objections.

- What dilemmas are evident in this situation?
- What are the value incongruencies?
- What are your values related to this situation?
- What factors should Maria consider in deciding whether to take the job?

Schoof notes that what one believes and how one thinks about a job is important, having a direct impact on job performance. Such internal belief systems tend to shape a person's thinking and direct them to do what they think is right regardless of the employer's philosophy. Schoof suggests that it is better to identify what is valued by the employer, that is, where they stand and what they pay attention to and reward, and then to decide if one can work in that environment. As an example he indicates that there are three primary ways to approach patient care: focus on meeting patient needs (intrinsic care), focus on doing all the tasks (extrinsic care), and focus on following the rules (systemic care) (personal communication, February 12, 1996). If there is a conflict between one's own values regarding patient care and the values of the institution, one may experience moral distress. **Moral distress** is the reaction to a situation in which there are moral problems that seem to have clear solutions, yet one is unable to follow one's moral beliefs because of external restraints. This distress is often evidenced in anger, dissatisfaction, frustration, and poor performance in the work setting.

One process for defining and making organizational values more explicit is described by Gingerich and Ondeck (1993). This process includes determining what is valued by staff, board members, management, and physicians regarding the elements of the organization's philosophy and identifying specific expectations for each group. Exercises focused on self-awareness, clinical priorities, and opinions about value-laden issues are conducted within each of the groups to develop awareness of and consensus around the values. This allows all involved to have an investment in the value system.

The Hartman Value Profile is another approach to looking at values within an organization (Hartman, 1967; Edwards & Davis, 1991; H. Schoof, personal communication, 1996). The process involves having the institution select a number of employees representing two groups within the organization: those considered to be the *shining stars*, and those considered least satisfactory. Those identified complete the profile, which is a forced ranking, from best to worst or most despicable, of eighteen items relating to how persons perceive the world around them and eighteen items related to how they perceive their inner selves. Patterns are identified by analyzing the participants' responses utilizing a computerized mathematical system that identifies how each item compares with the others that are ranked. The resulting information provides a profile of the underlying values within the organization. Decision makers can use this information to examine how prevailing belief systems are influencing performance and to seek potential employees whose values are most consistent with those of the organization.

CASE PRESENTATION

Differences in Personal and Organizational Values

Joan has been the nurse manager of her unit for the past ten years and is highly regarded by the hospital's administration. For the past several months, however, she has been feeling more frustrated and less satisfied with her work because of staffing cuts and other institutional decisions related to managed care. Attending to patient needs has always been the most rewarding part of her job. However, recently she feels that she has been forced to overlook these needs and attend more to the needs of the organization. She considers leaving, but she has seniority, good benefits, and two children to support. She is also aware that her distress at work is affecting her family because she carries a lot of the frustration home with her.

Think About It

How Values Affect Choices

- Identify values evident in this situation. Which of these reflect your personal values?
- What conflicts might arise from these values?
- What do you think Joan should do?
- If you were in Joan's position, what beliefs, ideals, or goals would guide you in making a decision to stay or leave? Identify potential consequences of each choice.

Clarifying Values with Patients

Values are an important consideration for nurses in patient care situations. Patients are the consumers of health care, so it is good to know what they expect or value. Patient and provider perceptions of what constitutes quality of care can be quite different. Great discrepancies in these perceptions may lead to patient dissatisfaction. This can have a variety of consequences, including affecting a patient's attitude and decisions regarding following recommendations for care and treatment (which may affect recovery), marring the reputation of the agency, or potentiating malpractice litigation. Allanach and Golden (1988) describe the process of a service audit aimed at identifying patient expectations and clarifying their opinions about the level of service. Nursing care behaviors identified as valued by patients in this study relate to the amount of care and time spent with patients and to the technical quality of nursing care. Consider the potential conflict of values when patients expect nurses to spend time with them and the institution puts more emphasis on getting the tasks done.

Ask Yourself

What Would You Do?

- You are busy and two call lights go on at the same time. What factors enter into deciding which one you respond to first?

- Consider that in the above situation one patient is in serious condition and has been verbally abusive to staff, while the other is not quite as serious and is someone you really enjoy being with. Who would you respond to first and why?

- Your patients let you know how much they appreciate the extra care and time you give them compared to the other nurses. At the same time, your evaluation is coming up and your supervisor has indicated that you need to be more efficient with your time. What would you do in this situation and why?

When working with patients regarding health care decisions, it is important for nurses to be aware of personal values and patients' values pertaining to health. When the health values of the nurse and those of the patient are different, the patient may become labeled as uncooperative, self-destructive, noncompliant, ignorant, or unwilling to take responsibility for her or his own health. Attentiveness to cultural and religious values is especially important in this regard. Refer to Chapter 18 for discussion of transcultural and spiritual issues.

Pender (1987; 1996) discusses the role of values in health promotion. She notes that knowing personal values is important, as is the need to avoid imposing one's values on patients. Consider, for example, an obese patient with terminal lung cancer and a prognosis of three to six months to live, who continues to smoke and is a confirmed agnostic. If priorities on the care plan include weight loss, smoking cessation, and facilitating the patient's making peace with God, one must consider whether nursing values are being imposed on the patient.

With self-awareness the nurse can be more effective in helping patients to identify their own values. Assisting patients to clearly articulate their values is important because a lack of clarity about values may result in inconsistency, confusion, misunderstanding, and inadequate decision making. The ability to make informed choices, including the process of informed consent, is enhanced by having clarity about one's values. "Assisting clients to clarify values; understand the personal and social consequences of acting on current values; achieve greater consistency among values, attitudes, and behaviors; and plan health-related experiences that may result in self-initiated changes in value hierarchies" are key nursing actions (Pender, 1987, p. 161).

Pender (1987) offers several instruments and processes that can facilitate exploring values in general and health values in particular. One example is a process that asks people to rank a list of ten health values from most important to least important. The list includes a comfortable life, an exciting life, a sense of accomplishment, freedom, happiness, health, inner harmony, pleasure, self-respect, and social recognition (Pender, 1987, p. 165). Pender notes that if health appears within the top four on the list, the person places a high value on health. However, definitions of health will vary, since each person defines health according to personal beliefs and values.

Another approach to analyzing health values described by Doyle (1994) asks people to identify from a list of ten health related behaviors, what they do and why they do it. Behaviors include activities such as exercising a minimum of three times per week, talking to a close friend or relative about worries, and practicing sex without using a condom. Doyle notes that the response to why a behavior is practiced provides insight into values surrounding the behavior, such as choosing not to exercise in order to have more time, or choosing to exercise because it helps in weight control.

SUMMARY

This chapter has discussed the importance of self-awareness regarding values and the valuing process. Values are learned and change in response to life situations as a person develops. The process of values clarification enables persons to begin to identify and choose their own values rather than merely act out of prior programming. The interaction of personal values with those of patients and organizations was presented as a consideration that can affect job satisfaction and patient care. The reader is encouraged to explore various processes that facilitate values clarification, both those presented in this chapter and those found in other resources.

CHAPTER HIGHLIGHTS

- Values are highly prized ideals, behaviors, beliefs, or qualities that are shaped by culture, ethnicity, family, environment, and education and are acquired in both conscious and unconscious ways.

- The process of incorporating values begins at an early age and continues throughout life. Some values remain consistent while others change in response to growth and life experiences.

- Awareness of personal values undergirds the ability to make clear and thoughtful decisions and enables one to acknowledge similarities and differences in values when interacting with others, thus promoting more effective communication, care, and facilitation of values clarification with others.

- Values clarification is not intended to instill values; rather, the aim is to facilitate awareness of personal values and the valuing process in order to move toward the point of choosing one's own values rather than merely reacting from prior programing.

- The valuing process includes prizing and cherishing, choosing, and acting on beliefs and behaviors.

- Dealing effectively with values conflict requires attention to personal values, the perceived values of others, and the ability to recognize both overt and covert expression of values in a situation.

- Congruence between personal values and those of an institution is an important consideration for a nurse seeking employment.

- Assisting patients to articulate their values and beliefs, an important part of nursing care, may help prevent deleterious consequences related to not addressing differences in values between patients and providers.

DISCUSSION QUESTIONS AND ACTIVITIES

1. A non-nursing classmate asks you what studying values has to do with nursing. How would you respond? Incorporate your understanding of the nature of values and how they are encoded into your response.

2. What values guide your personal life? How did you learn these values? Select something that you consider important in professional nursing practice and trace how you learned this value.

3. Discuss why values clarification is important both personally and professionally.

4. Identify the overt values of your health care agency and identify overt and covert values of nurses and others within the agency. Explain the importance of knowing about both.

5. Describe a situation in which you experienced someone (it could be you) reacting from values that were not conscious at the time. How did this affect the interaction?

6. Determine the health values of three patients or people you do not know well and discuss why nurses need to be attentive to what patients value.

7. Describe a situation in which you experienced values conflict and how you dealt with the conflict.

8. Find current examples of public or professional figures whose personal values seem at odds with their professional or public trust. Discuss your reaction to the discrepancy in values that you identify and the interplay between personal values and professional integrity.

REFERENCES

Adams, K. (1990). *Journal to the self—Two paths to personal growth*. New York: Warner Books.

Allanach, E. J., & Golden, B. M. (1988). Patients' expectations and values clarification: A service audit. *Nursing Administration Quarterly, 12,* 17–22.

Baldwin, C. (1991). *Life's companion: Journal writing as a spiritual quest*. New York: Bantam Books.

Banonis, B. C. (1997). *Principled behavior applied to everyday life*. Charleston, WV: Unpublished manuscript.

Chinn, P. L. (1995). *Peace and power: Building communities for the future* (4th ed.). New York: National League of Nursing Press.

Covey, S. R. (1990). *The seven habits of highly effective people*. New York: Simon & Schuster.

Davis, A. J., Aroskar, M. A., Liaschenko, J., & Drought, T. S. (1997). *Ethical dilemmas and nursing practice* (4th ed). Norwalk, CT: Appleton & Lange.

Doyle, E. I. (1994). Recognizing the value-health behavior connection: "What I do and why I do it." *Journal of Health Education, 25,* 116–118.

Edwards, R. B., & Davis, J. W. (1991). *Forms of value and valuation*. Lanham, MD: University Press of America.

Gingerich, B. S., & Ondeck, D. A. (1993). Values incorporation throughout the organization. *Caring Magazine,* 12, 18–23.

Hartman, R. S. (1967). *The structure of value*. Carbondale, IL: Southern Illinois University Press.

Kolkmeier, L. G. (1995). Self-reflection: Consulting the truth within. In B. M. Dossey, L. Keegan, C. E. Guzzetta, & L. G. Kolkmeier, *Holistic nursing: A handbook for practice* (2nd ed.). Gaithersburg, MD: Aspen.

Omery, A. (1989). Values, moral reasoning, and ethics. *Nursing Clinics of North America, 24,* 499–507.

Pender, N. J. (1987). *Health promotion in nursing practice* (2nd ed.). Norwalk, CT: Appleton & Lange.

Pender, N. J. (1996). *Health promotion in nursing practice* (3rd ed.). Norwalk, CT: Appleton & Lange.

Progoff, I. (1992). *At a journal workshop*. New York: Tarcher.

Seroka, A. M. (1994). Values clarification and ethical decision making. *Seminars for Nurse Managers, 2,* 8–15.

Simon, S. B., Howe, L. W., & Kirschenbaum, H. (1995). *Values clarification: A handbook of practical strategies for teachers and students*. New York: Hart.

CHAPTER 6

Values Development

What is firmly established cannot be uprooted.
What is firmly grasped cannot slip away.
It will be honored from generation to generation.
(Lao Tsu, *Tao Te Ching*)

OBJECTIVES

After completing this chapter, the reader should be able to:

1. Discuss influences of culture on values development.
2. Contrast theoretical approaches to moral development.
3. Describe and differentiate the ethic of care and the ethic of justice.
4. Evaluate personal phase of moral development.
5. Discuss gender bias and cultural bias regarding theories of moral development.

INTRODUCTION

Nurses frequently encounter situations that present ethical dilemmas. In some situations the "right" choice seems quite evident, while in other circumstances a considerable lack of clarity about what is "right" may exist. How does one come to know what is right or how to respond in a principled way in a given situation? This chapter reviews factors that influence values formation, theoretical perspectives related to stages of values development, and considerations for nursing regarding moral development.

TRANSCULTURAL CONSIDERATIONS IN VALUES DEVELOPMENT

Human values development, often referred to as **moral development,** is a product of the sociocultural environment in which one lives and develops. What is considered right and wrong within the culture are learned in formal ways such as by precept and admonition, through informal processes such as role modeling, and by technical learning in a teacher to student process (Hall, 1973). Norms for etiquette and ethical behavior that are "known" within the culture may be acquired by an outsider through technical learning; however, they are often appreciated by a neophyte only when a transgression has occurred and corrections to, or sanctions for, the behavior have been imposed. There is an innate human capacity for developing an ethical stance to life that emerges through this process.

Leininger (1978; 1984) and Tripp-Reimer (1987) speak of culture in terms of values, beliefs, customs, and behaviors that are learned within and shared by a group of interacting persons. Because values are *learned* within the context of a particular culture, moral values are culturally relative (Gostin, 1995). This suggests that a value such as individual autonomy may be regarded highly in a culture that prizes independence and individualism. However, the same value may be considered contrary to the norm in a society in which persons are defined by their relation to others. Fowler (1981) notes that "we are formed in social communities and that our ways of seeing the world are profoundly shaped by the shared images and constructions of our group or class" (p. 105). Understandings of principles such as justice and care may vary in different cultures. In the ensuing discussion regarding stages of values development, it is important to be aware that the norms described have been derived primarily from Anglo-American and Anglo-European populations. Although significant work has been done, there is a need for further validation of the models within a transcultural context.

Ask Yourself

How Did I Learn My Values?

Think about a professional or personal situation in which you were faced with an ethical dilemma.

- What made it a dilemma for you?

- How did you decide the best course of action?
- What factors did you consider in making your decision?
- What values or principles guided you in this process?
- When and how did you learn these values or principles?

THEORETICAL PERSPECTIVES OF VALUES DEVELOPMENT

Discussions of moral development found in current literature flow primarily from frameworks developed by Kohlberg (1981) and Gilligan (1982). An overview of the work of each of these scholars is presented in this section, followed by discussion of how they contribute to understanding moral reasoning within nursing. Fowler's (1981) work on faith development is briefly discussed regarding insights relative to values development. Kohlberg's theory, which suggests that cognitive development is necessary though not sufficient for moral development, draws upon Piaget's (1963) work on cognitive development in children. Thus, a brief review of Piaget's theory is included here. As you review the models highlighted here, remember that **theory** is a proposed explanation for a class of phenomena. A given theory is not necessarily truth or reality, but it does shed light on truth. Engage critical thinking and intuitive knowing as you read, being attentive to what rings true in your own experience.

Piaget's Stages of Cognitive Development

Piaget's (1963) description of stages of cognitive development addresses how the mind works, that is, the development of intellectual capacities through the time of childhood, from birth to about fifteen years of age. He notes that cognitive development progresses through four stages, provided there is an intact neurological system and appropriate environmental interaction and stimuli. Although Piaget suggests specific ages for each stage, there may be variation due to environmental factors or innate intellectual capacities. Piaget's stages are:

- Sensorimotor (birth to 24 months), includes six substages;
- Preoperational (age 2–7), includes preconceptual and intuitive stages;
- Concrete operations (age 7–11);
- Formal operations (age 11–15).

Piaget believes that there are no further quantifiable changes in cognitive abilities after age fifteen. According to his theory, cognitive development progresses from thought dominated by motor activity and reflex, through development and use of symbolic representations such as language, to logical thought applied to concrete and then to abstract situations.

Kohlberg's Theory of Moral Development

Kohlberg's (1981) theory of moral development was derived initially from interviews conducted with boys distributed in age from early childhood to late adolescence. In these interviews he asked participants to respond to hypothetical ethical dilemmas such as a man's considering stealing a drug to save his dying wife because he cannot afford the drug and has exhausted other possibilities of paying for it. The pattern of the responses that he observed, coupled with inferences about the reasoning behind the responses, suggested a progression in moral reasoning spanning three levels, each of which includes two stages. These levels and stages are summarized as follows:

Level I. The Preconventional Level has an egocentric focus and includes two stages. In Stage 1, *The Stage of Punishment and Obedience*, rules are obeyed in order to avoid punishment. In Stage 2, *The Stage of Individual Instrumental Purpose and Exchange*, conformity to rules is viewed to be in one's own interest because it provides for rewards. Fear of punishment is a major motivator at this level.

Level II. The Conventional Level is focused more on social conformity and includes two stages. In Stage 3, *The Stage of Mutual Interpersonal Expectations, Relationships, and Conformity*, concern about the reactions of others is a basis for decisions and behavior, and being good in order to maintain relations is important. In Stage 4, *The Stage of Social System and Conscience Maintenance*, one conforms to laws and to those in authority because of duty, both out of respect for them and in order to avoid censure. For persons in this level, fulfilling one's role in society and living up to expectations of others are important, and guilt is more of a motivator than the fear of punishment noted in Level I.

There is a transitional phase between Stages 4 and 5 in which emotions begin to be recognized as a component of moral reasoning. This transition includes an awareness of personal subjectivity in moral decision making and a recognition that social rules can be arbitrary and relative.

Level III. The Post-Conventional and Principled Level has universal moral principles as its focus. It includes two stages. In Stage 5, *The Stage of Prior Rights and Social Contract or Utility*, the relativity of some societal values is recognized, and moral decisions derive from principles that support individual rights and transcend particular societal rules such as equality, liberty, and justice. In Stage 6, *The Stage of Universal Ethical Principles*, internalized rules and conscience reflecting abstract principles of human dignity, mutual respect, and trust guide decisions and behaviors. Persons at this level make judgments based on impartial universal moral principles, even when these conflict with societal standards.

This model proposes a linear movement through hierarchical stages whereby each stage presupposes having completed the prior stage and is the basis for the subsequent stage. It is the pattern of a person's utilization of a particular level of reasoning that determines the stage, noting that each successive stage requires more advanced levels of moral reasoning. Research utilizing this framework indicates that not everyone moves through all the stages, and that few people actually progress to the postconventional level (Colby & Kohlberg, 1987). Within this framework women seem to plateau in Stage 3, and most men never move beyond Stage 4. Kohlberg's model is generally considered an **ethic of justice** because it is an approach to ethical decision making based on objective rules and principles in which choices are made from a stance of separateness.

Gilligan's Study of the Psychological Development of Women

Gilligan (1982; 1987; 1988), a former student of Kohlberg, studied the psychological development of women, arguing that women approach moral decision making from a different perspective than men. In contrast to the justice ethic described by Kohlberg, in which personal liberty and rights are prime, Gilligan noted that women utilize an **ethic of caring,** in which the moral imperative is grounded in relationship with and responsibility for one another. "Women's construction of the moral problem as a problem of care and responsibility in relationship rather than of rights and rules ties the development of their moral thinking to changes in their understanding of responsibility and relationship, just as the conception of morality as justice ties development to the logic of equality and reciprocity" (Gilligan, 1982, p. 73).

Gilligan's research suggests a progression of moral thinking through three phases, each of which reflects greater depth in understanding the relationship of self and others, and two transitions that involve critical reevaluation of the conflict between responsibility and selfishness. The sequence described proceeds from an initial concern with survival, to focusing on goodness, to reflectively understanding care as the most adequate guide for resolving moral dilemmas.

Phase 1. In this phase, *the concern for survival*, the focus is on what is best for the self and includes selfishness and dependence on others. The *transition* to Phase 2 involves an appreciation of connectedness and that responsible choices take into account the effect they have on others.

Phase 2. The phase of *focusing on goodness* includes a sense of goodness as self-sacrifice in which the needs of others are often put ahead of self and there is a sense of being responsible for others so that one is regarded positively. This focus on goodness reflects an awareness of relationship with others and may be used to manipulate others through a "see how good I've been to you" attitude. In the *transition* to Phase 3 there is a shifting from concern about the reactions of others to greater honesty about personal motivation and consequences of choices and actions. Responsibility to self is taken into account along with responding to needs of others.

Phase 3. The phase of *the imperative of care* reflects a deep appreciation of connectedness, including responsibility to self and others as moral equals, and a clear imperative to harm no one. One takes responsibility for choices, in which projected consequences and personal intention are the motivation for actions rather than concern for the reactions of others.

Although Gilligan does not clearly associate particular ages with each phase of development, she suggests a linear process moving from one phase to the next through the transitions. This process may be associated with cognitive and emotional development as they interface with experiences of connectedness. Gilligan's model is generally considered an ethic of care.

Fowler's Stages of Faith Development

Fowler's (1981) discussion of faith development incorporates reflections on the development of values. His insights offer another perspective on the process of moral development. Fowler refers to **faith** as "a generic feature of the human struggle to find and maintain meaning . . . a dynamic existential stance, a way of leaning into and finding or giving meaning to the conditions of our lives" (pp. 91–92). He notes that faith is not synonymous with religion and that it may or may not find religious expression. He suggests that faith development flows from an integration of ways of knowing and valuing. This perspective is different from the work of Piaget and Kohlberg who conceptually separate cognition or knowing from emotion or affection, suggesting that logical knowing is separate from other important modalities of knowing. Fowler writes that "in moral judgments the valuations of actions and their consequences as well as evaluations of self in relation to the expectations of the self and others are difficult to conceive, even in formal and structural terms, apart from inherent affective or emotive elements of knowing" (1981, p. 102).

Fowler (1981) proposes six stages of faith, beginning with an intuitive faith in early childhood and progressing to universalizing faith. He notes that movement through the stages may not be limited to a linear pattern, recognizing that spiraling back to earlier stages may occur in response to various life experiences.

Stage 1. Occurring after the undifferentiated faith of infancy, *Intuitive Projective* faith is image and fantasy filled. The child's understandings and feelings toward the ultimate conditions of life are intuitive and shaped by stories, actions, moods, and examples of those around them.

Stage 2. *Mythic-Literal* faith reflects beliefs and moral rules and attitudes that symbolize belonging within a community or family and that are taken on with literal interpretations. Story provides a major source of meaning, and a world view based on reciprocity and fairness is developed.

Stage 3. *Synthetic-Conventional* faith reflects a movement into a world beyond the family in which values and beliefs derive from experiences in interpersonal relationships. Expectations and judgments of significant others are very influential in determining the values one holds. Although a personal clustering of values and beliefs is emerging in this stage, reliance on those in traditional authority roles or on the consensus of a valued group for validation of beliefs and actions is common. Fowler notes that although this stage arises in adolescence, many adults remain in this stage.

Stage 4. In the stage of *Individuative-Reflective* faith, persons must begin to take responsibility for their own beliefs, values, and commitments, differentiating personal identity and world view from that of others. In this way one's own values become recognized as factors in judgments on and reactions to actions and decisions of self and others.

Stage 5. *Conjunctive* faith requires an opening to one's inner depths in which one is able to recognize values, beliefs, and myths developed within one's particular cultural, social, or religious tradition that separate one from others. This stage requires an attitude of openness to that which formerly might have been perceived as threatening, different, and *other*, appreciating that although one's own values provide a framework for ascribing meaning, they are only relative and partial apprehensions of transcendent reality.

Stage 6. With *Universalizing* faith, the imperatives of absolute love and justice become prime, and one focuses energy on transforming the present reality toward a transcendent actuality inclusive of all beings. Fowler notes that persons in Stage 6 are quite rare, frequently being honored more after death than in life.

Ask Yourself

Where Are You in Your Values Development?

- Where do you think you fit in each of the frameworks discussed?

- Where would you place your parents? Classmates? Friends? Government officials? People like Gandhi, Mother Teresa of Calcutta, or Martin Luther King, Jr.?

- Based on your critical thinking and intuitive knowing, which framework rings most true for you?

- What are the implications of a model that suggests that most members of a particular group are morally deficient?

Kohlberg and Gilligan suggest that values development moves from a focus on self and survival, through responding to external forces such as perceived authority or opinions of others, toward being motivated and guided by universal considerations. They also note that it is more common to find adults functioning in the middle phases of relying on external authority as guideposts for moral decisions than to find persons whose actions and decisions are based on internalized universal guides that transcend codified rules. Fowler's model acknowledges that both reason and emotional response are factors in moral decision making and includes the suggestion that development may follow a pattern more spiral than linear. Within this pattern it is conceivable that, in response to life-changing experiences, persons may spiral back to an earlier stage and move through the stages again from a renewed perspective.

CASE PRESENTATION

Three Nursing Students

Pat, Tanya, and Kuan are discussing experiences they had in clinical today. Tanya describes her distress because her dying patient wanted to see her six-year-old granddaughter, which she thought would be very therapeutic, but her preceptor said absolutely not because there were strict rules against children under twelve visiting that unit. Pat notes that she did not have time to even change her patient's bed, but that the sheets were clean so she just straightened them out and the instructor did not even notice. She said the nurses on that unit do that sometimes when they are busy, so it was okay. Kuan says she had gotten behind too, but decided she had better get everything done the right way so she would get a good grade and not get into trouble.

Think About It

Indicators of Values Development

- What insights into the values of each of these students can you glean from this discussion?
- How do you think the theorists noted above would describe the level of development of each of the students?
- How do you think you would have responded in the situations described by the students? What values would guide your response?

SOME NURSING CONSIDERATIONS

Gilligan (1982; 1987) and others (Gilligan, Ward, Taylor, & Bardige, 1988; Kittay & Meyers, 1987; Larrabee, 1993; Noddings, 1984) have suggested that there are gender differences in approaching moral decision making—that women tend to utilize a care or relational perspective, whereas men are more likely to use the justice perspective. These authors note that Kohlberg's perspective on moral development tends to portray women's choices as deficiencies in moral capacities. Other authors claim that research related to differences in ethical decision making based on gender is inconclusive and that the justice perspective is used by both women and men (Colby & Kohlberg, 1987; Duckett, Rowan-Boyer, Ryden, Crisham, Savik, & Rest, 1992; Walker, 1993). When considering developmental norms for moral development, it is important that nurses be alert for gender and cultural factors, norms, and bias so as to avoid erroneously classifying particular groups as lacking in moral capabilities.

The literature offers an ongoing deliberation about the ethic of care versus the ethic of justice. A comparison of the two perspectives reveals that the justice framework requires choices to be made from a stance of separateness, based on objective rules and principles, whereas the care perspective arises from natural relatedness in which the choice is contextually bound and requires responding to others in their terms, developing strategies that maintain connections when possible, and striving to hurt no one. Moral concern within the ethic of justice is with rights and responsibilities; in the ethic of care the concern is with competing needs and responsibility in relationship. Fowler's model suggests that both are important factors in making moral decisions. Although much of the discussion in the literature focuses on the dichotomy between the two, it is well to recognize that "the perspectives of justice and care do not negate each other but offer different foci for examination of the problem and collectively constitute a more comprehensive moral perspective" (Cooper, 1989, p. 13). Hekman (1995) suggests that a paradigm shift is occurring that requires a reconceptualization of morality and moral language away from the notion of universal morality toward a recognition of a plurality of moral voices.

Because of nursing's concern for relational caring, it has been argued that an ethic of care more faithfully reflects nursing's experience than a primary focus on justice (Cooper, 1989). It has also been suggested that nursing move beyond current models of biomedical ethics to a model that encompasses at least the concepts of care and justice (Cooper, 1990). One study exploring whether nurses deal with moral decisions using the justice or the care perspective found that both perspectives were utilized, with care being predominant overall (Chally, 1992). In this study, older nurses with more professional experience were more likely to utilize the care perspective than younger nurses with less experience. The author proposed a possible developmental process through which growth in experience leads from a reliance on rules to guide one's choices to a focus on the needs of patients and families, which is reflective of the care perspective.

It is important for nurses to understand that there are different perspectives from which moral decisions are made so that they can better appreciate their own and their patients' approaches to ethical dilemmas. Nurses need to honestly identify their own phases of values development and ethical perspective so as to better understand personal responses to situations and more effectively recognize how their approaches may be different than that of colleagues or patients. Acknowledging differences and similarities may prevent making inappropriate judgments about another's moral capabilities and potentiate better communication and collaboration in care.

 ## CASE PRESENTATION

A Difficult Decision

Reba's eighty-two-year-old father has been hospitalized with a stroke that has left him severely incapacitated, requiring total care. She has been informed that her father is ready for discharge, and the physician is suggesting that he go to a nursing home. Reba feels that she should take him home with her because her faith says to care for her parents, but the house is small and would need a bathroom added to the first floor. She also has concerns about performing her father's care because she works full time and has three small children. She has considered quitting her job, but the family needs her income because her husband's work is seasonal. When visiting her father, she tells the nurse, Moira, that she does not know what is best for him, noting that her sister in another state told her it is her duty to care for their father, but her husband says it is too much to take on with all her other family responsibilities. She asks Moira what she should do.

Think About It

Justice or Care—Is One Way Better?

- What factors and forces do you think weigh most heavily in this situation?
- What would you tell her if you were Moira?
- How would you approach this situation from the perspective of justice? From the perspective of care? Do you think one approach is better than the other? Explain.
- How would you describe Reba's phase of moral development? Her husband's? Her sister's?

SUMMARY

This chapter has presented an overview of theoretical perspectives related to values development, the importance of recognizing that values and beliefs are culturally relative, and nursing considerations related to moral development. Students are encouraged to explore and critique each model of values development so as to formulate a personal knowledge base to guide their own processes of development. Each perspective provides insight into what is true.

CHAPTER HIGHLIGHTS

- Human values development, which is a product of one's sociocultural environment, reflects the content and process of learning what is right and wrong within the culture.
- Values development moves from a focus on self, through responding to external forces, toward being guided by universal considerations.
- Moral values are culturally relative.
- Current models of values development need further transcultural and transgender validation.
- Kohlberg's model, often referred to as an ethic of justice, suggests that choices are based on objective rules and principles and are made from a stance of separateness.
- In Gilligan's model, often referred to as an ethic of care, the moral imperative is grounded in relationship and mutual responsibility. Choices are contextually bound, requiring strategies that maintain connections and a striving to hurt no one.

- The notion of a plurality of moral voices, which recognizes that perspectives of both justice and care are factors in moral decision making, is an important consideration for nursing.

- Understanding varying perspectives from which moral decisions are made enables nurses to appreciate their own and their patients' approaches to ethical dilemmas and to avoid making inappropriate judgments about another's moral capabilities.

DISCUSSION QUESTIONS AND ACTIVITIES

1. What does it mean to say that moral values are culturally relative?

2. What factors would you consider in determining a person's phase of moral development?

3. Explore the model that you think best reflects the process of values development. Discuss it with classmates, giving rationale for your choice.

4. Identify stages of values development of three patients of different ages.

5. Compare and contrast the ethic of care and the ethic of justice, and discuss this topic with classmates. Which perspective do you think is most appropriate for nursing? Why?

6. Why is it useful for nurses to be aware of phases of values development for themselves, patients, and colleagues?

REFERENCES

Chally, P. S. (1992). Moral decision making in neonatal intensive care. *Journal of Obstetrics, Gynecology, and Neonatal Nursing, 21*(6), 475–482.

Colby, A., & Kohlberg, L. (1987). *The measurement of moral judgment volume I: Theoretical foundations and research validation.* Cambridge, MA: Cambridge University Press.

Cooper, M. C. (1989). Gilligan's different voice: A perspective for nursing. *Journal of Professional Nursing, 5*(1), 10–16.

Cooper, M. C. (1990). Reconceptualizing nursing ethics. *Scholarly Inquiry for Nursing Practice, 4*(3), 209–221.

Duckett, L., Rowan-Boyer, M., Ryden, M. B., Crisham, P., Savik, K., & Rest, J. R. (1992). Challenging misperceptions about nurses' moral reasoning. *Nursing Research, 41*(6), 324–331.

Fowler, J. W. (1981). *Stages of faith: The psychology of human development and the quest for meaning.* San Francisco: Harper & Row.

Gilligan, C. (1982). *In a different voice: Psychological theory and women's development.* Cambridge, MA: Harvard University Press.

Gilligan, C. (1987). Moral orientation and moral development. In E. F. Kittay & D. T. Meyers (Eds.), *Women and moral theory* (pp. 19–33). Savage, MD: Rowman & Littlefield.

Gilligan, C., Ward, J. V., Taylor, J. M., & Bardige, B. (1988). *Mapping the moral domain.* Cambridge, MA: Harvard University Press.

Gostin, L. O. (1995). Informed consent, cultural sensitivity, and respect for persons. *Journal of the American Medical Association, 274*(10), 844–855.

Hall, E. T. (1973). *The silent language*. Garden City, NY: Anchor Press.

Hekman, S. J. (1995). *Moral voices, moral selves*. University Park, PA: Pennsylvania State University Press.

Kittay, E. F., & Meyers, D. T. (1987). *Women and moral theory*. Savage, MD: Rowman & Littlefield.

Kohlberg, L. (1981). *The philosophy of moral development*. New York: Harper & Row.

Lao Tsu. (1972). *Tao Te Ching*. (Gia-fu Feng & Jane English, Trans.). New York: Vintage Books.

Larrabee, M. J. (1993) (Ed.). *An ethic of care*. New York: Routledge.

Leininger, M. (1978). *Transcultural nursing: Concepts, theories and practice*. New York: John Wiley & Sons.

Leininger, M. (1984). *Transcultural care diversity and universality: A theory of nursing*. Thorofare, NJ: Slack.

Noddings, N. (1984). *Caring: A feminine approach to ethics and moral education*. Berkeley, CA: University of California Press.

Piaget, J. (1963). *The Origins of Intelligence in Children*. (M. Cook, Trans.). New York: Norton.

Tripp-Reimer, T. (1987). Cultural assessment. In J. P. Bellack, & P. A. Bamford (Eds.), *Nursing assessment: A multidimensional approach* (pp. 226–246). Boston: Jones & Bartlett.

Walker, L. J. (1993). Sex differences in the development of moral reasoning: A critical review. In M. J. Larrabee (Ed.), *An ethic of care* (pp. 157–176). New York: Routledge.

PRINCIPLED BEHAVIOR IN THE PROFESSIONAL DOMAIN

Part III examines various categories of issues that affect the profession of nursing and the everyday practice of individual nurses. Recognizing nursing as a profession, the chapters describe nurses' responsibility related to ethical, legal, professional, and practice issues. These issues are examined in light of ethics and contemporary nursing. Included in this part are chapters discussing legal issues affecting nurses; professional issues such as autonomy, authority, and accountability; issues related to the relationship between nurses and the health care system; issues related to technology and self-determination; and scholarship issues.

CHAPTER 7

Legal Issues

We are caught in an inescapable network of mutuality, tied in a single garment of destiny. Whatever affects one directly, affects all indirectly.
(Martin Luther King, Jr.)

OBJECTIVES

After completing this chapter, the reader should be able to:

1. Recognize the difference between ethics and the law and discuss the relationship of each to the other.
2. Describe sources of law.
3. Distinguish between constitutional law, statutory law, administrative law, and common law.
4. Describe the difference between public and private law.
5. Discuss instances in which nurses might be accused of breaches of public law.
6. Define tort and distinguish between unintentional and intentional torts.
7. Discuss recent legal trends in health care.
8. Discuss methods that nurses can use to limit liability.
9. Describe the role of the expert nurse witness.

INTRODUCTION

Up to this point, the focus of this book has been upon values, morals, and ethics. The reader will recall from Chapter 2 that moral thinking, though influenced in great measure by prevailing cultural tradition, is essentially an individual enterprise. Ethics are rules of behavior produced by moral thinking and may be either informal rules that guide individuals or formal rules of actions that guide groups of people. The American Nurses Association (ANA) *Code for Nurses with Interpretive Statements* is an example of a document outlining a formal set of ethical guidelines. These guidelines offer some general rules that are intended for use as a tool to guide professional behavior but are not, in themselves, fully enforceable. Laws, on the other hand, consist of enforced rules under which a society is governed. There are many laws that either directly or indirectly affect the practice of nursing. Highly publicized issues such as termination of life support and "no code" status indicate a recent trend toward involving the legal system in issues that were previously thought to be ethical in nature. This chapter discusses the relationship between ethics and the law, general legal concepts, areas of potential liability for nurses, and recent legal trends. The legal regulation of nursing is addressed in Chapter 8.

RELATIONSHIP BETWEEN ETHICS AND THE LAW

Law is the system of binding rules of action or conduct that governs the behavior of people in respect to relationships with others and with the government (Guido, 1997; Rhodes & Miller, 1984). Laws, meant to reflect the moral beliefs of a given population, are devised by groups of individuals serving in official capacity. Kozier and Erb outline four basic functions of the law in society:

1. To define relationships among the members of a society and to state which activities are permissible and which are not permissible
2. To describe what force may be applied to maintain rules and by whom it is to be applied
3. To provide solutions to problems
4. To redefine relationships between persons and groups when conditions of life change. (1988, p. 244)

The law establishes rules that define a person's rights and obligations and sets penalties for people who violate them. Laws also describe how government will enforce the rules and penalties. In the United States and Canada, there are thousands of state, provincial, federal, and local laws. Among others, these laws ensure the safety of citizens, protect property, promote nondiscrimination, regulate the professions, provide for the distribution of public goods and services, and protect the economic and environmental interests of society.

Laws are intended to reflect popular belief about the "rightness or wrongness" of particular acts and are, like ethics, built upon a moral foundation. In most countries laws represent an attempt to codify ethics. One would expect that laws would be congruent with the prevailing moral values of a society. Indeed, they usually are. For example, most people would agree that the murder of an innocent person is an immoral act. Laws that prohibit murder reflect this ethical standard. Murder of the innocent is both ethically and legally prohibited in every culture. As society's needs and attitudes evolve, laws emerge to reflect these changes. Occasionally, however, governments create and enforce laws that many people believe to be unjust. In a democratic society, constitutional law provides mechanisms to change or abolish unjust or unpopular laws.

Some authors of nursing ethics texts take the view that professional ethical standards are congruent with the law, that is, that which is legal is also ethical, and vice versa. These authors imply that following a set of ethical guidelines, such as the *ANA Code for Nurses with Interpretive Statements*, provides nurses a legal safety net. This is usually, but not necessarily, true. Laws exist that can be considered (by some at least) to be unethical. Some illegal acts are considered by many to be ethical.

There are many reasons for the possible discrepancy between that which is legal and that which is ethical. First, consider differences between ethical points of view. Deontology and utilitarianism, for example, offer quite opposite answers to some basic ethical questions. While the utilitarian perspective would allow consideration of abortion or euthanasia, for example, to provide for the good of many, deontological views might require that life be protected regardless of circumstance. Thus, a law thought to be ethical by the utilitarian might be considered unethical by the deontologist. Second, it can be argued that human behavior and motivation are more complex than can be fairly reflected in law. Think back to Chapter 6. Individuals may consider the same act either right or wrong, depending to some extent on their stage or level of moral development. For example, acts of civil disobedience such as those committed by Mahatma Gandhi and Martin Luther King, Jr., though unquestionably illegal, are generally considered to be motivated by high ethical standards. In his letter from the Birmingham Jail, Martin Luther King, Jr., wrote, "there are two types of laws: just and unjust. I would be the first to advocate obeying just laws. One has not only a legal but a moral responsibility to obey just laws. Conversely, one has a moral responsibility to disobey unjust laws" (1996, p. 574). Third, the legal system may seem to judge action rather than motivation. For example, nurses following personal moral convictions or professional ethical codes can find themselves at odds with policies or practices of employing institutions. In certain instances, the legal system may determine that an employing institution has the right to dismiss or discipline a nurse for laying aside institutional policy in favor of ethical considerations. Fourth, depending upon political climate and other variables, laws change. Recent examples of laws that have changed include those related to expanded roles of nurses, abortion, fetal tissue use, organ transplantation, self-determination, confidentiality for AIDS patients, informed consent, and legal definitions of death. As defined in Chapter 3, integrity is fidelity in adherence to moral norms sustained over time. One should be able to predict that nurses with integrity will not alter their basic moral beliefs in response to changes in the law. Thus, there are several valid circumstances in which there may be a discrepancy between that which is legal and that which is considered ethical.

GENERAL LEGAL CONCEPTS

Nurses need to familiarize themselves with the law and legal system for several reasons. First, the law authorizes and regulates nursing practice. Nurse practice acts of the individual states describe both the activity of nurses and the boundaries of nursing. Chapter 8 discusses the legal regulation of nursing in greater depth. Second, the legal system scrutinizes nursing actions and omissions. The profession is in a dynamic state of change: advanced practice nurses are expanding the traditional boundaries, critical care nurses are performing complex and vital tasks, staff nurses are caring for older and sicker patients, and many nurses are practicing in new settings. Recognizing that health care is experiencing a storm of litigation, nurses must have basic knowledge about law and the legal process. This knowledge will help to ensure that nurses' actions are consistent with legal principles and will help to protect nurses from liability. Third, knowledge of legal principles is a necessary component of ethical decision making. In order to make informed choices, nurses, physicians, patients, and families must be able to identify potential or real legal implications.

Sources of Law

There are at least four different sources of law that affect the practice of nursing: constitutional law, statutory (legislative) law, administrative law, and common law. Additionally, law can be divided into two main branches—private law and public law. Some laws are made by legislation, some by rule-making bodies, and some by judiciary precedent. Adding to an already confusing mix, there is frequent overlap between the sources and branches of the law.

Constitutional Law.   A constitution is a formal set of rules and principles that describe the powers of a government and the rights of the people. The principles laid out in a constitution, coupled with a description of how these principles are to be interpreted and carried out, form the basis of **constitutional law.** The *Constitution of the United States* is the preeminent source of this country's law. Ensuring legal rights and responsibilities of citizens and establishing the general organization of the federal government, constitutional law in the United States supersedes all other laws.

Nurses must be aware that the *Bill of Rights* of the *United States Constitution* guarantees each citizen the rights (among others) of privacy, equal protection, due process, freedom of speech, and freedom of religion. Nursing actions must take into account these basic rights. Rights guaranteed in the *Bill of Rights* are consistent with adherence to the ethical principles of autonomy, confidentiality, respect for persons, and veracity. The same rights that apply to patients also apply to nurses. As participants in the health care system, nurses cannot be forced to forfeit any constitutionally guaranteed rights.

Statutory/Legislative Law.   Formal laws written and enacted by federal, state, or local legislatures are known as **statutory** or **legislative laws.** Congress and the state legislatures pass thousands of laws each year. These are added to the hundreds of volumes of federal and state statutes already in force. Because many people think that every problem in society can be solved by passing a law, legislatures make more and more laws to satisfy the demands of society and special-interest groups. Changes in Medicare and Medicaid laws, statutory recognition of nurses in advanced practice (including prescriptive authority), and proposed health care reform legislation are all examples of statutory or legislative law.

Administrative Law. **Administrative law** involves the operation of government agencies. National, state, and local governments set up administrative agencies to do the work of government. These agencies regulate such activities as education, public health, social welfare programs, and the professions. Administrative law consists mainly of the legal powers granted to administrative agencies by legislative bodies and the rules that the agencies make to carry out their powers. State boards of nursing are examples of this type of agency. These boards are granted the authority to execute the intent of state statutes by creating, implementing, and enforcing comprehensive and appropriate rules and regulations. As administrative bodies, the role of boards of nursing is to protect the public rather than advocate for nurses. Rules promulgated by the individual states' boards of nursing carry the same weight as other law.

Common Law. The United States (except Louisiana), Canada (except Quebec), Great Britain, and other English-speaking countries have a **common law** system. Constituting the basis of the judicial system, this type of law is also known as case law. In the common law system, decisions are based upon earlier court rulings in similar cases. These are also known as **precedents.** Over time, precedents take on the force of law.

Types of Law

Law can be divided into two different types: public and private. Recall that law is a system of enforceable principles and processes that governs the behavior of people in respect to relationships with others and with the government. In general, legal problems related to the relationship between people and the government are the domain of public law, and problems occurring as a result of relationships between people are the domain of private law.

Public Law. **Public law** defines a person's rights and obligations in relation to the government and describes the various divisions of government and their powers. One important branch of public law is **criminal law.** Criminal law deals with crimes—that is, actions considered harmful to society. Even though a crime might be committed against a particular person, the government considers the commission of a serious act, such as murder, to be harmful to all of society. In the United States, each state, as well as the federal government, has its own set of criminal laws. Nevertheless, the criminal laws of each state must protect the rights and freedoms guaranteed by the federal Constitution. Crimes range in seriousness from public drunkenness to murder. Criminal law defines these offenses and sets the rules for the arrest, the appropriate procedures to ensure due process, and the punishment of offenders.

In the course of practice, nurses can be accused of a variety of criminal offenses. For example, nurses can be accused of directly injuring a patient, either intentionally or unintentionally. Nurses can also be accused of crimes related to their actual relationship with the government. These include such actions as falsifying narcotic records, failure to renew license, and fraudulent billing. Crimes are delineated according to seriousness as either felonies or misdemeanors.

Felonies are serious crimes that carry significant fines and jail sentences. Examples of felonies include first and second degree murder, arson, burglary, extortion, kidnaping, rape, and robbery. These crimes are punishable by jail terms. Nurses are rarely accused of felonies in the course of practice. However, this can occur. For example, it is possible that those participating in the unauthorized removal of life support from a terminally ill patient could be accused of first degree murder because of the intentional nature of the act which resulted in death. This could occur even though the act might be viewed as beneficent by a majority of people. A nurse who unintentionally causes the death of a patient by administering a medication to which a patient is allergic could be charged with second degree murder (manslaughter).

A **misdemeanor** is a less serious crime, usually punishable by a fine, a short jail sentence, or both. Examples of misdemeanors include disturbing the peace, solicitation, assault, and battery (assault and battery are also considered intentional torts and can be decided by private or civil law). A nurse slapping a patient or giving an injection without consent can be accused of the misdemeanor of battery.

Think About It

Institutional Versus Individual Negligence

Occasionally nurses find themselves in situations in which institutional policies and practices are inconsistent with public law. In these instances nurses and other staff members can be accused of crimes. In 1986 members of the staff of a nursing home in Louisiana were charged with cruelty, neglect, and mistreatment of the infirm. In the *State of Louisiana v. Brenner* (1986), the staff was charged for the following reasons:

1. Failure to adequately feed and care for the patients

2. Failure to properly train the staff

3. Failure to provide adequate medical supplies

4. Failure to supply adequate staff

5. Failure to maintain a sanitary nursing home

6. Failure to maintain patients' records

7. Failure to see that the appropriate and necessary health services were performed.

• Ethics and the law are usually, but not always, consistent. Think about each of the seven accusations listed above in terms of breaches of ethical principles. What is the relationship between the accusations and ethical principles?

- Imagining that you live in a small community and are employed by a nursing home with similar problems, how do you think you would deal with the problems in a manner that is both legal and ethical? How do you think you would deal with the situation if you feel compelled to maintain your employment at the nursing home?

- Do you believe that individual nurses should be punished for actions that are clearly caused by institutional negligence? Substantiate your answer with ethical arguments.

Private Law.   **Private law** is also called **civil law.** It determines a person's legal rights and obligations in many kinds of activities that involve other people. These activities include everything from borrowing or lending money to buying a home or signing a job contract. More than a million civil suits are tried in the United States courts each year. There are six branches of private law that include: contract and commercial law, tort law, property law, inheritance law, family law, and corporation law. The branches of private law that are most applicable to nursing practice are contract law and tort law. Noncompliance with private law generally leads to monetary compensation granted the injured or complaining party (**plaintiff**).

Contract Law.   **Contract law** deals with the rights and obligations of people who make contracts. A **contract** is an agreement between two or more people that can be enforced by law. Contracts may be either written or oral; however, in the presence of both a written and oral contract, the written contract takes precedence. In health care, contracts may be either expressed or implied. Expressed contracts occur when the two parties agree explicitly to its terms, as in an employment contract. Implied contracts occur when there has been no discussion between the parties, but the law considers that a contract exists (Kozier & Erb, 1988). The nurse-patient relationship is essentially an implied contract with which the nurse agrees to give competent care.

Tort Law.   A **tort** is a wrong or injury that a person suffers because of someone else's action, either intentional or unintentional. The tortious action may cause bodily harm; invade another's privacy; damage a person's property, business, or reputation; or make unauthorized use of a person's property. The victim may sue the person or persons responsible. Tort law deals with the rights and obligations of the persons involved in such cases. Many torts are unintentional, such as damages that occur as a result of accidents. But if a tort is deliberate and involves serious harm, it may also be treated as a crime. The purpose of tort law is to make the person whole again—primarily through the award of monetary damages. Because it involves negligence and malpractice, tort law is the branch of law with which nurses are most familiar.

Unintentional torts occur when an act or omission causes unintended injury or harm to another person. Nurses are familiar with the unintentional torts of negligence and malpractice. **Negligence** is "the omission to do something that a reasonable person, guided by those ordinary considerations which ordinarily regulate human affairs, would do, or doing something which a reasonable and prudent person would not do" (Creighton, 1986, p. 141). As part of ensuring the safety of citizens, the law requires that every person is accountable for behaving in a reasonable way, particularly if the welfare of others is jeopardized. For example, there is certainly no law against throwing rocks into the air. However, within a crowd of people, this is not the act of a reasonable person. Though the person throwing rocks may enjoy the beauty of the arc or the distance of the throw and has no intention of harming others, a resultant injury would be the outcome of negligence. A nurse who pours liquid on the floor in a patient's room would be held to the same standard: that is, a reasonable person would recognize that wet floors often cause falls and would immediately clean the floor and warn people who may be walking in the vicinity. Negligence can also occur as a result of an omission. The nurse in the situation above may have walked into the room and found that the patient had spilled water. Had she ignored the spill, the nurse would be responsible for the results of her negligence in omitting the action of removing the danger, even though she did not actually cause the spill. Acts of negligence in nursing can be judged upon the criteria of the knowledge and abilities expected of a reasonable and prudent nurse (as opposed to a reasonable and prudent person). Because the knowledge base of nursing is broad, technical, and specific to the profession, these criteria go far beyond those required of the ordinary person.

The term **malpractice** is the form of negligence in which any professional misconduct, unreasonable lack of professional skill, or nonadherence to the accepted standard of care causes injury to a patient or client. Creighton (1986) also includes lack of fidelity, evil practice, and illegal or immoral conduct in the definition of malpractice (p. 141). Malpractice is the segment of the tort law of negligence that is specifically reserved for the professional person. To be held liable for malpractice, the nurse must fail to act as other reasonable and prudent professional nurses who have the same knowledge and education would have acted under similar circumstances (Catalano, 1991, p. 69). There are four components that are required to prove liability for malpractice: first, it must be established that the nurse has a duty owed to the patient; second, there must be a breach of standards of care or failure to carry out that duty; third, actual harm or injury must be suffered by the patient; and, fourth, there must be a causal relationship between the breach of duty and the injury suffered. (See Figure 7–1.)

Figure 7–1 **Components of Malpractice**

1. Duty owed to the patient
2. Breach of standards of care or failure to carry out duty
3. Actual harm or injury suffered by the patient
4. Causal relationship between the breach of standards of care or duty and the injury

There are several areas that are traditional sources of malpractice litigation. Medication errors, falls, loss or damage to patients' property, incorrect sponge counts, intentional infliction of emotional distress, and burns are examples of actions that have resulted in malpractice litigation against nurses.

The most common area for nursing liability relates to medication errors. There are many ways that nurses can make errors of medication preparation and administration. The nurse can give the wrong medication, in the wrong dose, by the wrong route, at the wrong time, or to the wrong patient. Because of the frequency and likelihood of medication error and the potentially serious consequences that can result, nurses need to be especially careful in administering medications. Nurses are responsible for safe and appropriate administration of medication, regardless of physician orders, workload, unusual circumstance, or institutional policy. There are many examples of medication errors cited in the literature. It is not unusual for damages to be awarded to victims or families when medication errors occur. Creighton (1986) discusses a particular case in which a nurse, in an attempt to assist on a busy pediatric unit, administered a lethal dose of digitalis to an infant. This nurse did not usually work with pediatric patients and was unfamiliar with pediatric doses. Even though the nurse thought the dose ordered seemed high, she did not check the literature, discuss the dose with a pharmacist, or question the physician. The parents in this case recovered substantial damages because the nurse's actions were determined to constitute malpractice.

Falls, particularly in nursing homes, are another frequent subject of malpractice litigation. Nurses must be attentive to patients' ambulatory abilities, cognitive and emotional states, and medications that will affect alertness. Nurses must always use professional judgement, common sense, and institutional policy when relying on such devises as side-rails and restraints. Nurses' responsibility in preventing falls goes beyond direct care of patients. Fiesta (1988) describes the case of *Washington Hospital Center v. Butler*:

> Before admission to the hospital, a patient had been suffering from dizziness, blackouts, and weakness. A pyelogram was ordered. The form to be completed by the nurse required a summary of the patient's history and complaints. The nurse wrote "diabetic complications" but made no reference to the patient's dizziness. During the examination, the x-ray table was placed in a vertical position. When the patient stood up, she fell over and broke her cheekbone.
>
> The court held that expert testimony was not needed to prove her case. Since the chart clearly indicated that the patient was prone to fainting spells, the court ruled that the nurse was negligent in not notifying the radiologist of that fact. The court also held that the radiologist, who knew that the patient was a diabetic, should have known that she was quite likely to be unsteady. The court said there was sufficient evidence for the jury to conclude that a reasonably prudent person in the circumstances would have provided this particular patient with some form of safeguard from falling. (p. 60)

Loss or damage of patients' belongings is another frequent area of liability for nurses. Jewelry, favorite blankets and pillows, dentures, and money are belongings that are frequently lost or damaged. Though many institutions have policies in place that reduce liability in case of loss or damage, nurses are expected to take reasonable precautions to protect patients' property.

Another area of frequent liability for nurses is sponge counts. Sponges and other small items can inadvertently be left in patients' body cavities. This can be a cause for serious postoperative complications. The nurse responsible for counting the sponges is often held liable for malpractice. Creighton (1986) discusses a particular case of a sponge being overlooked:

> Out of an award of $36,000, a scrub nurse and a circulating nurse had to pay $4,000 apiece in a case in which a laparotomy sponge was left in a patient during abdominal surgery although they had reported the sponge count correct. Since the surgeon had ordered the metal rings removed from the sponges, which was a safeguard provided by the employer, he became the nurses' special employer during the surgery and was liable with them. (p. 144)

In a similar case, a surgeon left a large surgical sponge in a patient's abdomen after a hysterectomy. The jury in the initial trial found both the hospital and the physician to be negligent, and further that the nurses involved were agents of the hospital and not the physician. On appeal, the court found that it was a reasonable inference from the evidence that the sponge count done before surgery was performed negligently or that the procedure for counting sponges was below the standard of care. The court ordered a new trial unless the physician agreed to a $125,000 damage award divided between the defendants (*Truhitte v. French Hospital*, 1982).

Intentional infliction of emotional distress can also be claimed as negligence for nurses. There are certain contractual relationships, such as in the transmission and delivery of telegrams announcing the death of a close relative and services incident to a funeral and burial, that carry with them deeply emotional responses. Legal claims have been recognized that require a duty to exercise ordinary care to avoid causing emotional harm in such situations. Furrow, Johnson, Jost, & Schwartz (1991) argue that this duty also applies to the delivery of medical and nursing services. They describe an interesting and complex case involving several instances in which nurses and other health care workers contributed to the emotional distress of Larry and Susan Oswald. In *Oswald v. LeGrand* (1990) the plaintiffs describe a sequence of events preceding the premature birth of their third child. Just prior to her five-month checkup, Susan began experiencing bleeding and painful cramping. Her physician, Dr. Smith, ordered an ultrasound subsequent to which Susan was examined by Dr. Smith's associate, Dr. LeGrand. Finding no explanation for the problems, Dr. LeGrand instructed Susan to go home and stay off her feet. Later the same day, Susan began bleeding heavily and was taken by ambulance to Mercy Health Center. The bleeding having spontaneously stopped, Dr. Smith discharged Susan with instructions to take it easy. The following day, with symptoms worsening, and fearing a miscarriage, Larry drove Susan to the Mercy emergency room. Another associate of Smith and LeGrand, Dr. Clark, examined Susan and advised her that there was nothing to be done and she should go home. Larry insisted that Susan be admitted and Dr. Clark honored the request. Susan was transferred to the labor and delivery ward where her first contact was with a nurse who said, " 'What are you doing here? The doctor told you to stay home and rest' " (Furrow et al., p. 166). Later, another nurse told Susan that if she miscarried there would not be a baby but rather a "'big blob of blood'" (Furrow et al., p. 166). Susan reports that she was scared. The next morning Susan overheard a loud argument outside her door in which Dr. Clark was heard to yell, "'I don't want to take that patient. She's not my patient and I am sick and tired of Dr. Smith dumping his case load on me'" (Furrow et al., p. 166). Urged by Larry, Dr. Clark apologized and assured Susan that he would care for her until he left for vacation at noon that day, at which time Dr. LeGrand would take over. Susan began experiencing a great deal of pain at around 9:00 A.M., and Dr. Clark instructed the staff to schedule her for an ultrasound and amniocentesis. After viewing the ultrasound, Dr. Clark told the Oswalds that the situation was unusual and left without further explanation one-half hour before his scheduled off-time. Confused, distressed, in extreme pain, and still in the hallway outside the x-ray lab, Susan began giving birth. Summoned by Larry, two nurses delivered a one-pound baby girl who they determined to have no pulse or respiratory activity. They wrapped the baby in a towel, placed her on an instrument tray, and told the parents she was stillborn. After having called relatives to break the sad news, Larry touched the baby's hand and was startled when his grasp was returned. The nurses rushed the infant to the neonatal intensive care unit where she died several hours later.

Ask Yourself

Emotional Harm

- In the above case, do you think there was negligence on the part of any of the health care providers? If so, explain your thinking.

- If you believe there was negligence, do you think the premature birth or death of the infant was directly caused by the negligence?

- Larry and Susan contend that they have suffered severe emotional distress as a result of alleged breaches of professional conduct. Think about the several instances in which either the physicians or nurses may have contributed to the Oswalds' emotional distress.

- Do you feel there should be a duty to exercise ordinary care to avoid causing emotional harm? Was that duty breached in this instance?

- What are the ethical implications of the nurses' behavior?

Nurses can also be found liable if a patient sustains burns in the process of nursing care. Burns can occur as a result of fires, baths, showers, hot water bottles, or heating pads. Patients who are comatose or have diminished sensitivity are especially prone to burns. In one case a three-month-old infant suffered second and third degree burns on his buttocks after an operating room nurse placed him on a heating pad at the instruction of the anesthesiologist. The purpose of the heating pad was to help the child maintain body temperature during surgery. Though neither the nurses nor the surgeon noted anything unusual after surgery, arriving at home, the parents found the infant to have blisters draining bloody fluid. The child required subsequent skin grafting.

Although admitting liability in this case, the defendants attempted to exclude from evidence the manufacturer's warning to avoid use on an infant, invalid, or sleeping or unconscious person. The manufacturers warned that burns could result from improper use (*Smelko v. Brinton*, 1987). In another case, a patient received a judgment against a hospital after he was seriously burned. The patient was paralyzed and had a speech impediment. He was left alone while smoking his pipe. The pipe fell from his mouth and set the bed on fire (Creighton, 1986, p. 145). Clearly a reasonable and prudent nurse would not leave a paralyzed person alone with a lit pipe in his mouth.

Intentional torts are "willful or intentional acts that violate another person's rights or property" (Catalano, 1991, p. 69). A tort must include three elements to be considered intentional: the act must be intended to interfere with the plaintiff or his property, there must be intent to bring about the consequences of the act, and the act must substantially cause the consequences. There is no legal requirement that damages or injury actually result from the act; proof of the defendant's intention is sufficient (Catalano). (See Figure 7–2.) Examples of intentional torts include fraud, invasion of privacy, assault, battery, false imprisonment, slander, and liable.

Figure 7–2 **Components of Intentional Torts**

1. The defendant's act must be intended to interfere with the plaintiff or his property.
2. The defendant must intend to bring about the consequences of the act.
3. The act must substantially cause the consequences.
4. There is no legal requirement that the act causes damages or injury—proof of intention is sufficient.

Fraud is a deliberate deception for the purpose of securing an unfair or unlawful gain. Though nurses are seldom accused of fraud, when this occurs it is usually prosecuted as a crime. Examples of potential areas of nurses' fraud include falsification of information on employment applications, untruthful billing procedures, false representation of a patient's physical condition in order to induce contracts for services, and falsification of patient records to cover up an error or avoid legal action. As is true with some other intentional torts, fraud can lead to both civil and criminal proceedings. Because of the deliberate nature and potential harm of fraudulent acts, court decisions tend to be harsh.

The **right of privacy** is the right to be left alone or to be free from unwanted publicity. Individuals have the right to withhold themselves and their lives from public scrutiny. The intentional tort of **invasion of privacy** occurs when a person's privacy is invaded. Fiesta (1988) outlines four types of invasions of privacy: intrusion on the patient's physical and mental solitude or seclusion, public disclosure of private facts, publicity that places the patient in a false light in the public eye, and appropriation for the defendant's benefit or advantage of the patient's name or likeness (p. 160). There are many cases involving invasions of privacy. In *Bethiaume v. Pratt*, a dying patient being treated for cancer of the larynx was repeatedly photographed at the direction of his surgeon. On the day of his death the patient asked not to be photographed, but nevertheless the physician photographed him after lifting his head to place a pillow under it. A court decided that the physician be held liable for invasion of privacy (Fiesta, 1988, p. 160). In another invasion of privacy case, Earl Spring, a senile seventy-eight-year-old man was residing in a nursing home where he was undergoing kidney dialysis. In an attempt to discontinue dialysis treatments, his legal guardians, his wife and son, were involved in a prolonged court battle. In opposition to the family's position, and without their consent, the nursing home staff permitted right-to-life advocates to interview the senile man. Interviews with the patient and four nurses were published. After winning a Superior Court ruling regarding discontinuing the dialysis, Mrs. Spring sued the nursing home and the four nurses for $80 million in damages. She claimed that her husband's right to privacy had been violated. Although the attorney for the nursing home maintained that the patient had become a "public figure," the jury found in favor of Mrs. Spring, awarding her $2.5 million.

The terms *assault* and *battery*, though usually used together, have different legal meanings. Both are intentional torts. **Assault** is defined as the unjustifiable attempt or threat to touch a person without consent that results in fear of immediately harmful or threatening contact (Bernzweig, 1990). Touching need not actually occur. **Battery** is the unlawful, harmful, or unwarranted touching of another or the carrying out of threatened physical harm. Battery includes any willful, angry, violent, or negligent touching of a person's body or clothes, or anything held by or attached to the person (Creighton, 1986, p. 185; Guido, 1997). In the course of everyday activities, nurses have been accused of both assault and battery. For example, if a nurse threatens to give an injection to an unruly or noncompliant adult patient without consent, actionable assault has occurred. Battery is often thought of as such actions as slapping, shoving, or pinching, but the courts have upheld battery charges in actions that were much more subtle. Regardless of intent or outcome, touching without consent is considered battery. Even when the intention is beneficent and the outcome is positive, if the act is committed without permission, the nurse can be charged with battery. Surgical procedures that are performed without informed consent are the most common example of battery occurring in the hospital setting.

The case of *Robertson v. Provident House* (1991) illustrates an example of battery involving nurses. Although having an order for an "as needed" indwelling catheter, a quadriplegic patient objected when nurses tried to insert one. He had experienced pain and complications with indwelling catheters in the past. The nurse reportedly told the patient to "shut up" and then proceeded to insert the catheter. The catheter was removed after repeated requests from the patient and family. Subsequently, ignoring the patient's objections, the nurse reinserted the catheter. Injury occurred when a nurse forcefully pulled the catheter out. The family eventually sued for damages and recovered $25,000. The Louisiana Supreme Court found that battery occurs when a nurse ignores the objections of the patient and performs an invasive procedure like the insertion of an indwelling catheter.

Fiesta (1988) cites a case in which a patient was involuntarily committed to a mental hospital. A practicing Christian Scientist, the patient refused medications and other treatment. Apparently the patient was forced to take medication. Not having been shown to be a danger to herself or others, mentally ill, or incompetent, the court allowed her to recover for both assault and battery.

Creighton (1986) offers an exception to the requirement of consent from competent adults. In some states nurses are permitted to obtain blood and other specimens, without consent, at police request from persons under arrest.

False imprisonment is the unlawful, unjustifiable detention of a person within fixed boundaries or an act intended to result in such confinement (Creighton, 1986, p. 197). Such acts can include physical restraint of the person or acts intended to accomplish confinement such as refusing the patient clothing or car keys. If false imprisonment is accompanied by forcible restraint or the threat of restraint, assault and battery may also be charged. However, each state has legal procedures granting authorization to detain, for a limited period of time, specific categories of persons who are disoriented, mentally ill, or substance abusers or who have contagious diseases. Generally, these persons can be held without consent while the hospital reports them to authorities and obtains commitment or custody orders (Rhodes & Miller, 1984).

Nurses have been accused of false imprisonment for restraining patients, locking patients in rooms, and detaining patients for payment of bills. An example of false imprisonment is seen in the case of *Big Town Nursing Home, Inc. v. Newman* (1970) in which a sixty-seven-year-old man was kept against his will for nearly two months. Having been brought to the nursing home by his nephew, the man attempted to leave several times and was forcibly detained. The staff of the nursing home restrained him in a chair and denied him the use of a telephone and his clothing. The court found that the staff of the nursing home acted recklessly, willfully, and maliciously in unlawfully detaining him. In the case of *Blackman for Blackman v. Rifkin* (1988), the court held that some circumstances justify detainment. In this instance the court upheld the hospital's duty to prevent further harm by detaining a highly intoxicated patient with a head injury despite her insistence that she be allowed to leave. The court ruled that the hospital could assume that the patient would have consented to the treatment had she not been intoxicated.

Defamation occurs when one harms a person's reputation and good name, diminishes others' value or esteem, or arouses negative feelings toward the person in others by the communication of false, malicious, unprivileged, or harmful words. Only those remarks or statements that might arouse derogatory opinions about a person are considered defamation. Additionally, defamation only occurs when the words are communicated to a third person—two persons directing remarks and epithets to each other are not liable for defamation. In most states there are two distinct forms of defamation, slander and libel. **Slander** occurs when one defames or damages the reputation of another by speaking unprivileged or false words. Slander can occur in nursing practice when nurses make cruel, false, or unsubstantiated claims against patients. By making value judgments or voicing the opinion that a patient is uncooperative, malingering, unintelligent, or drug-seeking, a nurse may be committing actionable slander. Nurses may also be accused of slander as a result of inappropriate defamatory remarks voiced against another professional. **Libel** consists of printed defamation by written words and images that injure a person's reputation or cause others to avoid, ridicule, or view the person with contempt. Nurses risk accusations of libel, for example, when writing information in patients' charts that can be damaging. Judgmental, critical, or speculative statements made in patients' charts such as, "The patient is drug-seeking," or "The patient is rude," can lead to charges of libel, particularly if the patient has reason to believe that the words adversely affect care given by others.

If the defamatory remarks have the potential of harming the business prospects of the person, proof of damage is not needed. An example of this can be seen in the case of *Schessler v. Keck* (1954). In this case an unmarried female caterer had a false positive test for syphilis. Though the patient had never had the disease, a nurse seeing her catering at a party told the hostess that the woman was being treated for syphilis. This resulted in destroying the patient's business. The appeals court found that there was a valid basis for her claim of slander.

Nurses have also been the object of defamatory remarks. A physician accused his office nurse of having mixed up reports on a patient's chart and lying about it. He fired her the next day and called a meeting of his office employees. He told his staff that he couldn't work with anyone who was a liar, untrustworthy, and disloyal. A jury awarded the nurse $125,000 in damages (Creighton, 1986).

There are certain instances in which derogatory remarks may not constitute defamation. Two defenses to defamation include truth and privilege. In fact, there may be a legal or moral duty to pass on defamatory information in certain circumstances. For instance, a nurse has the duty to report suspected child abuse, a director of nursing service has a duty to truthfully report the character and qualifications of nurses to potential employers, and peer review groups are required to discuss privileged information for the purpose of improving services, disciplining providers, and so forth. Additionally, nurses are ethically obligated to report the illegal or incompetent practice of others. To avoid charges of defamation, prudent nurses will take care to observe appropriate channels of communication when making reports of this nature. In the absence of privileged communication, truth is a good defense for defamation.

RECENT LEGAL TRENDS

The combination of an evolving health care delivery system, increased public awareness, and a vigorous legal system have led to changes in the delivery of care, exposure to potential sources of liability, and changing legal trends. The public has begun to subject both the individual provider and the health care system to intense legal scrutiny. Litigation involving managed care organizations, increasing numbers of malpractice claims against nurses, and movement toward criminalization of negligence are three recent legal trends.

Legal Trends Involving Managed Care Organizations

Promising efficiency and economy of health care delivery, managed care organizations (MCOs) have begun to supplant traditional fee-for-service providers of care. As a result of policies that encourage restrictions of expensive services, MCOs are experiencing significant financial corporate liability losses (Fiesta, 1996b). Being both the insurer and provider of care, MCOs have a vested interest in providing the most cost-efficient services. This can sometimes lead to diminution of the quality of care. Fiesta cites a recent case in Georgia in which a jury awarded $45 million to a family whose son had his hands amputated as a result of Kaiser Permanente's efforts to minimize health care costs. The malpractice occurred when the child's mother called the MCO's emergency line to report that her infant son was lethargic and had a temperature of 104 degrees. The nurse on duty first told the mother to place the child in a tepid bath and, after checking with a physician, instructed her to take the child to an approved Kaiser Permanente affiliate, even though there was a closer hospital. The child's heart stopped en route to the hospital and gangrene resulted from lack of circulation to his extremities. The family's lawyer argued that this was an example of what happens when cost-conscious managed care providers try to cut corners.

Another potential source of liability for MCOs is the fact that they choose the clinicians who provide care to members. Having a duty to investigate provider credentials and expertise and to offer competent and qualified providers, MCOs take on potential liability under the corporate negligence doctrine (Fiesta, 1996b). Courts have concluded that by limiting members' choice of providers to a select group, there is an unreasonable risk of harm if the clinicians are unqualified or incompetent. MCOs must be careful that decisions regarding quality and availability of care are not negatively affected by financial considerations.

Malpractice Claims Against Nurses

As the health care system changes, nurses are becoming the target of a growing number of malpractice charges. According to Fiesta (1996a), though many of the current issues point toward examples of corporate liability, cases involving the actions of individual nurses are also increasing. Traditional errors such as burns, falls, and medication errors seem to be more common than in the past. This leads to the speculation that negligent actions are a direct result of increased stress in the workplace and decreased morale, which together lead to the overall effect of distracting nurses from focusing clearly on individual patients. "As the health care delivery system undergoes monumental change, it is apparent that the traditional areas of liability exposure continue to exist while simultaneously new areas of risk exposure are evolving" (1996a, p. 22). Validated trends in malpractice litigation include the following:

1. Nurses continue to appear as named defendants, emphasizing the fact that nurses are professionally accountable for their own actions.

2. Telephone call situations continue to indicate high levels of liability exposure because of the potential for miscommunication and the lack of documentation supporting the defendant's version of the conversation.

3. Failure to communicate and to access the chain of command continues to be a major liability risk for nurses.

4. Obstetrical cases continue to present high monetary losses when negligence is established. (Fiesta, 1996a, pp. 22–24)

Criminalization of Nurses' Professional Negligence

Traditionally, nurses who make errors that cause harm to patients have been charged with the unintentional tort of professional negligence (malpractice). Either heard in civil court or settled out of court, charges of negligence against nurses have not resulted in criminal prosecution. It appears, however, that there may be a disturbing legal trend toward charging nurses with criminal negligence in particular cases. Cathy A. Klein, a nurse practitioner and practicing defense attorney, reports on one such case:

> Until recently, the risk of criminal prosecution for nursing practice was non-existent unless nursing action arose to the level of criminal intent, such as the case of euthanasia leading to murder charges. However, in April, 1997, three nurses were indicted by a Colorado grand jury for criminally negligent homicide in the death of a newborn. Public records show that one nurse was assigned to care for the baby. A second nurse offered to assist her colleague in caring for the baby. A third nurse was a nurse practitioner working in the hospital nursery. Because the baby was at risk for congenital syphilis, the physician ordered that the nurses give 150,000 units of intramuscular penicillin—which would have required five separate injections. In relation to other problems the same day, the baby was subjected to a lumbar puncture which required six painful attempts. To avoid inflicting further pain, Nurse Two asked the nurse practitioner if there was another route available for administration of the penicillin. Nurse Two and the nurse practitioner searched recognized pharmacology references and determined that IV administration would be acceptable. The nurse practitioner had the authority to change the route and directed Nurse Two to administer the medication intravenously rather than intramuscularly. Unrecognized by the nurses, the pharmacy erroneously delivered the medication prepared and ready to administer in a dose ten times greater than was ordered—1.5 million units. As Nurse Two was administering the medication intravenously, the baby died. The Colorado Board of Nursing initiated disciplinary proceedings against Nurse Two and the nurse practitioner, but not against Nurse One. The grand jury indicted all three nurses on charges of criminally negligent homicide, but did not indict the pharmacist. (C. A. Klein, personal communication, May, 14, 1997)

This case is an ominous reminder of the days of witch hunts—when bad outcomes of childbirth led to the execution of nurse midwives. It is a frightening example of the devastating and unpredictable consequences that can occur when a nurse makes a serious error. At this writing, the case has not come to trial.

Ask Yourself

Criminal Negligence Versus Malpractice

- What feelings are evoked as you consider the example above?
- Should the courts take into consideration the fact that the nurses' error occurred because they wanted to avoid causing the baby unnecessary pain? Discuss your thinking.
- Can you think of other occupations in which the consequences of unintentional errors have greater legal implications? Discuss your answer with classmates.
- How should the profession respond to this frightening new legal threat?

RISK MANAGEMENT

Recognizing the litigious state of today's society, how can nurses limit the risk of lawsuits? Much of today's litigation occurs as a result of events over which nurses have little control. Unfortunate outcomes can result from institutional circumstances, errors or incompetence of other professionals, or unpredictable or intractable physical phenomena. Other litigation occurs as a result of thoughtless or negligent actions on the part of nurses or other professionals. Though it is impossible to completely eliminate the risk of litigation, attention to a number of critical factors may reduce the threat of malpractice suits. Critical factors include maintaining open communication with patients, conscientious practice, and autonomy. (See Figure 7–3.)

Figure 7–3 **Reducing the Risk of Malpractice Litigation**

I. Maintain Good Communication
- Be courteous, show respect, and take time to listen attentively
- Do not belittle patients or make value judgments
- Involve patients in decision making
- Assess patients' level of understanding
- Explain in language that patients can understand
- Clarify and verify telephone orders; whenever possible, avoid accepting telephone orders or giving advice over the telephone

II. Maintain Expertise in Practice
- Keep up-to-date in both knowledge and skills
- Do not attempt any task or give any medication that is unfamiliar
- Practice within the professional and statutory scope of practice

- Be familiar with and follow institutional and professional standards of care
- Be attentive to patients' changing health status
- Pay close attention to detail, avoiding distraction
- Document objectively, thoroughly, and in a timely fashion

III. Maintain Autonomy and Empowerment
- Challenge questionable physician orders
- Seek attention for patients with changing health status
- Challenge bureaucratic structures that threaten patient welfare
- Avoid institutional settings that produce systematic and persistent threats to patient welfare

Maintaining Communication with Patients

On many occasions, nurses could have prevented malpractice lawsuits had they paid careful attention to interpersonal relationships and good communication techniques. Patients tend to become angry if they believe they are not being taken seriously, are not being listened to, are being belittled, or are denied involvement in the decision making process. Regardless of the professional's knowledge or ability, angry patients are more likely to file lawsuits. One of the most important factors in reducing the risk of litigation is a genuine regard for others. This quality produces nurses who are courteous, honest, and caring. They maintain open lines of communication, spend the time that is required to show respect, have genuine interest and patience, and listen to understand. The value of untiring listening cannot be overemphasized. Anecdotal information reveals that a professional's lack of listening is a key element for patients who are inclined to file lawsuits. In addition to the psychosocial benefits, listening with a discerning ear can lead to clues of health status that might otherwise have gone undetected. Good communicators listen objectively, avoid making value judgments, and include patients in health care decisions.

Patients may also sue when there are negative outcomes resulting from a lack of understanding of self-care, treatment options, potential outcomes of treatments, side effects of drugs, and so forth. In addition to listening skills, good communication techniques include assessing patients' level of understanding and finding ways to help patients to understand important information. Nurses with a genuine regard for others are more likely to be aware of patients' level of understanding. They will teach and explain, being respectful, yet using language that patients understand. They will ensure that informed consent is truly informed. They will continue to check and recheck patients' level of understanding, involving other family members when appropriate. Because lawsuits are frequent and it is particularly difficult to assess patients' level of understanding, nurses need to be especially careful about giving advice or patient teaching over the telephone.

Maintaining Conscientious Practice

There are many factors related to conscientious practice. Recall that expertise in practice is not only one hallmark of a professional but is also a legal and ethical imperative.

There have been monumental advances in knowledge and technology in the past several years. With the advent of health insurance in the post World War II era and malpractice litigation in recent years, standards of care have become very stringent. Society's expectations of nurses' knowledge and abilities are high. Consequently, prudent nurses strive to maintain up-to-date knowledge and technical skills. Lack of knowledge is no defense in a court of law. It is, in fact, tantamount to an admission of negligence. It is important that nurses know and uphold institutional, professional, and legal standards of practice and work within their scope of practice—never attempting to perform any task or administer any medication that is unfamiliar. Nurses' actions are examined in light of current knowledge levels that are expected of all nurses, professional or statutory scope of practice, and institutional and professional practice standards. Statements such as "Everyone does it that way," "That is what I learned in school 20 years ago," or "I did the best I could" will not protect a nurse from being found negligent.

Conscientious practice also includes close attention to detail. Nurses make serious errors when they become overly tired or distracted, are called away from tasks, are inattentive to patients' changing health status, or do not take the time to document thoroughly. Attention to detail will eliminate many errors that result in charges of negligence. Ethics and the law are closely related in regard to attention to detail. Recall from Chapter 2 that deontological ethics requires that each person is seen as an end and not as a means only, and that one is compelled to fulfill one's duty to others, thus implying that nurses must focus clearly upon each patient and each task. Attention to detail will serve to improve patient outcomes and protect the nurse against lawsuits.

Maintaining Autonomy and Empowerment

As examples in this chapter have illustrated, the courts demand that nurses practice autonomously. Time and again, court decisions have indicated that society expects nurses to be courageous in questioning physicians' orders (particularly those given over the telephone), vigorous in seeking attention for patients with changing health status, and active in challenging bureaucratic structures that threaten patient welfare. The courts know that nurses have in-depth knowledge in areas such as pharmacology and pathophysiology and expect nurses to protect patients from harm. Facing institutional situations that systematically present threats to patient safety and welfare, and being unable to bring about change, nurses may find they can protect themselves from liability only by leaving the situation.

Liability Insurance

Despite efforts to reduce the risk of liability, nurses are increasingly vulnerable to claims of malpractice. Regardless of nurses' level of expertise, patients can be injured. Even if a claim has no merit, the process of defense is time consuming, emotionally exhausting, and costly. Liability insurance is an important risk management strategy that protects assets and income and affords nurses peace of mind. Professional liability insurance provides for payment of lawyer fees and settlement or jury awards. It also provides nurses a mechanism of accountability in that they have the ability to pay should their actions cause injury (Guido, 1997). Nurses should never be without liability coverage.

Choosing a particular type of malpractice policy can be confusing and intimidating. How much coverage is appropriate? Are occurrence-based or claims-made policies better? Do nurses need individual policies if they have employer-sponsored coverage? Is it important that nurses be knowledgeable about their unique malpractice risks?

There are two basic types of insurance coverage. *Occurrence-based* policies provide broad coverage. These policies cover the nurse for claims arising from incidents that occur during the period of time that the policy is in effect. Occurrence-based policies protect the nurse when lawsuits are filed after the policy has expired, even if the policy was not renewed. In particular, nurses who work with children or infants run the risk of lawsuits being filed many years after an injury occurs. *Claims-made* policies provide coverage only in instances in which both the injury and the claim are made during the time in which the policy is in effect. This type of coverage is adequate if the nurse maintains continuous coverage and purchases a *tail* to provide uninterrupted extension for a period of time after the policy period. Occurrence-based policies are preferable for most nurses.

Another distinction is made between malpractice policies and professional liability policies. Generally speaking, *malpractice policies* offer coverage exclusively for claims of malpractice. Though specific coverage differs from policy to policy, *professional liability* insurance offers protection against various injuries that are not directly related to malpractice (Mitchell & Grippando, 1993).

Nurses also question whether they need individual coverage if their group or employer provides insurance. *Individual coverage* is purchased by the individual and offers the policy holder twenty-four-hour protection against liability claims for actions that fall within the scope of professional nursing practice, either paid or volunteer services (Guido, 1997). Individual coverage pays lawyer fees and monetary damages (in relation to limits of the specific policy) and offers the nurse some control over details of the defense strategy. Infrequently used by nurses, *group coverage* is purchased by professionals who have essentially the same job descriptions and covers only those activities performed during office hours. This is particularly attractive as a less expensive choice for nurse practitioners in group practice. *Employer-sponsored coverage* is purchased by the employing agency for the purpose of protecting business concerns. Though nurses have coverage under employer-sponsored policies, the protection is limited to activities performed within the scope of employment. Though employers may claim that employer-sponsored coverage is adequate, it is actually the most limited type of liability insurance. In fact, if found negligent, nurses may be required to repay the employer a portion of the loss. Guido (1997) reports that nurses who rely solely on hospital policies have a greater chance of inadequate monetary protection and legal counsel.

NURSES AS EXPERT WITNESSES

The role of expert witness is relatively new to the nursing profession. Because of the complex and highly technical nature of nursing, attorneys require the assistance of knowledgeable and experienced expert witnesses. These witnesses may be hired by either the plaintiff or the defendant. Serving the legal system, expert witnesses are neither parties to the dispute nor patient advocates. Ideally, they remain honest and give objective opinions to the court.

Serving as an expert witness involves a complex and extensive process of examining evidence, reviewing pertinent nursing literature, giving depositions, and testifying in court. The expert witness is expected to be familiar with the following: all medical records of the patient during the time of the incident; pertinent written policies and procedures of the institution; the nursing care plan, including nursing assessment, diagnosis, plan, interventions, and evaluation; the state nurse practice act; the Joint Commission on Accreditation of Healthcare Organizations manual; applicable nursing standards; current professional literature outlining accepted practice at the time of the incident; and opinions from the state board of nursing (Dyke, 1989). The witness must describe the standards of care to the court, evaluate the nurse's actions against them, and discuss conclusions relative to the accusation of malpractice. Effectiveness of the expert witness is influenced by the breadth of experience, degree of preparation, depth of knowledge, and confident delivery.

The use of expert witnesses gives strength to the argument that nursing is a true profession. It supports the autonomy of nursing in that no other professional can appropriately judge the practice of nurses. Strickland and Fishman (1994) suggest that nursing leaders should collaborate with members of the legal profession to establish professional standards for the role and develop educational programs for interested and qualified nurses.

SUMMARY

As the enforceable system of principles and processes that govern the behavior of people, laws reflect moral and ethical tradition. Though there is sometimes disagreement regarding the rightness or wrongness of certain laws, the laws are generally consistent with popular beliefs.

Laws in the United States are either constitutional, statutory, or administrative and are divided into public and private realms. Public law deals with the relationship between persons and the government, and private law deals with the relationship between people. Nurses and other health care providers are more likely to be involved in liability cases related to tort law, a division of private law. Tort law includes unintentional torts, such as negligence and malpractice, and intentional torts, such as fraud, invasion of privacy, assault, battery, false imprisonment, and defamation.

Recent trends in health care delivery systems have both created new areas of liability and increased instances of traditional negligence. Managed care organizations, while assuming the roles of both insurer and provider of health care, are frequently charged with corporate negligence. Perhaps because of increased stressors in the workplace, nurses are experiencing an increasing number of malpractice claims related to the traditional kinds of errors.

With the increase in malpractice litigation, nurses are wise to take certain precautions to limit the risk of lawsuits. Critical factors include maintaining open lines of communication with patients through the use of good listening techniques, accepting demeanor, and attention to patients' level of understanding; maintaining conscientious practice, including retaining expertise and ensuring attention to detail; maintaining autonomy through courageous and vigorous patient advocacy; and maintaining continuous professional liability insurance. When patients charge nurses with malpractice, expert nurse witnesses can serve the court by describing standards of care, evaluating the nurse's action against standards, and discussing conclusions relative to the accusation of malpractice.

CHAPTER HIGHLIGHTS

- Ethics is the foundation of law; however, because laws are created by individuals and there are differences in beliefs among people, ethics and the law are not always congruent.
- Constitutional law is based upon the Constitution and supersedes all other law.
- Statutory law is created through the lawmaking process in state or federal legislatures and is also called legislative law.
- Administrative law consists mainly of the legal powers granted to administrative agencies by the legislature and the rules that the agencies make to carry out their powers.
- Common law, also known as case law, is a system of law based largely on previous court decisions.
- Public law defines a person's rights and obligations in relation to government and describes the various divisions of government and their powers.
- Private law, also called civil law, determines a person's legal rights and obligations in many kinds of activities that involve other people.
- A tort is a wrong or injury that a person suffers because of someone else's action, either intentional (willful or intentional acts that violate another person's rights or property) or unintentional (an act or omission that causes unintended injury or harm to another person).
- Changes in health care financing and delivery have caused litigation related to corporate liability.
- Nurses can limit the risk of liability through maintaining open communication with patients, expertise in practice, attention to details, and autonomy.
- Supporting the autonomous nature of nursing, expert nurse witnesses serve the court through the process of examining evidence, applying nursing standards, reviewing pertinent nursing literature, and explaining conclusions.

DISCUSSION QUESTIONS AND ACTIVITIES

1. Find examples of recent court cases related to issues such as termination of life support, fetal tissue use, genetic engineering, and patient self-determination.

Discuss your ethical beliefs related to the court decisions. What ethical principles are applicable?

2. Discuss with classmates their opinions about the courts becoming involved in issues that have traditionally been considered ethical in nature.

3. Read the *Bill of Rights* of the *United States Constitution*. How do the rights guaranteed in the *Bill of Rights* relate to patient care? How do they relate to nurses' employment?

4. Discuss recent examples of state or federal legislation that create changes in the health care delivery system or in the practice of nursing.

5. In the common law system, how do previous court decisions affect the outcome of current cases?

6. Discuss instances in which nurses can be charged with crimes of public law, even though acts were committed without malice in the process of giving nursing care.

7. Discuss specific examples of unintentional torts of which nurses have been accused.

8. How can you protect yourself from being accused of an unintentional tort?

9. In what instances can nurses be charged with intentional torts, even though they follow a professional code of ethics?

10. Discuss areas of potential liability for nurses and the present health care delivery system.

REFERENCES

Bernzweig, E. P. (1990). *The nurse's liability for malpractice* (5th ed.). St. Louis, MO: Mosby.

Big Town Nursing Home, Inc. v. Newman, 461 S.W.2d 195 (Tex. Civ. App. 1970).

Blackman for Blackman v. Rifkin, 759 P.2d 54 (Colo. App. 1988), *cert. denied* (1989).

Catalano, J. T. (1991). *Ethical and legal aspects of nursing*. Springhouse, PA: Springhouse.

Creighton, H. (1986). *Law every nurse should know* (5th ed.). Philadelphia: Saunders.

Dyke, R. M. (1989). The nurse expert witness: Professional implications. *Neonatal Network, 8*(3), 3–39.

Fiesta, J. (1988). *The law and liability: A guide for nurses* (2nd ed.). New York: John Wiley & Sons.

Fiesta, J. (1996a). Legal update, 1995: Part 1. *Nursing Management, 27*(5), 22–24.

Fiesta, J. (1996b). Legal update, 1995: Part 2. *Nursing Management, 27*(6), 24–25.

Furrow, B. R., Johnson, S. H., Jost, T. S., Schwartz, R. L. (1991). *Liability and quality issues in health care*. St. Paul, MN: West.

Guido, G. W. (1997). *Legal issues in nursing* (2nd ed.). Norwalk, CT: Appleton & Lange.

King, M. L., Jr. (1996). Letter from the Birmingham jail. In J. Feinberg (Ed.), *Reason and responsibility: Readings in some basic problems of philosophy* (9th ed., pp. 572–580). Belmont, CA: Wadsworth. (Reprinted from M. King, Jr., *Why we can't wait*, 1963, John Davis Agency).

Kozier, B., & Erb., G. (1988). *Concepts and issues in nursing practice*. Menlo Park, CA: Addison-Wesley.

Mitchell, P., & Grippando, G. (1993). *Nursing perspectives and issues.* (5th ed.). Albany, NY: Delmar.

Oswald v. LeGrand, 453 N.W.2d 634 (Iowa 1990).

Rhodes, A. M., & Miller, R. D. (1984). *Nursing and the law* (4th ed.). Rockville, MD: Aspen Systems.

Robertson v. Provident House, 576 So. 2d 992 (La. 1991).

Schessler v. Keck, 271 P.2d 588 (Cal. Ct. App. 1954).

Smelko v. Brinton, 740 P.2d 591 (Kan. 1987).

State of Louisiana v. Brenner, 486 So. 2d 101 (La. 1986).

Strickland, O., & Fishman, D. (1994). *Nursing issues in the 1990's.* Albany, NY: Delmar.

Truhitte v. French Hospital, 180 Cal. Rptr. 152 (Cal. Ct. App. 1982).

CHAPTER **8**

Professional Issues

[A]s we stand on the threshold of a historic event in nursing, let us repeat that we join to accomplish for nursing those objectives impossible to do so singularly. We are living in a very complicated world and with the pressures of science, technology, and societal demands, nursing must foster its image, determine its goals, and plan its direction, or the outside forces will indeed obliterate this profession.

(Zschoche, 1983)

OBJECTIVES

After completing this chapter, the reader should be able to:

1. Discuss the meaning of the term *professional,* including traits commonly associated with professional status and the historical debate regarding the professional status of nursing.

2. Relate codes of ethics to professional status.

3. Discuss the relationships among the concepts of expertise, ethics, and professional status.

4. Discuss autonomy in terms of both the individual nurse and the profession of nursing.

5. Discuss the relationship between professional autonomy and ethics.

6. Discuss the term accountability, including various mechanisms of nursing accountability.

7. Explain the relationship between accountability and professional status.

8. Define the term *authority,* differentiating between professional and personal authority.

9. Discuss the concept of unity and its relationship to professional status in nursing.

INTRODUCTION

In discussing the role of ethics in nursing, one is inevitably led to a discussion of the professional status of nurses. Any discussion of nursing ethics presupposes the professional nature of nursing. To some, a systematic code of ethics is a defining criterion—separating professions from occupations. This chapter begins by examining the meaning and historical context of the term *professional* and then discusses the professional status of nursing and the selected characteristics of expertise, autonomy, accountability, authority, and unity in nursing.

PROFESSIONAL STATUS

Professions exist for the purpose of meeting the needs of society. It is the larger society that determines its needs and authorizes certain people to meet those needs. There is a uniform process by which professionals develop the values that lead to a type of social responsibility and desire to meet the needs of society (Aydelotte, 1990). Professionals contract with society by promising to meet a set of identified needs better than any other group of people. In turn, society grants the profession a monopoly over these particular services. Historically, professions have attempted to instill in their members a somber recognition of the profound nature of their responsibility through the reciting of pledges and oaths such as the Hippocratic Oath for physicians and the Nightingale Pledge for nurses.

Since before the turn of the century, there have been discussions about the professional status of nursing. Professions have been described in a number of ways. Gruending (1985) describes a **profession** as a complex, organized occupation preceded by a long training program. Professional education is geared toward the acquisition of exclusive knowledge necessary to provide a service that is either essential or desired by society. These attributes lead to a monopoly that provides autonomy, public recognition, prestige, power, and authority for the practitioner. Many other distinguishing attributes of professions have been proposed over the years. Among others, these include expertise, accountability, the presence of systematic theory, ethical codes, a professional culture, an altruistic service orientation, competence testing, licensure, high income, credentialing, the description of a scope of practice, and the establishment of standards.

Ask Yourself

Is Nursing a Profession?

Most nursing programs have course content that is geared toward identifying the professional status of nursing through the use of identified traits or functions.

- Do you recall discussions in earlier courses about the professional status of nursing? If so, what do you recall from those discussions?
- What (or whose) criteria were used to judge professional status?

> • Based upon what you recall, would you identify nursing as a profession, an emerging profession, a quasi-profession, or an occupation struggling to become a profession?

Perhaps the most frequently quoted source describing the criteria of professionals is Abraham Flexner. An educator, Flexner was well known for his 1910 evaluation of the professional status of medical schools. In 1915, Flexner listed traits that he observed in the established professions of medicine, law, and the clergy. He then proposed that in order to be recognized as professions, all occupations must meet these criteria. Following are six criteria that he utilized to identify professions:

1. professions involve essentially intellectual operations;
2. they derive their raw materials from science and learning;
3. this material they work up to a practical and definite end;
4. they possess an educationally communicable technique;
5. they tend to self-organization;
6. they are becoming increasingly altruistic in motivation. (Flexner, 1915, pp. 901–912)

Unsolicited by the nursing community, Flexner evaluated nursing according to his criteria and judged that nursing was not a profession. Optimistically, he proposed that occupations could alter their status by developing these traits.

Subsequently, in 1945 and 1959, two educators, Genevieve and Roy Bixler, published landmark articles in the *American Journal of Nursing* (AJN) evaluating the professional status of nursing. These articles utilized criteria similar to those proposed by Flexner. They listed the following seven criteria of a profession:

1. A profession utilizes in its practice a well-defined and well-organized body of specialized knowledge which is on the intellectual level of the higher learning;
2. A profession constantly enlarges the body of knowledge it uses and improves its techniques of education and service by the use of the scientific method;
3. A profession entrusts the education of its practitioners to institutions of higher education;
4. A profession applies its body of knowledge in practical services which are vital to human and social welfare;
5. A profession functions autonomously in the formulation of professional policy and in the control of professional activity, thereby;
6. A profession attracts individuals of intellectual and personal qualities who exalt service above personal gain and who recognize their chosen occupation as a life work; and
7. A profession strives to compensate its practitioners by providing freedom of action, opportunity for continuous professional growth, and economic security. (Bixler & Bixler, 1959, pp. 1142–1146)

Predictably, the Bixler evaluations came to the same conclusion as Flexner: Nursing was deficient as a true profession.

Though both Flexner and the Bixlers had a tremendous lasting impact on nursing, none were nurses. Even though their lists of traits seem to have been chosen arbitrarily, their approach assumes that true professions will demonstrate all of the essential attributes. Fowler (1990) calls their lists of characteristics "an untidy aggregation of overlapping, arbitrarily chosen, or undifferentiated elements, lacking a unifying theoretical framework that explains their interrelationship" (p. 24).

Prior to the Flexner report, American nurses were secure in their identity as professionals. Even physicians and the judicial system had recognized nursing as a profession. However, following the Flexner report and the subsequent Bixler articles, nurses began to question their status as professionals (Parsons, 1986). Like sixteenth century women who came to believe the myth that women were intrinsically evil, nurses accepted the idea that nursing was not a true profession (Newman, 1990; Sleicher, 1981). The process of examining and evaluating, though, resulted in many positive changes for nursing. Striving to meet the criteria set by Flexner and the Bixlers, nurses became involved in research to create a unique body of knowledge for nursing, to move "professional" nursing education to the university setting, to become politically involved, to increase the autonomy of nursing, and to extend practice boundaries.

There are those who argue that the process used to identify traits of professions was flawed from the inception (Achterberg, 1990; Ehrenreich & English, 1973; Parsons, 1986). There are even those who suggest that the term *professional* is sexist, elitist, and racist. At the turn of the century, the three "professions" that were said to be universally accepted as such—medicine, law, and the clergy—were overwhelmingly male and Caucasian. As a result of the cultural and religious influences discussed in Chapter 1, by the time Flexner wrote his report, women had been systematically purged from both professional education and practice. Examining and describing traits of the male dominated "professions," and subsequently using those findings as criteria to judge the professional status of other occupations, may have effectively excluded all predominately female groups.

Nurses as Professionals

For lack of a better word, nurses continue to discuss their occupation in terms of a profession. Recognizing that there are a myriad of sources claiming to define the term *professional* by describing traits, attributes, functions, or characteristics, there will likely never be agreement about the professional status of nursing. Notwithstanding the importance of these discussions, for the purposes of this chapter, the assumption is made that nursing is a true profession.

In many ways nurses, as professionals, are connected to each other and set apart from others. Professionals are connected to each other by common experiences, language, and body of knowledge. They are set apart from others by virtue of the prestige and mystique offered members of a profession and by the knowledge that comes from personal, intimate, and spiritual experiences surrounding the beginning and the end of life (Nathaniel, 1994).

Beletz describes a professional as "one bound by values and standards other than those of his or her employing organization, setting one's own rules, seeking to promote standards of excellence, and being evaluated and looking for approval from one's own professional peers" (1990, p. 18). Jameton further suggests that being a professional is similar to having a calling. He describes a calling as "something one feels called upon to do, perhaps by God, by some deep need in one's being, or by the demands of historical circumstance. A calling is central to one's life and gives it meaning" (1984, p. 18).

EXPERTISE

Expertise relates to the characteristic of having a high level of specialized skill and knowledge. It is a "composite of a knowledge base, gained through long years of study in an academic setting, and superior skill. Expertise is the primary distinguishing difference between professionals and nonprofessionals" (Beletz, 1990, p. 17). Professionals must have the knowledge base and functional skills that are required to meet the needs of society and thereby fulfill the purpose of the profession. Regarding expertise, Jameton (1984) writes:

> Professions maintain their autonomy partly through their claim to maximal competence [expertise]. So long as people believe that the professionals are the only ones who fully understand their work, it is very hard to supervise or criticize them. (p. 21)

Expertise can be established in a variety of ways. Extensive educational requirements, intense guided practice, examination for licensure, certification, and mandatory continuing education are ways that nurses either attain, maintain, or assert expertise. Florence Nightingale recognized the importance of an education consisting of depth and breadth of general knowledge combined with a very specific nursing focus. Nurses today are in possession of a knowledge base that is continually expanded through research and enhanced by the knowledge gained through the study of nursing and other disciplines. Having completed basic nursing education and successfully demonstrated a minimum level of competence through licensure examination, nurses are further required (either ethically or legally) to continue the learning process and maintain up-to-date knowledge and technical proficiency. Continuing education programs assist individuals in this process. The expertise of nurses is also advanced through graduate nursing education, specialty preparation, and the certification process.

Merely claiming expertise is not enough. Through the various mechanisms of accountability, professionals must prove to society that they are faithful to the promise the profession makes. In response, society grants professionals the authority to practice with a certain measure of autonomy. Thus, the professional realms of expertise, accountability, autonomy, and authority are interrelated.

Ask Yourself

When the Bottom Line Becomes Personal

Imagine that one of your loved ones becomes gravely ill and needs to be hospitalized. Your third party payer determines the hospital and provider you must use. Because of your background, you are familiar with the nursing skills and knowledge that are required to adequately care for your loved one. You recognize many instances in which the nurses demonstrate poor knowledge and lack of basic skills—potentially leading to threats to the well-being of your family member.

- How would you feel in this circumstance?
- What do you think nurses' responsibilities are regarding their ability to adequately care for your loved one?
- Discuss your beliefs concerning an ethical requirement to maintain expertise in the area of practice.
- Does the profession have an obligation to society in this regard?

AUTONOMY

In terms of a profession, the word **autonomy** literally means "self-governing." The concept of nursing autonomy can be discussed on two levels: autonomy of the profession and autonomy of the individual practitioner. Self-regulation is the mark of collective professional autonomy. Individual autonomy involves self-determination, responsibility, accountability, independence, and a willingness to take risks. Autonomy is generally considered to be an important criterion in judging professional status of an occupation. People who are considered to be professionals have the power and authority to control various aspects of their work including goals toward which to work, whether to work and with whom, details of how the work is to be done, choice of clientele, and so forth (Jameton, 1984). Whether or not nurses have autonomy has been a much debated topic for many years.

Inasmuch as the profession of nursing is self-regulating, it can be said to be autonomous. Unlike the early years of this century, most state boards of nursing are now made up predominately of nurses. By virtue of the authority granted by statutory law, the boards of nursing enforce the individual states' nurse practice acts, thereby ensuring the autonomy of the profession within each state. Among other tasks, boards of nursing oversee the schools of nursing within the states, control licensure, and discipline nurses.

Jameton (1984) implies that the profession of nursing maintains autonomy through the combination of a claim to maximal competence and a continuing monopoly over their work. He writes:

> Professions also maintain their autonomy by means of monopoly
> over their work. In our competitive culture, people do not achieve

autonomy simply by declaring it or believing in it. Professions maintain their control over their work partly by keeping people with other skills and other ideas from doing the same work. Only nurses may legally practice nursing. Licensure, educational requirements, certification of schools, and the like help nurses maintain control over nursing practice. This control is strengthened when nurses—rather than physicians and nonprofessionals—control the processes of licensure and certification. (p. 21)

No other group has the ability to do the work of nurses; consequently, there is a legal restriction barring non-nurses from practicing nursing. The legally sanctioned monopoly over the domain of nursing helps to establish autonomy for nurses.

In recent years non-nurse groups and organizations have attempted to undermine the autonomy of the profession of nursing in various ways. The American Medical Association's effort in the 1980s to institute a new category of bedside health care provider, the Registered Care Technician (RCT), can be viewed as an attempt to gain access into the domain of nursing, and thereby threaten the autonomy of the profession. Recognizing the implications of this proposal, in an unprecedented joint effort, a number of disparate nursing organizations banded together to successfully oppose this plan. In the mid-1990s, hospital associations moved to gain some control over the profession of nursing. These groups targeted specific states in which to attempt drastic changes in nurse practice acts (*State Scan*, 1996). These efforts included proposals to legislate changes in the membership and responsibility of the state boards. In at least one state, this effort included replacing an essentially all-nurse board with a new board consisting of physicians, hospital administrators, consumers, and nurses. Recognizing a threat to the integrity of the profession, nurses in various states continue to work to defend against opening of nurse practice acts by non-nursing groups. As competition for health care dollars becomes more fierce, nurses will be acutely aware of outside efforts that threaten the autonomy of the profession.

Nurses are both legally and ethically required to practice autonomously. Autonomous practice serves as a safeguard for the patient, nurse, physician, and institution. At least three points of the ANA *Code for Nurses with Interpretive Statements* (1985) strongly imply the ethical imperative of autonomous practice. These include:

Point 3. The nurse acts to safeguard the client and the public when health care and safety are affected by the incompetent, unethical, or illegal practice of any person.

Point 4. The nurse assumes responsibility and accountability for individual nursing judgments and actions.

Point 6. The nurse exercises informed judgement and uses individual competence and qualifications as criteria in seeking consultation, accepting responsibilities, and delegating nursing activities to others. (p. 1)

Each point requires autonomy of the nurse in exercising independent judgment in regard to nursing care. The purpose of autonomy as described in the ANA Code is to protect the patient from harm and allow for the full benefit of professional nursing care.

Questions often arise about autonomy as related to the practice of nursing by individual nurses. Does each nurse have autonomy? Can nurses say that they are autonomous even though they are required to follow physicians' orders? Lyon (1990) defines autonomous nursing practice as "the diagnosis and treatment of phenomena that nurses have the self-directed authority to treat" (p. 270). Furthermore, she writes that nursing has a social mandate for two different scopes of practice: the medical scope that requires physician authorization to initiate treatment, and the autonomous nursing scope that requires no authorization.

As a practical necessity, hospitals and other health care institutions, having physicians as their clients, must provide qualified staff to carry out physicians' orders. Combined with the provision of nursing care, carrying out of the medical plan of care is an essential service of many institutions. When nurses seek employment at these institutions, they are implicitly agreeing to perform the functions for which they are hired. Accepting a position implies this contract. Nevertheless, nurses are legally and ethically required to use independent judgment in making nursing decisions. The exercise of independent nursing judgment should be welcomed by institutions because of the safeguards that are afforded. It is not unusual to hear about a nurse who refuses to carry out a physician's order that is later found to be incorrect. Such actions protect patients from physician negligence and thus prevent litigation against the nurse, the physician, and the institution. The fact that nurses are often found legally negligent for following questionable physicians' orders, or failing to follow through with the hierarchical chain of command when questioning or disagreeing with acts or omissions of physicians or others, proves that the courts not only recognize, but expect, nursing autonomy.

Ask Yourself

Judgments About Physicians' Orders

Nurses are frequently asked to give medication with which they are not familiar. Unable to quickly determine the appropriateness or safety of a given drug, nurses may decide to refuse to administer a particular drug.

- What feelings, emotions, and values are involved in the nurse's decision to refuse to follow a physician's order?

- What are some predictable reactions of the nurse's coworkers, supervisors, and physicians when a nurse refuses to follow a physician's order?

- What ethical principles can be used to guide such decisions?

- How is the nurse empowered in these types of situations?

- How would it affect the nurse if the drug in question is later found to be safe and appropriate? How should this affect future decisions?

Autonomy does not mean that one has absolute control of every facet of practice. Accepted as one of the three prototype professions, medicine, for example, no longer retains the measure of control it once enjoyed. Government regulations now guide such facets of medical care as reimbursement levels and length of hospital stays. Managed care organizations limit expensive procedures, referral networks, and formulary medications. Consequently, physicians, though continuing to maintain professional status, are experiencing less absolute control over patient care than ever before. In the past, some (including Abraham Flexner) based the argument that nurses were not autonomous on comparisons between the independent decision making capacities of medicine and nursing. That comparison no longer illustrates a great degree of distinction.

It is clear that nurses do not always feel autonomous, and, in fact, some may not practice autonomously. Certainly there are nurses who spend each workday complying with physicians' orders and completing various nonautonomous tasks—never exercising independent nursing functions nor making nursing diagnoses and initiating self-directed treatment. In the truest sense, these nurses are only marginally practicing professional nursing and cannot be said to be autonomous. Practicing in this manner, nurses fail to fulfill their ethical duty to utilize independent nursing judgment.

ACCOUNTABILITY

According to the American Nurses Association (1985), "**Accountability** refers to being answerable to someone for something one has done. [It is] grounded in the moral principles of fidelity and respect for the dignity, worth, and self-determination of clients" (p. 8). Safe, autonomous practice is ensured through various processes of nursing accountability. Accountability is related to both responsibility and answerability (Leddy & Pepper, 1989). Because of the trust accorded nurses by society (gained through recognition of nurses' expertise) and the right given the profession to regulate practice (autonomy), individual practitioners and the profession must be both responsible and accountable.

Related to the concepts of autonomy and authority, accountability is an inherent part of everyday nursing practice. Each nurse is responsible for all individual actions and omissions. The ANA *Code for Nurses with Interpretive Statements* makes it clear that each nurse has the responsibility to maintain ethical and competent practice regardless of circumstances, stating that "neither physicians' orders nor the employing agency's policies relieve the nurse of accountability for actions taken and judgments made" (1985, p. 9). As has been previously noted, the courts have tended to support this claim.

Mechanisms of Accountability

Accountability is based upon the implicit contract between nursing and the larger society. Donabedian (1976) writes that self-regulation to ensure quality in performance is at the heart of the relationship between society and the professions—in fact, accountability is the "hallmark of a mature profession" (p. 8). The profession of nursing has developed several mechanisms through which this relationship between nursing and society is made explicit, thereby acknowledging to both the professional and the public the areas of nursing accountability. These mechanisms include codes of nursing ethics, standards of nursing practice, nurse practice acts, nursing theory and practice derived from nursing research, educational requirements for practice, advanced certification, and mechanisms for evaluating the effectiveness of nurses' performance of nursing responsibilities (ANA, 1985). In both a professional and a legal sense, it is necessary that nurses are familiar with both formal and informal mechanisms of accountability.

Codes of Nursing Ethics.   Nearly universally accepted as one criterion of a profession, a code of ethics is profoundly important to nursing. A **code of nursing ethics** is an explicit declaration of the primary goals and values of the profession that indicates the "profession's acceptance of the responsibility and trust with which it has been invested by society" (ANA, 1985, p. iii). Like other professions, nursing has developed and enforces specific obligations to ensure that members of society will find them to be competent and trustworthy. These obligations are correlative to the rights of individual patients and society as a whole (Beauchamp & Childress, 1994). Upon entrance into the profession, nurses make an implicit moral commitment to uphold the values and moral obligations expressed in their code. Nurses are called upon to base professional judgment upon consideration of consequences and the universal moral principles of respect for persons, autonomy, beneficence, nonmaleficence, veracity, confidentiality, fidelity, and justice (ANA, 1985). Examples of professional codes of ethics for nurses include the American Nurses Association *Code for Nurses with Interpretive Statements* (1985), the International Council of Nurses *Code for Nurses* (1989), and the Canadian Nurses Association *Code of Ethics for Registered Nurses* (1997) (see Appendices).

Standards of Nursing Practice.   **Standards of nursing practice** are written documents outlining minimum expectations for safe nursing care. Standards may describe in detail specific acts performed by nurses or may outline the expected process of nursing care. Standards are used to guide and evaluate nursing care. Courts look to standards of nursing practice for guidance when malpractice cases are deliberated. The two basic types of standards of nursing practice are internal and external standards (Fiesta, 1988).

Internal standards of nursing practice are those developed within the profession of nursing for the purpose of establishing the minimum level of nursing care and standardizing expectations for nursing. They help to ensure that nurses are competent and safe to practice (Kozier & Erb, 1988). These documents guide nurses in giving nursing care and can be used as a yardstick to measure the practice of individual nurses. Like other types of standards, internal standards can be used to determine whether or not the actions of nurses accused of malpractice are consistent with reasonable minimum expectations. An example of internal standards is the American Nurses Association *Standards of Nursing Practice*. These comprehensive standards utilize the nursing process. They make nurses accountable for ensuring that each step of the process is followed in the delivery of nursing care. The ANA also publishes standards of care for nurses in advanced or specialty roles such as nurse practitioners, maternal-child nurses, geriatric nurses, psychiatric nurses, community health nurses, and others.

External standards of nursing practice consist of guides for nursing care that are developed by non-nurses, the government, or institutions. These standards are usually developed to describe the specific expectations of agencies or groups that utilize the services of nurses. They serve the same function as internal standards—guidance and evaluation. Examples of external standards include such documents as the nurse practice act of each state, guidelines by the Joint Commission on Accreditation of Healthcare Organizations, and formal policies and procedures for individual agencies. Nurses are responsible and accountable to know and follow the standards of care for the profession, the specialty (if applicable), the geographic area, and the institution.

Often nurses in administrative or advisory capacities are responsible for developing institutional standards. These nurses sometimes develop standards that describe ideal nursing care. This type of standard may actually create a risk by placing both practicing nurses and the employing institution in jeopardy of malpractice litigation. Because standards are used to judge nursing actions, they should reflect reasonable expectations for safe nursing care, rather than optimal or ideal care. While ensuring safe patient care, nursing standards must be practical and reasonable.

 ## CASE PRESENTATION

When Standards Are Difficult to Meet

Linda Luaces is a registered nurse in charge of a large psychiatric unit. At any given time her unit houses an average of twenty-two patients with a variety of diagnoses ranging from drug dependence to acute psychoses. The unit is usually staffed by one registered nurse, two licensed practical nurses, and two attendants. Hospital policy requires that the registered nurse evaluate each patient's physical and mental status at least twice per shift, supervise the administration of all psychotropic medication, participate in group activities, supervise the implementation of each patient's plan of care, and be available to individual patients for one-to-one interaction. There are additional standards that describe the appropriate care for patients who are potentially suicidal: "Patients who are identified as suicidal will be isolated in private rooms and continuously monitored by a registered nurse." On one particular day two of the patients are identified as potentially suicidal, six geriatric patients with dementia need to be fed and ambulated, one patient is exhibiting violent behavior, and all the patients need individual assessment. Linda calls the supervisor for assistance but is told that there is no one available to help her. The reader will no doubt have noticed that in addition to the other duties, Linda is required to simultaneously and continuously monitor two patients in separate rooms—a physical impossibility. Linda tries to meet all of her obligations under these very strict standards, yet while she is answering a question raised by one of her staff members, one of the suicidal patients manages to injure herself attempting to jump out of a window.

Think About It

Problems Posed by Unreasonable Institutional Standards

- What dilemmas are posed by these standards?
- What were Linda's alternatives?
- What is the purpose of the standards that Linda is required to follow?
- What do you see as the legal liability created by the standards?
- Do you think the institution shares the legal blame for the situation?
- What is the effect of the standards on Linda's practice?
- Is there any way that Linda can meet the standards?
- What do you think you would do in similar circumstances?
- What are the ethical implications for the institution and for Linda?

Nurse Practice Acts. As the foremost legal statute regulating nursing, the **nurse practice act** of each state protects the public, defines nursing practice, describes the boundaries of practice, establishes standards for nurses, and protects the domain of nursing. Nurse practice acts are considered a form of nursing standard. Utilized by courts in determining the appropriateness of nursing actions, violations can result in either civil or criminal prosecution.

Each of the fifty states independently develops, updates, and interprets the individual nurse practice acts. Though both the ANA and the National Council of State Boards of Nursing, Inc., have developed model nurse practice acts in the past, the laws continue to be different in each state. Some nurse practice acts are very general and somewhat vague in describing parameters of the professional role. These laws are considered to be permissive, allowing nursing practice to change and grow in a dynamic way. Others list each act that nurses are permitted to perform. As nursing continues to evolve, these very specific nurse practice acts, while originally applauded as recognizing nurses' legitimate authority to perform certain advanced tasks, have become restrictive. Murphy says, "Specificity in the statute is not without its costs. Specifically worded statutes tend to freeze the status quo rather than accommodate evolving roles" (1990, p. 33). With nurses continually expanding the domain of nursing, very specific, restrictive nurse practice acts have become a barrier to advanced nursing practice. Reflecting this concept, the ANA document *Nursing's Social Policy Statement* (1996) states:

> Nursing's scope of practice is dynamic and evolves with changes in the phenomena of concern, in knowledge about various interventions' effects on patient or group outcomes, or in the political environment, legal conditions, and cultural demographic patterns in society. (p. 12)

Because nurses are legally accountable to follow the standards set by the nurse practice acts within their states, they must be particularly attentive to the language describing the definition of nursing and the scope of nursing practice. Nurses are accountable to know and follow their states' nurse practice acts. Because legislatures meet and pass laws regularly, nurse practice acts can be changed often. Nurses are responsible for knowing even the most recent changes in their states' nurse practice acts and for implementing these changes in practice.

Moreover, nurses are called upon to be active in promoting needed changes in nurse practice acts. The *Code for Nurses with Interpretive Statements* specifically speaks about this responsibility, "The nurse participates in the profession's efforts to implement and improve standards of nursing" (ANA, 1985, p. 13). Recent changes in the health care delivery system, financing mechanisms, and roles of other health care professionals require careful study of existing nurse practice acts and judicious implementation of well-thought-out changes.

Nursing Theory and Practice Derived from Research. A frequently cited characteristic of professions is the existence of a unique body of knowledge derived from research. Recall that Genevieve and Roy Bixler's first two characteristics of a profession relate to a unique body of knowledge. The Bixlers' second characteristic actually calls for professions to constantly enlarge the body of knowledge by use of the scientific method (1959). In the past, authorities debated whether nursing's body of knowledge was unique to the profession or was borrowed from behavioral and physical sciences and medicine. It seemed clear to some that nursing knowledge had been derived from the combination of experience and intuition and by borrowing from other disciplines (Leddy & Pepper, 1989). Responding to arguments that nursing was not a true profession because of this lack of a clearly unique body of knowledge, nurses in academic and clinical settings began gathering data and doing legitimate research. The process of theory building and research in nursing continues to increase the unique body of nursing knowledge. The benefit of this process is twofold. First, the expanded knowledge base allows nurses to more knowledgeably and skillfully respond to the needs of society. Second, the presence of a clearly unique body of knowledge aids in validating nursing as a true profession.

AUTHORITY

The term **authority** relates to the state of having legitimate power and sovereignty. The authority to practice nursing is granted by statute based upon the contract the profession has with society. The granting of authority acknowledges the professional's rights and responsibilities and in turn requires that there be mechanisms for public accountability (ANA, 1996). Authority assumes a certain measure of autonomy. Donabedian (1976) relates authority to both autonomy and accountability:

> Society grants the professions authority over functions vital to itself and permits them considerable autonomy in the conduct of their affairs. In return, the professions are expected to act responsibly, always mindful of the public trust. Self-regulation to assure quality

in performance is at the heart of this relationship. It is the authentic hallmark of a mature profession." (p. 8)

In a practical sense, authority is granted by society in the form of the permission for the profession to exist, coupled with the privilege granted to individuals to practice the profession. Thus, as with autonomy, authority for nurses is two-tiered. State legislatures create laws designed to protect the public's health and safety. The establishment of nurse practice acts is the exercise of this type of power. Nurse practice acts define nursing, describe the scope of practice, and grant the state boards of nursing the power to oversee the licensure of nurses and the practice of nursing in the states. Thus, the state boards of nursing have the legitimate authority to regulate the practice of nursing within each state.

Having specified requirements for entry into practice, defined nursing, and described the scope of nursing practice, nurse practice acts empower state boards of nursing to grant individual nurses the authority to practice. This authority is granted through the process of examination and licensure. Licensure benefits both the public and the professional. It protects the public from the unqualified, and it protects professionals' job territory by establishing a monopoly. The legal protection afforded by licensure enhances nurses' status by authenticating the profession (Beletz, 1990). Having met all requirements for entry into practice, nurses are granted the legal authority to practice nursing.

The authority given each nurse to practice is contingent upon the nurse continuing to uphold the established standards of nursing. State boards of nursing have the power and responsibility to discipline nurses who do not follow established standards or who violate provisions of licensure law. Discipline can take several forms, including suspension or revocation of license.

UNITY

There is general agreement that one of the defining characteristics of a profession is a sense of unity among its members. This unity is multifaceted and based on what Aydelotte (1990) calls moral uniformity and class ideology among its practitioners. Unity relates to the ability of nurses to organize for the purpose of fulfilling the profession's promises and the relationships that nurses have with one another.

It is only through unity of the profession's leaders and members that nursing is able to coherently standardize the professional characteristics of competence, autonomy, authority, and accountability. Through political and policy processes, nurses work together to meet the health care needs of society and to improve the status of the profession. The structural component of a professional community is realized through a professional association. The professional association provides a collective identity and serves as the voice of the profession to both the profession and society (Beletz, 1990). It fulfills four basic functions: to standardize services provided by its members, to provide a professional hub for members, to assist with educational needs of members, and to perform political, advisory, and policy functions. There is an expectation that professionals will be active members of their professional association.

Though systematic organization of professional groups is necessary in fulfilling the professions' responsibilities, there is also a need for unity among individual members. Unity involves showing sympathy, care, and reciprocity to those with whom one appropriately identifies, working closely with others toward shared goals, keeping promises, making mutual concerns a priority, sacrificing personal interests to the relationship, and attending to these over a period of time (Jameton, 1984). Beletz eloquently describes this type of unity:

> The professional's bond with colleagues emanates from relationships established by shared mysteries of a common technical language, educational background, rites of passage, styles of work, attire, and a consciousness of being set apart and insisting on being set apart from other occupational categories. Colleague relationships are expected to be cooperative, equalitarian, and supportive vis-a-vis clientele and peers. (1990, p. 19)

Though loyalty is a virtue, there are certain risks inherent in professionals experiencing a strong sense of loyalty to each other. Jameton (1984) warns that nurses must be careful that their loyalty to each other does not supersede that owed to patients. For example, mistakes that nurses or doctors make should be reported to patients. Because of a sense of loyalty and friendship that exists between coworkers, there is a risk that nurses' duty to patients will be neglected. Nurses are required to closely examine and prioritize conflicting loyalties. Jameton identifies nurses' main priorities as: patients, nurses and the nursing profession, physicians, hospitals, other health professions, and society. Questioning which of these priorities should be central and which should be peripheral, he suggests that the best choices for first priority are patient, nursing, and society.

Ask Yourself

Are Nurses Loyal to Nursing?

Nurses who are politically active in a particular state nurses' association report an incident that led them to question nurses' loyalty to the profession. At the prompting of hospital and physicians' lobbying groups, a number of nurse administrators participated in writing proposed legislation that would dismantle the all-nurse board of nursing in favor of one composed of hospital administrators and physicians.

* How would you characterize the loyalty of these nurses to the profession and to other nurses?
* What circumstances could justify prioritizing employer loyalty above loyalty to patients or to other nurses?
* What are the ethical implications of the actions of the nurses described in this situation?
* What should the role of nurses' associations be in these situations?

SUMMARY

Because ethics is a commonly cited criterion for judging the professional status of an occupation, the study of ethics must include a discussion of nursing's professional status. In order to rationally discuss professional issues in nursing, one must examine the meaning and historical context of the term *professional*. Beginning with Abraham Flexner's 1915 opinion that nursing did not meet his criteria for professional status, there has been continuing debate about this topic. Striving to create professional status for nursing, nurses have worked to solve the deficiencies that were identified by Flexner and others. There are those who believe that the original methods of determining professional status were flawed by a cultural background of sexism, racism, and elitism. Though this debate will continue, there are a number of traits that are nearly universally accepted as belonging to professional groups. Expertise, autonomy, accountability, authority, and unity were discussed as professional characteristics of nursing.

CHAPTER HIGHLIGHTS

- Acknowledgment of professional status is dependent upon meeting particular criteria that include, but are not restricted to, expertise, autonomy, authority, accountability, and unity.

- Historical and cultural influences have affected the trait definitions commonly used for the term *professional*.

- A system or code of ethics is generally accepted as one trait of professions.

- Because society allows professionals a monopoly over the services they provide, ethics demands that those services must be provided with expertise.

- Because it is self-regulating, the profession of nursing can be said to be autonomous.

- There are legal and ethical imperatives for individual nurses to practice autonomously.

- Autonomy does not mean full and absolute control over every aspect of practice.

- Grounded in the moral principle of fidelity, accountability refers to being answerable to someone for something one has done.

- Mechanisms of accountability include, but are not restricted to, codes of nursing ethics, standards of nursing practice, nurse practice acts, and nursing theory and practice derived from nursing research.

- Authority for nurses to practice is granted through the legal processes of society.

- Nursing unity relates to the profession's ability to organize for the purpose of fulfilling the promises made to society.

DISCUSSION QUESTIONS AND ACTIVITIES

1. Write your own definition of the term *professional*.

2. List ten different occupations and compare their common characteristics. Which occupations meet your criteria for professional status?

3. Discuss the relationship between historical and cultural influences and Flexner's method of identifying professions.

4. Discuss the relationship between the concepts of fidelity, professionalism, and expertise.

5. Discuss the statement, "To be less than maximally competent is unethical."

6. Find recent examples of case law that relate to court opinions regarding autonomy in nursing.

7. Observe a registered nurse at work. List tasks that the nurse performs and categorize them as autonomous or dependent.

8. Read the nurse practice act in your state. Evaluate your state's law in terms of its usefulness as a mechanism of accountability.

REFERENCES

Achterberg, J. (1990). *Woman as healer.* Boston: Shambhala.

American Nurses Association. (1985). *Code for nurses with interpretive statements.* Washington, DC: Author.

American Nurses Association. (1996). *Nursing's social policy statement.* Washington, DC: Author.

Aydelotte, M. (1990). The evolving profession: The role of the professional organization. In N. L. Chaska (Ed.), *The nursing profession: A time to speak* (pp. 16–23). St. Louis, MO: Mosby.

Beauchamp, T., & Childress, J. (1994). *Principles of biomedical ethics* (4th ed.). New York: Oxford University Press.

Beletz, E. (1990). Professionalization: A license is not enough. In N. L. Chaska (Ed.), *The nursing profession: Turning points* (pp. 16–23). St. Louis, MO: Mosby.

Bixler, G. K., & Bixler, R. W. (1959). The professional status of nursing. *American Journal of Nursing, 59*(8), 1142–1147.

Donabedian, A. (1976). Foreword in M. Phaneuf, Ed., *The nursing audit: Self-regulation in nursing practice* (2nd ed.). Norwalk, CT: Appleton & Lange.

Ehrenreich, B., & English, D. (1973). *Witches, midwives, and nurses: A history of women healers.* New York: The Feminist Press.

Fiesta, J. (1988). *The law and liability: A guide for nurses.* New York: John Wiley & Sons.

Flexner, A. (1915). Is social work a profession? *School Society, 1*(26), 901–911.

Fowler, M. (1990). Social ethics and nursing. In N. L. Chaska (Ed.), *The nursing profession: A time to speak* (pp. 24–31). St. Louis, MO: Mosby.

Gruending, D. L. (1985). Nursing theory: A vehicle of professionalization. *Journal of Advanced Nursing, 10,* 553–558.

Jameton, A. (1984). *Nursing practice: The ethical issues.* Englewood Cliffs, NJ: Prentice-Hall.

Kozier, B., & Erb, G. (1988). *Concepts and issues in nursing practice.* Menlo Park, CA: Addison-Wesley.

Leddy, S., & Pepper, J. M. (1989). *Conceptual bases of professional nursing* (2nd ed.). Philadelphia: Lippincott.

Lyon, B. (1990). Getting back on track; nursing's autonomous scope of practice. In N. L. Chaska (Ed.), *The nursing profession: A time to speak* (pp. 267–274). St. Louis, MO: Mosby.

Murphy, J. D. (1990). The legal perspective of nurse autonomy. In N. L. Chaska (Ed.), *The nursing profession: A time to speak* (pp. 32–39). St. Louis, MO: Mosby.

Nathaniel, A. K. (1994, October). *The promise of nursing.* Keynote speech at the Sophomore Nursing Convocation of Alderson-Broaddus College, Philippi, WV.

Newman, M. A. (1990). Professionalism: Myth or reality. In N. L. Chaska (Ed.), *The nursing profession: A time to speak* (pp. 49–52). St. Louis, MO: Mosby.

Parsons, M. (1986). The profession in a class by itself. *Nursing Outlook, 34,* 270–275.

Sleicher, M. N. (1981, April). Nursing is not a profession. *Nursing & Health Care,* 186–218.

State Scan. (1996, March/April). *Nurse Practitioner World News, 1,* 22–23.

Zschoche, D. (1983). Letter calling for a national nurses' congress. In M. M. Styles, The anatomy of a profession. *Issues in Critical Care, 12,* 570–575. (Original letter December 29, 1972)

CHAPTER 9

Issues Involving Nurses and the System

*These virtues we acquire by first exercising them ...
Whatever we learn to do, we learn by actually doing
it ... By doing just acts we come to be just; by doing
self-controlled acts, we come to be self-controlled; and
by doing brave acts, we become brave....*
(Aristotle, *Nicomachean Ethics*)

OBJECTIVES

After completing this chapter, the reader should be able to:

1. Identify relationships and potential conflicts that nurses face in the professional realm.
2. Characterize the nature of various conflicts.
3. Examine beliefs about the relative strength of various obligations.
4. Identify nurses' primary obligation.
5. Discuss issues related to nurses' relationships with other nurses, institutions, physicians, and subordinates.
6. Discuss issues related to racial discrimination, sexual harassment, and discrimination against persons with disabilities.

INTRODUCTION

Armed with knowledge about the physical, psychological, social, and spiritual realms of nursing care, and proudly possessing a wide range of coveted technical and professional skills, new nurses expectantly enter the workforce. Anticipating respect for their opinions and encouragement to focus their efforts on giving excellent care, nurses soon realize that their attention must be divided between giving patient care and dealing with problems among providers and within the institutional system. This dichotomy can present a confusing and frustrating challenge, forcing nurses to examine conflicting loyalties, question previously held values, make decisions based upon both practical and moral considerations, and test skills of negotiation.

The nurse continually affirms that each person is a moral agent, an autonomous being worthy of respect having the duty to pursue solutions to problems of a moral nature. It is important that solutions consistently honor the uniqueness and value of each person and faithfully adhere to ethical principles. This process requires that nurses critically examine their own particular values and determine an ethically sound method of conflict resolution, even before conflict arises.

Recognizing that the profession of nursing struggles to overcome contextual barriers with cultural and historic overtones, nurses must enter professional relationships with attentiveness and skill. Rather than attempting to offer solutions to a comprehensive list of system-related problems, this chapter provides the opportunity to critically examine selected problems related to nurses' relationships within the health care delivery system. It is suggested that students further prepare themselves to deal with conflict by learning morally sound skills of negotiation and conflict management.

PROBLEM SOLVING IN THE PROFESSIONAL REALM

Practical and ethical dilemmas are part and parcel of everyday nursing practice. Though many dilemmas involve patient centered issues such as self-determination, confidentiality, and the like, nurses frequently encounter troubling moral questions re-lated to professional relationships, conflicting role expectations, and patterns of inter-action within the institutional setting. In the long run, problems of this nature can both directly and indirectly affect patient well-being and are, therefore, important to nurses on a professional level. These problems are often more troubling to the nurse than problems directly involving patients. Recognizing that dilemmas of this sort are fre-quent and troubling, nurses are well advised to consider rational methods of solving problems before they occur. In fact, failing to pursue resolution to conflict results in furthering the harm that such problems create.

Though there is no absolute formula with which to solve conflicts, there are some general guidelines that can be helpful. First, the nurse must maintain attentiveness to personal values and beliefs. Firm and consistent adherence to personal values allows the nurse to approach problems with integrity. Second, the nurse should construct a hierarchy of loyalty or obligation based upon both personal and professional values and beliefs. For example, does the nurse owe a primary obligation to the physician, the institution, or the patient? Third, when conflicts arise, the nurse should determine the nature of the problem. Is the dilemma ethical or practical in nature? Is it a conflict of loyalty, obligation, duty, values, principles, and so forth? Fourth, it is important to thoughtfully consider and weigh alternatives, including the degree of immediate harm or potential for harm as well as the long range effects that could occur with any given alternative. Although some alternatives may seem attractive initially, there may be long term effects that are undesirable. Fifth, it is imperative to develop solutions that recognize each person as an autonomous being, worthy of respect. Utilization of these steps will help the nurse resolve most conflicts in the professional arena.

Attentiveness to Personal Values

Prior to other considerations, nurses must maintain their own personal values and beliefs. This attention to integrity is unrelated to self-interest and predicates action based upon coherent and integrated moral values. Integrity ultimately leads to trustworthiness and the respect of others. Beyond questions of loyalty or duty, the nurse is compelled to maintain integrity in seeking always to do that which is right. This is sometimes referred to as attention to matters of conscience. Childress (1978) distinguishes between **appeals to conscience** and appeals to self-interest or convenience in that appeals to conscience are personal and subjective beliefs, founded on a prior judgment of rightness or wrongness, that are motivated by personal sanction rather than external authority. Institutions, in turn, must recognize the nurse as a person and encourage ethical autonomy. This enables nurses to act in ways that are rational, free from coercion or manipulation, and consistent with personally held values and principles (Benjamin & Curtis, 1986).

In addition to enhancing professional relationships, nurses' integrity is necessary to attaining patient well-being. Gadow (1980) asserts that only those nurses who act out of self-unity can truly assist patients in reaching decisions that express their complex totality as individuals. Integrity is required of nurses, then, since the welfare of patients is their primary obligation.

Obligation

Even nurses in possession of a high level of integrity do not escape a sense of conflicting loyalty on occasion. When this happens, how does the nurse determine the best course of action? One can be prepared by examining **obligations** and devising a rational and consistent hierarchy. An obligation signifies being required to do something by virtue of a moral rule, a duty, or some other binding demand. Some obligations derive from a particular role or relationship (Honderich, 1995). The nurse may believe an obligation is owed to any of the following: the patient for whom care is currently being given, other patients who may be affected in the future by problems that occur in the present, the employer with which the nurse has an implied or expressed contract, the profession of nursing, peers and other coworkers, physicians, the broader society, family, and self.

Obligation to Patients.   As a part of professional nursing practice, nurses have an obligation to patients above all others. Because nurses are professionals, they have a moral obligation to maintain fidelity—they must be faithful to the promises made to society, and thus give priority to meeting the needs of each patient. The International Council of Nurses *Code for Nurses* clearly makes the point that the nurse's primary responsibility is to the patient (see Appendix D). By following established professional codes of ethics and maintaining integrity and loyalty to patients, the nurse also fulfills related obligations to the broader society, the profession, and self.

Obligation to the Institution.   The nurse's secondary obligation is to the institution. By accepting and maintaining terms of employment and payment for services, the nurse has both a legal and moral obligation to the institution. This obligation, however strong, does not suggest that the nurse should jeopardize personal integrity or subordinate loyalty to the patient. To succeed in the age of technological advancement, competition, and litigation, institutions need the services of nurses who express the professional characteristics of autonomy, integrity, and ethically based practice. Conflicts arise when the institution's goals are focused more upon "bottom-line" economics than moral responsibility and patient welfare. Conflict is inevitable when nurses, whose primary loyalty is to the welfare of patients, are employed by institutions that eliminate important programs, employ poorly qualified staff or inadequate numbers of staff, and are otherwise ill-equipped to meet the needs of patients.

 CASE PRESENTATION

When Economy Replaces Excellence

Community Hospital is a large metropolitan hospital that boasted the reputation of maintaining excellent nursing care services for many years. As a result of fierce competition and increasing financial strain, the hospital Board of Trustees decided to affiliate with a large hospital corporation. Television and radio advertisements describing the hospital corporation as having state-of-the-art equipment and services were far from reality. Immediately after the official affiliation was finalized, the hospital began dismissing nurses, cutting back supplies, eliminating unprofitable patient care services, and increasing patient charges. It was soon clear to nurses that patients would no longer receive the excellent nursing care that had been the hallmark of that hospital for many years. Nurses who remained on staff were faced with a changing environment that was no longer patient centered, did not encourage autonomous nursing practice, and fostered ethical and practical dilemmas related to "bottom-line" orientation. Many felt trapped because of a shrinking job market and years of investment in the hospital retirement program. They also felt powerless to change impersonal policies that were created by faceless bureaucrats hundreds of miles away.

Think About It

How Do Nurses Respond to Bottom-Line Economics?

- What kinds of dilemmas are likely to occur in this situation?
- Recognizing that a nurse's primary responsibility is to patients, how does the new hospital arrangement affect the nurse-patient relationship?
- Can nursing practice maintain a patient-centered, ethically sensitive focus in this type of setting? Discuss your thinking.
- What alternative solutions to potential problems faced by nurses in this situation can you suggest?

Determine Nature of the Problem

It is important that the nurse is able to clearly determine the nature of the problem. Is this a problem of a practical or ethical nature? Ethical considerations should carry more weight than matters of self-interest, though, clearly, nurses owe some consideration to their own needs. For example, with changing patient demographics and increasing hospital bed vacancies, nurses face being asked to "float" to unfamiliar settings. This practice redistributes the workload and offers the promise of improved nursing care. However, nurses frequently object to the prospect of being asked to float. Nurses complain, "I've never worked there; I would be unsafe to practice in that setting!" They are tempted to refuse to float to unfamiliar settings. These nurses are faced with a moral dilemma. Recall that the nurse has obligations to both ensure the welfare of the patient and meet the needs of the institution. In either case—in assigning a nurse to float or in accepting the assignment—one must be guided by the principles of nonmaleficence and beneficence: the actions that the nurse is expected to perform must be relatively certain to do good and do no harm. In that regard, neither the nurse, the patient, nor the institution will benefit from requiring a nurse to perform tasks for which there is no preparation. To do so would be unethical. The ANA *Code for Nurses with Interpretive Statements* is very specific about the nurse's duties in situations of this sort:

> If the nurse concludes that he or she lacks competence or is inadequately prepared to carry out a specific function, the nurse has the responsibility to refuse that work and to seek alternative sources of care based on concern for the client's welfare. In that refusal, both the client and the nurse are protected. (1985, p. 11)

Nevertheless, it could also be said that to refuse an assignment is unethical on a number of levels. The nurse must not abandon patients in need of care. If there is no one else available to care for the patients, the nurse is obligated to give care, albeit only the type of care for which the nurse is prepared and competent. For example, nurses temporarily assigned to specialty units can be asked to give basic, supportive nursing care but should not be asked to perform technical tasks for which they are unprepared. To do so is both ethically wrong and legally risky. In the same regard, nurses should not attempt tasks for which they are not prepared: to do so is to compromise fidelity. Nurses should not, however, refuse to accept float assignments simply because there is a fear of the unknown, because familiarity is comfortable, or for other self-interested reasons.

CASE PRESENTATION

Facing a Dilemma in the Newborn Nursery

Maggie Corin is a nurse employed in the newborn nursery of a small hospital. She is working toward completing her bachelor's degree and has an important exam at 4:30 P.M. Though she is scheduled to leave work at 3:00 P.M., by 4:00 P.M. the nurse from the next shift has not yet arrived. There is an LPN who is capable of caring for the newborns, but hospital policy requires the presence of an RN in the unit at all times. The supervisor is unable to give her any assistance. All the babies are quiet; she expects the evening shift RN to arrive soon and feels the LPN can handle the nursery for a short time. Maggie is torn between honoring her duty to patients versus leaving to take her exam.

Think About It

What Should the Nurse Do?

- Is this a practical or an ethical dilemma? What factors make this either a practical or an ethical dilemma?
- Do you think Maggie's duty to stay outweighs her obligation to take the exam?
- What is the harm that could occur if she leaves before the evening shift RN arrives?
- What is the harm that could occur if she stays and misses her exam?

The situation in the previous example constitutes a practical dilemma. Moral and nonmoral claims are in conflict. Based upon the principles of beneficence, nonmaleficence, and fidelity, Maggie has a moral obligation to the patients committed to her and to the institution for which she works. On the other hand, her obligation to attend class is a matter of self-interest and is not based upon moral principle. There is the potential for harm to the newborns if she leaves the unit inappropriately staffed. An emergency could arise for which the LPN is not prepared. Possibly the evening shift RN will not arrive at all. If Maggie utilizes Kant's moral imperative—one should do only that which could become a rule for all people—a decision to leave the unit unattended by an RN would be untenable. By leaving, she would create a situation that should not become a rule for all nurses in all situations. A rule suggesting that all nurses should leave patients improperly attended would harm many patients in the future and as a result would harm society's faith in the profession of nursing. Based upon a comparison of moral versus practical considerations and the potential harm that could result if Maggie left the unit improperly attended, it seems clear that she should not leave. This is not meant to imply that nurses should always subjugate personal needs to patient or institutional ones. Staying at work later than scheduled as a result of an occasional, unpredictable circumstance is one thing; being required to stay repeatedly is something entirely different.

NURSES' RELATIONSHIPS WITH INSTITUTIONS

Nurses enter the workforce with very different perceptions than those held by employing institutions. Having learned that autonomy and accountability are valuable components of the nursing role, nurses believe they owe primary loyalty to patients. They also expect that their beliefs will be honored and that their opinions and knowledge will be respected. Hospitals and other health care institutions, on the other hand, tend to be sharply hierarchical and bureaucratic institutions that expect nurses' and other subordinates' primary loyalty to be toward the institution (Jameton, 1984). In the only country that openly calls the health care delivery system an industry, institutions' motives sometimes seem to be geared more toward profit and control than compassion and care (Kritek, 1994). Moreover, institutions expect nurses' actions to be directed toward attaining the goals of the system: goals that focus strongly upon ensuring the well-being of the institution itself and sustaining patterns of power and control. Difficulties arise when there is conflict between the goals of nurses and patients and those of the institution.

Problems arise, in part, because the institution's demands for loyalty are often inequitable (Jameton, 1984). Though requiring employees to accede to certain requests, institutions rarely reciprocate with similar loyalty to nurses. For example, due to budget constraints, most institutions are fairly rigid about nurses' work hours. Nurses are expected to arrive ready to begin and complete work according to a set schedule. They are sometimes directed to complete more work than can reasonably be expected in that time period. Nurses, loyal to the institution and to the duty that they feel toward the patients in their care, are often willing to skip meals and breaks and complete work after "clocking out." In essence these practices, though very stressful for nurses, are financially appealing to institutions.

Nurses need to balance professional obligation and the ideal of compassionate service with basic personal commitments. The ANA *Code for Nurses* (1985) supports nurses' professional role, which may include working overtime and attending meetings on one's own time and expense in order to improve patient care or to establish and maintain conditions of employment conducive to high quality nursing care. However, consistently repeated, self-sacrificing, altruistic behavior on the part of nurses is self-defeating and does not establish conditions of employment conducive to high quality nursing care. It tends to support and perpetuate a flawed system—as long as nurses continue to work selflessly, the system (rather than the patient) benefits. Nurses willing to work for free devalue the work of nurses and perpetuate the expectation that this type of one-sided self-sacrifice will continue. Of course, on rare occasion this sort of problem can occur in any institution, but when nurses repeatedly accept workloads that are unreasonable, they become complicit in continuing the wrongs. Though working extra appears to fulfill both professional obligations and the ideal of compassionate service, it "may only superficially meet obligations to clients and may actually lead to a less desirable state of affairs not only for nursing colleagues and the nursing profession, but ultimately for clients" (Benjamin & Curtis, 1986, p. 137). In the long run, this type of behavior is harmful to both patients and nurses. Jameton (1984) says:

> A basic choice is forced on those who work in hospitals by the existence of prevalent and systematic problems in health care. If one fails to resist exploitation, incompetence, and corrupt practices, one becomes responsible for them. If one resists them, one enters into conflict with conventional conceptions of behavior for employees and thereby risks reprisals. One has to choose between complicity and self-sacrifice. . . . (p. 289)

Jameton's term *self-sacrifice* is related to the willingness of some nurses to risk reprisals for resisting exploitation in the health care system. He does not suggest that nurses sacrifice all issues of self-interest in favor of institutional interests.

In some instances, nurses base the motivation for altruism on misguided beliefs about duty. Some believe that altruism is necessary to fulfill their duty to patients. Though many philosophers consider altruism and sacrifice a virtue, Ayn Rand (1996) suggested that altruism has a dehumanizing effect. Rand believed that those who are altruistic have a nightmare view of existence—believing that people are trapped in a malevolent universe. Using the term *self-sacrifice* in a fashion nearly opposite that of Jameton, Rand viewed a persistent willingness to sacrifice as flowing from poor self-esteem and inappropriate priority-setting. Moreover, she believed that those with poor self-esteem have difficulty valuing others. Because genuine regard is partially a product of sympathy (imagining oneself in the situation of another), one must value oneself in order to value others. Additionally, nurses who repeatedly sacrifice for the good of an institutional system fail to assume the power to change the wrongs that are committed.

 CASE PRESENTATION

When Patients Suffer from Lack of Nursing Care

Tim, an RN, works weekends on the skilled nursing unit of a small rural hospital. Recently purchased by a large corporation, the hospital was forced to dismiss nearly one-third of the staff of the skilled nursing unit. Lately, when Tim comes to work, he feels totally overwhelmed. Although he always considered himself efficient, Tim is distressed because he rarely has enough time to complete his work. He knows that many of the patients suffer because of lack of attention. Those who are bedfast are not turned on a regular schedule, they often wait for assistance with eating until their food is cold, and medications are rarely given on time. Suffering from expressive aphasia and hemiplegia secondary to a CVA, Mrs.

Wallace was admitted to the skilled nursing unit after two weeks in the intensive care unit. Mrs. Wallace has been on the skilled nursing unit for three weeks when her daughter, Nina, notices a large reddened area surrounding a small gray ulcer over her mother's coccyx. Concerned, Nina asks Tim what caused this problem. Even though Mrs. Wallace's nursing care plan calls for attention to activity including frequent turning and sitting in a chair twice daily, Tim suspects that this was not consistently done the previous week. He recognizes that the reddened area is the beginning of a large pressure ulcer, a problem that might have been prevented with proper attention to activity and good nutrition. Tim hesitates to tell Nina that the problem is a potentially serious one that might have been prevented by good nursing care measures. He believes she has a right to know but is hesitant to implicate himself or the other nurses, and he is afraid that he will lose his job if he whistle-blows.

Think About It

How Do Nurses Make Decisions When Loyalties Conflict?

- What are the ethical principles implicit in this situation?
- What are Tim's conflicting loyalties?
- The staff on the unit is efficient and hard-working—skipping lunch and staying overtime to complete their work. Do you believe the staff is responsible for the apparently poor nursing care that Mrs. Wallace is getting?
- Do you believe Tim should tell Nina the truth about the pressure sore?
- Should Tim risk losing his job by whistle-blowing?
- Is this an ethical or practical dilemma?
- What harm can result from either option?
- What would you do?

The previous case presentation is another example of a practical dilemma. The conflict that Tim is experiencing is between the principle of beneficence (the desire to do good for the patient) and a sense of loyalty to the institution or the other nurses with whom he works. There may also be an element of self-interest—Tim may not want to be implicated in the harm that the patients are experiencing as a result of the staff cutbacks. Tim's primary loyalty is owed to the patients—Mrs. Wallace, other patients suffering from the shortage of staff, and future patients who could be harmed by perpetuation of the problem. There are strong arguments that he should act to correct the situation. He may choose to take any number of actions: he can work through the administrative hierarchy to improve staffing; he can answer Nina's questions honestly; though his job will certainly be jeopardized, he can inform the media of the problems that were created by the drastic staffing shortages. In any case, if Tim fails to act to solve the problem, he will be complicit in its perpetuation and the subsequent harm to patients.

Another example related to institutions' inequitable demands for loyalty is seen in the customary practice of requiring nurses to complete incident reports. In an effort to prevent litigation, institutions discourage nurses from talking to patients about mistakes that have been made. They much prefer that nurses file incident reports. These documents, geared toward institutional goals, are filed and kept for use in the event the hospital needs a legal defense, in firing or disciplining workers, or in reorganizing services to prevent future incidents (Jameton, 1984). Thus, patient-centered goals based upon the principles of autonomy, fidelity, veracity, and respect for persons are subordinated to institutional subgoals of employee control and risk management.

Nurses' loyalty to the institution is an important mode of control. Without loyalty, administrators cannot manage institutions (Jameton, 1984). For this reason supervisors and administrators react negatively to egalitarian cooperation and loyalty among staff. The ensuing perception of nonsupportive supervisors is a contributing factor for job stress and dissatisfaction (Moore, Kuhrik, Kuhrik, & Katz, 1996). In the end this can be harmful to nurses and patients alike. Jameton says, "Where institutions as a whole fail to serve patients well, this demand for loyalty can interfere with the nurses' expressions of loyalty to nurses and patients" (1984, p. 121).

NURSES' RELATIONSHIPS WITH OTHER NURSES

In close proximity, nurses work together day in and day out. No other profession is so intimately connected with the essence of life. The knowledge gained from the intimate experiences of birth, illness, life, and death are both powerful and mysterious. Nurses are connected to each other and set apart from others: connected by common experience, language, and knowledge; set apart through professional mystique. Nurses work closely together, identify with each other, and supervise or are supervised by other nurses. The practice of one affects that of others.

Loyalty is a natural product of long-term acquaintance and close working relationships. Some view loyalty among members as a distinguishing characteristic of a profession. Jameton (1984) defines loyalty as:

> showing sympathy, care, and reciprocity to those with whom we appropriately identify; working closely with others toward shared goals; keeping promises; making mutual concerns a priority; sacrificing personal interests to the relationship; and giving attention to these over a substantial period of time. It supports showing respect for persons. And it resolves potential conflicts in autonomy by making values and goals that I see as my own more like values and goals of those who work with me. (p. 118)

Promoting faithfulness and commitment, loyalty is very limited and exclusive in its scope. Though normally viewed as admirable, loyalty is seldom regarded as a cardinal virtue because of the potential for fanaticism and blind injustice (Honderich, 1995).

In practical matters, loyalty is a productive virtue. It enhances unity, strength, and power. Facing bureaucratic, economic, and political forces, nurses' loyalty to each other and to the profession adds strength to the voice calling for improved patient care, public welfare, nursing autonomy, and optimum employment conditions.

 CASE PRESENTATION

Nurses' Loyalty to the Profession

A few years ago, politically active nurses in a small state lobbied for a bill mandating nurse representation on government bodies charged with considering health related issues. Positions included membership on committees, task forces, advisory panels, and so forth. There was also a stipulation that required each public hospital to include one nurse on its governing board. As the largest group of health care professionals, nurses believed their knowledge and experience would be a welcome addition. Though there was strong and unified nursing support, the bill was fiercely opposed by both the state hospital association and individual hospitals. When public hearings were held, the politically active nurses found themselves testifying for the bill in opposition to commanding and articulate nurse administrators. Representing individual hospitals, nurse administrators cited everything from nurses' lack of economic expertise to a gossipy tendency to spill industry secrets as reasons to oppose nurse members on hospital governing boards. The bill failed.

 Think About It

Examining Differences in Loyalty

- Can you think of moral justification for the diverse positions of nurses?
- To whom is each group of nurses loyal?
- How would you characterize each group's stance in relation to the professionalization of nursing?
- How would you account for the diverse positions of the nurses?

While having the potential to strengthen the profession of nursing and improve the welfare of patients, loyalty among nurses can also be harmful. Misguided or fanatical loyalty can lead to a confused sense of obligation. Though nurses' primary obligation is to patients, those who are overly loyal to other nurses might act in ways that are harmful to patients' health status. For example, a nurse having blind loyalty to another might cover up a coworker's incompetent practice, illegal drug use, or other actions that have the potential to harm present or future patients. For this reason nurses must be careful to maintain objectivity in balancing loyalty to nurses and the profession against the obligation owed to patients.

NURSES' RELATIONSHIPS WITH PHYSICIANS

Nurses' relationships with physicians are an important factor in the quality of the care that is given to patients. Ideally, the work of nurses and physicians should be complementary and synergistic. Because both professions hold claim to the primary goal of patient well-being, one would expect a sense of collegiality and collaboration between nurses and physicians. When this type of relationship exists, it is rewarding and productive. When there is conflict between nurses and physicians, the relationship is stressful and damaging to nurses, physicians, and patients alike. Because nurses and physicians work in close proximity, conflict that occurs between them is a strong contributor to the lack of satisfaction of nurses.

Nurse-physician relationships have generally reflected the prevailing gender roles in society. For centuries these roles were well defined. The traditional nurse was expected to obey the physician, much as the wife was expected to obey her husband. Physicians demanded obedience, and nurses hesitated to disagree with physicians even if there was good reason to do so. Unfortunately, these "time-worn attitudes" linger in both professions (Benjamin & Curtis, 1986, p. 86).

Given the bureaucratic nature of most health care institutions, particularly hospitals, the relationship between physicians and nurses today is complex and peculiar. Generally, nurses are employees of the institutions while physicians are independent practitioners who have the privilege of institutional practice. Physicians, who are not employees of the institutions, have no formal chain-of-command relationship with the nurses who care for their patients. Curtin and Flaherty (1982) write, "This tradition of self-employed 'guest practitioners' in health care institutions having so much power over the large groups of 'full-time employees' of the institutions defies explanation, but it is a fact of life in health care" (p. 144). Though they issue orders directly to nurses, physicians are not employed by, subordinate to, or even responsible to the institutional administration. These dual lines of authority are confusing and have the potential to severely limit the autonomous decision making role of the nurse (Benjamin & Curtis, 1986, p. 82). Because most nurses are employees with either expressed or implied contracts with institutions, they have an obligation to perform the tasks required by the institutions. One of the major tasks that most institutions require of nurses is the implementation of physicians' orders. When nurses question or disagree with physicians, they may feel distressed, believing they are being disloyal to both the physician and the institution.

Another contributor to conflict in the nurse-physician relationship is the rapid advent of advanced practice nursing. Having an expanded knowledge base and a scope of practice that includes many functions once the sole domain of physicians, advanced practice nursing can contribute to the tensions that exist between nurses and physicians. The outmoded tradition of the nurse who obeys the physician is in direct conflict with the autonomous nurse who thinks independently, makes nursing diagnoses, and implements independent nursing actions (Benjamin & Curtis, 1986).

What actions should be taken by the nurse who questions or disagrees with an order or action of a physician? The nurse must remember that the primary obligation is owed the patient, not the physician. Nurses are autonomous practitioners. They have the knowledge and experience, and the legal and ethical responsibility, to make independent judgments related to carrying out physicians' orders. If medical care constitutes incompetent, unethical, or illegal practice, the nurse is clearly obligated to disobey orders (American Nurses Association, 1985). When deciding what course to take in situations in which nurses disagree with physicians' orders, Benjamin and Curtis (1986) suggest that nurses apply the test of the **spectrum of urgency.** At one end of this spectrum are problems that are minor and may be solved at a leisurely pace. At the other end are problems that are urgent and require quick solutions and immediate actions. The low-urgency end of the spectrum includes situations in which there is little risk of serious harm or significant time available to examine all aspects of the situation. The high-urgency end of the spectrum consists of emergencies in which lifesaving actions must be carried out at once. Nurses may have time to discuss and negotiate satisfactory solutions to problems at the low-urgency end of the spectrum. Problems at the high-urgency end of the spectrum require quick, sometimes drastic action.

 CASE PRESENTATION

Making a Decision in an Urgent Situation

Marta is night shift charge nurse in the emergency department. She has advanced certification and twenty-five years of experience. Marta works well with the other members of the emergency room staff and is comfortable and efficient in situations of extreme urgency. The emergency department in which she works is usually staffed by board certified emergency physicians. Because one of the regular physicians recently moved to another state, there has been a series of physicians with various preparation and ability moonlighting in the department, particularly on night shift. During an unusually busy shift, an ambulance arrives with a middle-aged man having severe chest pain and dyspnea. His condition quickly deteriorates, and after a few minutes he experiences cardiac and respiratory arrest. The physician on duty, Dr. Andrews, is a family practice physician moonlighting after his regular shift at a local community health center. Marta perceives Dr. Andrews as nervous and hesitant. During the first phase of the "code," Dr. Andrews seems uncertain of every detail. As the nurse in charge, Marta begins instituting a seldom used protocol that was developed for use in the event that the nurses are faced with a cardiac arrest when no physician is present. All the nurses are trained in intubation techniques, but hospital policy prohibits their performing that particular procedure. Marta suggests to Dr. Andrews that he intubate the patient. After several clumsy attempts, Dr. Andrews angrily orders Marta to call an anesthesiologist at home to come and intubate the patient. Marta realizes that the patient's chances of survival are best if he is intubated quickly. She asks the unit clerk to call the anesthesiologist. Over his angry objections, Marta removes the laryngoscope and endotracheal tube from Dr. Andrews's trembling hands and proceeds to quickly and successfully intubate the patient. The patient responds to resuscitation attempts and is discharged five days later.

Think About It

Was Marta's Decision Correct?

- What is your immediate response to the situation in which Marta finds herself?
- Where would you place this situation on the "spectrum of urgency"?
- What are the arguments in favor of Marta's actions?
- What are the arguments in favor of Marta's following Dr. Andrews's orders?
- Do you consider Marta's actions to be based upon ethical principle?
- Did Marta place herself at risk of reprisal or legal action?
- What would you have done?

Nurses are charged with making thoughtful, fair, and knowledgeable decisions in relation to questioning physicians' orders, being careful to consider the overall harm that can result from any given action. Recognizing that the physician's goal, like that of the nurse, is the welfare of the patient, the nurse must be mature and objective when questioning orders. Nurses have an ethical obligation to protect the patient from medical incompetence. Nevertheless, they must be careful in this regard, keeping in mind the overall harm that can result from the practice of constantly and inappropriately questioning insignificant aspects of physicians' orders.

NURSES' RELATIONSHIPS WITH SUBORDINATES

While maintaining an awareness of the primary obligation owed to patients, nurses must be sensitive to those who work beside them. Each person is a moral agent and must be recognized as worthy of dignity and respect. As the coordinator of patient care, the professional nurse is accountable for the quality of nursing care rendered to patients. This accountability includes supervision, delegation of nursing care functions, and disciplining of other health care providers. The inherent practical, moral, and legal implications of these functions are facets of the role of professional nurse that must be undertaken with sensitivity and respect.

The structure of health care delivery in some institutional settings renders the professional nurse responsible for delegating a number of nursing functions to subordinate staff members. The nurse has a moral obligation to ensure that each patient receives excellent nursing care, to respect the value of each individual, and "to establish and maintain conditions of employment conducive to high quality nursing care" (ANA, 1985). Following is an excerpt from the *Code for Nurses with Interpretive Statements* regarding the nurse and delegation of nursing activities:

Inasmuch as the nurse is accountable for the quality of nursing care rendered to clients, nurses are accountable for the delegation of nursing care activities to other health workers. Therefore, the nurse must assess individual competency in assigning selected components of nursing care to other nursing service personnel. The nurse should not delegate to any member of the nursing team a function for which that person is not prepared or qualified. Employer policies or directives do not relieve the nurse of accountability for making judgments about the delegation of nursing care activities. (ANA, 1985, p. 11)

As the coordinator of patient care, the nurse is accountable for all nursing care that patients receive, whether from the nurse or subordinates.

In addition to delegation, the supervisory role of professional nurses occasionally includes disciplining of subordinates. Disciplining is a difficult task that must be done with insight, respect, compassion, and logic. The nurse must be keenly aware of the effect of disciplinary action upon others and must focus on the intended goal. The traditional methods of discipline, such as punishment and chastisement, are damaging to the spirit and counterproductive in practice. Quoting the great teacher, Maria Montessori, Leah Curtin (1996) writes, "'Our aim is to discipline for activity, for work, for good; not for immobility, not for passivity, not for obedience'" (p. 51). Curtin suggests that the most meaningful method is self-discipline, which corrects the problem, strengthens the character of the worker, and improves performance. She defines self-discipline as a process by which the rules are internalized and become a part of the individual's personality. This process is possible only if the person knows the rules, understands their purpose, and agrees that they deserve compliance. To achieve this result the nurse must model the expected standard daily and have few rules—all of which are applied consistently, change infrequently, and apply equally to all personnel. The nurse has a moral obligation, to both patients and personnel, to uphold rules that protect the health or safety of patients, other employees, the institution, and oneself as leader (Curtin, 1996, p. 51).

DISCRIMINATION AND HARASSMENT

Claims of discrimination or harassment in the workplace are becoming more frequent. In fact, millions of Americans have experienced employment discrimination. Swart, Wendt, and Slonaker (1996) report that twenty-seven percent of workers believe they have experienced discrimination on the job. Discrimination is ethically prohibited. Because this prohibition entails treating others fairly and equitably, the ethical principle of justice is a key point when discussing issues of discrimination. In their 1991 position statement on human rights, the ANA wrote, "Actions that are termed 'unjust' are of three basic types: first, discrimination or arbitrarily unequal treatment in legislating, administering, or enforcing rules; second, exploitation, taking advantage of another person to gain unfairly; and third, making false or derogatory statements about people or their work that aren't fair" (p. 1). Discrimination is also legally prohibited. The *Bill of Rights* of the *United States Constitution*, the Civil Rights Act of 1964, the Americans with

Disabilities Act of 1990 (ADA), and the Civil Rights Act of 1991 provide legal protection against discrimination in the workplace.

Racial Discrimination

The Civil Rights Act of 1964 made it unlawful for an employer to fail or refuse to hire or to discharge any individual, or to otherwise discriminate against any individual, because of the person's race, color, religion, sex, or national origin. Unlawful acts include discrimination in terms of compensation or payment, conditions of employment, or privileges of employment. Considered one of America's strongest civil rights laws, the Civil Rights Act of 1964 primarily protects the rights of African-Americans and other minorities. Attempting to correct a long tradition of racial discrimination, this act ensures that minorities receive fair and equal treatment from government, other persons, and private groups, including schools and employers. Enforced by the Equal Employment Opportunity Commission (EEOC), the act also specifically forbids discrimination by any program that receives money from the federal government.

The Civil Rights Act of 1964 enjoins employers to provide equal employment opportunities to individuals from the initial recruitment or application process through termination of employment. When considering claims of discriminatory practices, the legal system looks at two discriminatory outcomes—disparate treatment and disparate impact. *Disparate treatment* occurs when an individual is treated differently by a superior or by organizational policy. For example, if a supervisor passes over all Hispanic nurses who apply for promotion, regardless of their qualifications or abilities, disparate treatment exists. *Disparate impact* occurs when employers consistently apply policies that appear to be fair to all employees but actually adversely affect one group. For example, job interviews that ask questions about illegal drug use could inadvertently have an adverse impact on a group that is more statistically likely to have used illegal drugs (Swart, Wendt, & Slonaker, 1996).

Because stereotypes are slow to change, it can be very difficult for nonmajority group members to enter and succeed in any occupational group. Though the landmark civil rights legislation was passed decades ago, there is some indication that discrimination continues to exist in the health care system. Swart, Wendt, and Slonaker (1996) studied a group of nurses who had filed discrimination claims. Among nurses reporting discrimination, forty-seven percent based their claims on race discrimination.

Another source of race discrimination may be a lack of recruitment and retention of minority nursing students. According to Dowell (1996), student, faculty, and administrative populations in many schools of nursing still reflect uniformity and homogeneity. Citing several studies, Dowell identifies barriers to recruitment of minority groups, including the following: lack of full scholarships, scarcity of minority groups in certain geographic areas, lack of effective minority recruitment strategies, a negative attitude from administrators, and a lack of minority role models.

Discrimination Against Persons with Disabilities

The Americans with Disabilities Act of 1990 (ADA) was signed into law on July 26, 1990. Seen by some as the most significant piece of legislation since the Civil Rights Act of 1964, this act provides comprehensive protection to Americans with disabilities. Challenged to combine the legal concepts of disability and equality, the aim of Congress in drafting this legislation was to ensure equality for the disabled without creating "undue" hardships on employers (Guido, 1997). The ADA considers one to have a covered *disability* if there is record of physical or mental disability that causes an impairment substantially limiting one or more of the major life enjoyments of the person, and if the person actually has such an impairment. *Major life enjoyments* include such activities as the average person can perform with little or no difficulty, such as caring for oneself, performing manual tasks, walking, seeing, hearing, speaking, learning, and working. A *physical impairment* includes any physiologic disorder or condition, cosmetic disfigurement, or anatomical loss affecting any body system. A *mental impairment* includes any mental or psychological disorder such as mental retardation, organic brain syndrome, emotional or mental illness, and learning disabilities. Mental or psychological conditions that result from such conditions as diabetes, cancer, AIDS, alcoholism, and drug abuse qualify under this definition (Guido, 1997).

Related to the Civil Rights Act of 1964, the ADA has several provisions. The act ensures that people with disabilities are not excluded from job opportunities or adversely affected in other aspects of employment unless they are unqualified or unable to perform the job. This protection extends to application, salary, promotion, discharge, transfer, and all other aspects of work. The ADA prohibits the practice of requiring medical examinations before employment except for drug testing, which may be performed. Medical examinations may be done only after a job offer has been extended. Employers may question individuals about their educational qualifications, experience, and their ability to perform the job safely with or without accommodation. To avoid the suggestion of discrimination, the prospective employer may not ask questions about disabilities, past medical problems, or previous workers' compensation claims. Upon request from disabled employees, employers must make necessary physical accommodations to the workplace, such as wheelchair accessibility, telephone systems for the hearing impaired, and so forth, but may be exempted from hiring persons with disabilities if the necessary accommodations cause *undue hardship* because they are extremely expensive or difficult to implement. The employer must have investigated the required accommodations and offer data proving the hardship. Undue hardship is based on cost, numbers of employees, and type of business (Guido, 1997).

The ADA does not require employers to hire individuals with disabilities. It demands, however, that employers base employment decisions solely upon job qualifications and ability, without regard to physical or mental disabilities. It also protects employers from financial ruin in the case of undue hardship related to making workplace accommodations for disabled persons.

Sexual Harassment and Discrimination

Sexual discrimination and harassment is not new in nursing. In the nineteenth century certain occupations were redefined as feminine. Nursing and teaching, for example, became accepted as feminine lines of work, and women in these occupational groups were seen and treated as "ladies." Florence Nightingale struggled with this identity; "In effect, she violated the gender norms of the day and threatened male power. Very much aware of her threat to the men, she continually emphasized that she was doing only what a proper lady should do—extending the role by accepting what society said women were especially qualified to do" (Bullough, 1990, p. 6). While allowing women to function as nurses, this attitude sustained the social order. Defined today as sexual harassment, there was an effort to sustain male power by treating women as sexual objects and inferiors.

According to Friedman (1992), "sexual harassment refers to conduct, typically experienced as offensive in nature, in which unwanted sexual advances are made in the context of a relationship of unequal power or authority" (p. 9). Recognizing sexual harassment as a significant problem, federal and state courts have struggled with the issue for the past several decades. In October of 1991, the problem was brought to the attention of the public with the Senate confirmation hearings of Supreme Court nominee Clarence Thomas. A direct result of these hearings, the Civil Rights Act of 1991 was signed into law on November 21, 1991. This act defines sexual harassment and identifies two categories of the offense—quid pro quo sexual harassment, and hostile work environment sexual harassment.

When submission to or rejection of the sexual conduct of an individual is used as a basis for employment decisions, *quid pro quo sexual harassment* is said to occur. There are four requirements to prove quid pro quo sexual harassment. The employee must show first that there was unwelcome harassment in the form of sexual advances or requests for sexual favors; second, that the harassment was based on sex; and third, that submission to the unwelcome sexual advances was required for receiving job benefits or that refusal to submit to the advances resulted in job detriment. Fourth, the individual who claims to be a victim of sexual harassment must be a member of a group that is lower on the chain of command than the person making the unwelcome advances. In quid pro quo harassment suits, employers are liable for the conduct of supervisory personnel (Guido, 1997).

Hostile work environment sexual harassment occurs when the employee is subjected to sexual innuendos, remarks, and physical acts that are so offensive as to create an abusive work environment. The two factors that must be shown in claims of hostile work environment are that the harassment unreasonably interfered with work and that the harassment would affect a reasonable person's work. The employer is only liable in such an instance when it can be shown that there was knowledge of the harassment. In hostile work environment sexual harassment cases, it is not necessary that the conduct be directed toward the individual who files the complaint, merely that the employee's psychological well-being was affected because the conduct was observed or known. This can occur, for example, with the unwanted posting of pornographic pictures or cartoons, sexually explicit comments or jokes, or sexual propositions. It is not necessary to prove that terms of employment are attached to this type of sexual harassment (Guido, 1997).

Although ninety percent of sexual harassment claims are filed by women (Wolfe, 1996), men can also be the object of real or perceived sexual harassment or discrimination. Kelly, Shoemaker, and Steele (1996) discuss the problem of underrepresentation of men in schools of nursing. Male student nurses in the study reported that they experienced a fear of being perceived as unmanly, felt isolated, and were excluded from activities and discussions. In addition to the same type of sexual discrimination experienced by women, there are potential areas for sexual discrimination targeted specifically against men. These might involve such behaviors as stereotyping all male nurses as being gay or as assigning an inequitable portion of tough patients to men because of perceived physical stamina or strength.

SUMMARY

In the professional realm, nurses are faced with the dichotomy of striving to meet their primary obligation to patients while dealing with problems among providers and within the institutional system. Nurses must be prepared to examine personal beliefs, prioritize obligations, and devise morally sound solutions to problems. Solutions must reflect an overall respect for persons and recognize the moral agency of individuals. Nurses are guided in this endeavor by personal values and beliefs and by professional codes of ethics.

CHAPTER HIGHLIGHTS

- As a moral agent each person has the duty to pursue solutions to moral problems.
- Solutions to practical and ethical problems in the professional realm must be sensitive to personal values and beliefs.
- Nurses must be able to identify and prioritize conflicting obligations.
- It is important for nurses to determine the nature of conflicts in the professional realm.
- Problem resolution requires thoughtful consideration and weighing of alternative solutions.
- In solving problems, nurses must recognize that each person is an autonomous being, worthy of respect.
- Nurses must seek solutions to moral problems related to conflicting role expectations in the institutional setting.
- Nurses must seek solutions to moral and practical problems related to relationships among nurses, physicians, and subordinates.
- Discrimination is prohibited by the ethical principle of justice because it entails claims related to fair and equitable treatment of persons.

DISCUSSION QUESTIONS AND ACTIVITIES

1. Describe potential problems in the professional realm that fall into each of the following categories:

   - Conflicts of obligation
   - Conflicts of principle
   - Practical dilemmas
   - Conflicts of loyalty

2. With your classmates discuss situations that could reasonably occur in the work setting that would constitute an appeal to conscience.

3. Review the ANA *Code for Nurses with Interpretive Statements*. List each statement that applies to problems related to nurses' relationships with other professionals. Discuss the practical application of each of these statements.

4. Interview nurses who have been in practice one year or less. Ask them to compare their expectations of the work environment with the reality that they faced upon graduation.

5. Discuss the conflict that results as shrinking institutional budgets require cutbacks in nursing staff.

6. List the positive and negative aspects of loyalty. Do you feel loyalty is a virtue?

7. Describe the ideal professional relationships that can occur between nurses and physicians.

8. Role-play a situation in which a nurse is sensitive and respectful in disciplining a subordinate—focusing on the goal of improving performance rather than punishing.

9. Discuss racial discrimination, discrimination against persons with disabilities, and sexual harassment in terms of ethical principles and legal mandate.

REFERENCES

American Nurses Association. (1985). *Code for nurses with interpretive statements*. Washington, DC: Author.

American Nurses Association. (1991). Philosophical statement on ethics and human rights. Position paper, Kansas City, MO: Author.

Americans with Disabilities Act of 1990, Pub. L. No. 101-336, § 2, 104 Stat. 328 (1991).

Benjamin, M., & Curtis, J. (1986). *Ethics in nursing* (2nd ed.). New York: Oxford University Press.

Bullough, V. (1990). Nightingale, nursing and harassment. *Image: Journal of Nursing Scholarship, 22,* 4–7.

Childress, J. (1978). Appeals to conscience. *Ethics, 89,* 316–321.

Civil Rights Act of 1964, 41 U.S.C.A. § 2000e *et seq.*

Civil Rights Act of 1991, P.L. 102-166, 105 Stat. 1071 (1991).

Curtin, L. (1996). Ethics, discipline and discharge. *Nursing Management, 27*(3), 51–52.

Curtin, L., & Flaherty, M. J. (1982). Nursing ethics: Theories and pragmatics. Bowie, MD: Brady.

Dowell, M. (1996). Issues in recruitment and retention of minority nursing students. *Journal of Nursing Education, 35*(7), 293–297.

Friedman, J. (1992). *Sexual harassment.* Dearfield, FL: Health Communications.

Gadow, S. (1980). Existential advocacy: Philosophical foundation of nursing. In S. F. Spicker and S. Gadow (Eds.), *Nursing: Images and ideals, opening dialogue with the humanities* (pp. 90–91). New York: Springer.

Guido, G. (1997). *Legal issues in nursing* (2nd ed.). Norwalk, CT: Appleton & Lange.

Honderich, T. (Ed.). (1995). *The Oxford companion to philosophy.* New York: Oxford University Press.

Jameton, A. (1984). *Nursing practice: The ethical issues.* Englewood Cliffs, NJ: Prentice-Hall.

Kelly, N., Shoemaker, M., & Steele, T. (1996). The experience of being a male student nurse. *Journal of Nursing Education, 35*(4), 170–174.

Kritek, P. B. (1994). *Negotiating at an uneven table: A practical approach to working with difference and diversity.* San Francisco: Jossey-Bass.

Moore, S., Kuhrik, M., Kuhrik, N., & Katz, B. (1996). Coping with downsizing: Stress, self-esteem and social intimacy. *Nursing Management, 27*(3), 28–30.

Rand, A. (1996). The ethics of emergencies. In J. Feinberg (Ed.), *Reason and responsibility: Readings in some basic problems of philosophy* (9th ed., pp. 541–545). Belmont, CA: Wadsworth.

Swart, J., Wendt, A., Slonaker, W. (1996). Employment discrimination experiences of registered nurses. *JONA, 26,* pp. 37–43.

Wolfe, S. (1996). If you're sexually harassed. *RN 5*(2), 61–64.

CHAPTER 10

Practice Issues Related to Technology

There is an appointed time for everything,
and a time for every affair under the heavens.
(Ecclesiastes 3:1)

OBJECTIVES

After completing this chapter, the reader should be able to:

1. Discuss the impact of technology on nursing and health care.
2. Apply beneficence and nonmaleficence to decisions about technology.
3. Discuss issues and dilemmas related to current technology and to life-sustaining interventions.
4. Relate the concept of medical futility to health care decisions.
5. Relate economics to decisions regarding health technology.
6. Discuss considerations in decisions about cardiopulmonary resuscitation and artificial sources of nutrition for patients.
7. Describe legal issues associated with health care technology.
8. Discuss issues and dilemmas associated with technologies affecting reproduction, genetics, and organ transplantation.
9. Describe nursing considerations for patient care in the midst of technology.

INTRODUCTION

Nursing care is inextricably intertwined with ever expanding advances of scientific knowledge and technology. Few would deny the benefits of medical advances, often referred to in terms such as *wonders* or *miracles*. However, the many benefits brought to the health care arena by technology are often accompanied by serious dilemmas for both practitioners and patients. Technology brings to the fore many questions related to issues of living and dying, and the changing definitions of both that are brought on by scientific advances. Dilemmas include availability of technologies, what patient situations warrant the use of available technologies, and who decides when to initiate and when to withdraw particular interventions. Additionally, nurses must be concerned about the amount of nursing energy and attention that technology requires. As much as we say that nursing focuses on holistic caring for the patient, nurses are faced with increasing demands to focus attention to technology rather than on their patients.

This chapter focuses on common issues related to technology encountered in today's health care settings. Issues of technology, patient self-determination, and economics are intertwined. It is important that nurses who are directly involved in dilemmas, and those who are more on the periphery, are aware of considerations regarding the effect of technology on patient care. These considerations include values, attitudes, communication, and attention to the humanistic caring role. The term *technology* includes the vast range of scientific advances that affect health and health care. Changing technologies bring with them the challenge of dealing with new issues, and nurses need to be prepared to face this challenge.

BENEFITS AND CHALLENGES OF TECHNOLOGY

Scientific advances in the past one hundred years have been phenomenal. They include medications, surgical techniques, machines and equipment, diagnostic procedures, specialized treatments, expanded understanding of cause and progression of disease, and greater insight into what is required for people to stay healthy. New interventions have saved lives, improved quality of life, alleviated suffering, and significantly decreased the incidence of some diseases. Before the advent of many modern health related technologies, people experienced illness and death as an inevitable part of the cycle of their lives. Although death was not necessarily welcomed, it was expected as the natural outcome when the body could no longer ward off the effects of certain diseases or injuries. If someone was born with or developed a deformity, it may have been seen as a curse but was also considered part of who the person was. Life began when the infant started breathing, and life ended when heart and breathing stopped.

Current technology makes it possible to restart arrested hearts, use machines to breathe for people, correct deformities, assist the body in dealing with disease through use of medications and other interventions, eliminate diseased parts through surgery, and even to replace malfunctioning or diseased vital organs. The many ways to prolong life, or at least to extend the functioning of the physical being, have prompted the necessity of dealing with some very important issues. One dilemma relates to questions of quality of life and whether physical existence is synonymous with living. Another issue relates to whether the availability of certain technologies means they should always be used. Many issues relate to decisions about how and for whom technologies will be used.

Quality of Life

The ability to keep people alive and physically functioning through use of technology has led to much reflection and discussion about what constitutes life and living. Some people believe that biological life must be preserved regardless of the effect on the person whose body is being kept alive. A frequently asked question is whether a person is truly alive in situations where there is merely physiological functioning without awareness of oneself or others. Many suggest that living implies a quality that goes beyond physical existence. **Quality of life,** a subjective appraisal of factors that make life worth living and contribute to a positive experience of living, means different things to different people. It is difficult to find a clear and concise definition of quality of life because of the multidisciplinary usage and variable cultural understanding of the concept. Farquhar (1995) points out that definitions of quality of life derive from both lay and "expert" sources and range from global understandings of the concept, such as satisfaction with life, to focused definitions used for research, for example, health or functional ability. Ideas incorporated in understandings of the concept include fulfillment, satisfaction/dissatisfaction, conditions of life, happiness/unhappiness, experiences of life, and factors such as comfort, functional status, socioeconomic status, independence, and conditions in one's environment.

Farquhar (1995) suggests that deciding what weight to give different dimensions of the concept presents problems in defining quality of life. For instance, does one consider functional status, such as the ability to get around and do for oneself, or happiness more important when evaluating the quality of one's life? Nurses need to understand patient perspectives of what constitutes quality in their lives in order to incorporate these factors into goal setting and care planning.

Quality of life is a personal perspective that is determined by each individual. Recognizing this, it is important not to judge the quality of another's life based on one's own values. If judgments are made about a person's worth and quality of life based on factors such as contributions to society, age, mental capacity, or ability to function, discrimination against those who are judged to have a lesser quality of life may easily follow. Perceptions of quality of life often change with age and life experiences. For example, persons with debilitating health concerns may rate the quality of their lives quite positively, although others might feel that they could never live with such limitations. When patients and families are confronted with technological options, nurses need to help them clarify their perceptions regarding quality of life and discuss not only how life might be extended, but also how quality of life may be affected by various options.

Principles of Beneficence and Nonmaleficence

When dealing with issues of technology, the principles of **beneficence** and **nonmaleficence** may be in conflict. A particular technology, which may be implemented with the intention of *doing good* (beneficence), may result in much suffering for the patient. Inducing such suffering is counter to the maxim of *do no harm* (nonmaleficence). In some circumstances this is accepted as part of the treatment process, such as pain associated with surgery or side effects of chemotherapy. One is willing to endure the discomfort because there is an expectation of recovery, that one will ultimately be or feel more healthy. In circumstances in which there is little or no expectation of recovery or improved functioning, the question of import is whether the harm imposed by technology outweighs the good intended by its use. Suffering associated with technology may include physical, spiritual, and emotional elements for both patient and family. Making decisions required by technology may cause pain, and there is suffering in living with unknown results of ongoing decisions. Relief of suffering, a goal of healing from its earliest days, needs to be addressed in all patient encounters.

CURRENT TECHNOLOGY—ISSUES AND DILEMMAS

Current technologies related to organ and tissue transplantation, genetic engineering, reproduction, and sustaining life have profound potential for affecting our lives and health in positive ways. Their use also presents dilemmas for patients, families, professionals, and society. Nurses generally do not make the decisions regarding implementing or withdrawing particular technologies (except perhaps in situations like initiating cardiopulmonary recuscitation following specific protocols), yet they are involved as the caregivers of recipients of interventions and in many levels of care involving technology. A primary responsibility of nurses is to help patients and families deal with the purposes, benefits, and limitations of the specific technologies. This section focuses primarily on the issue of withdrawing or withholding treatment in situations of medical futility as a prime example of a dilemma related to technology. Other issues related to technology are discussed briefly, and the reader is encouraged to further explore particular areas as the need or interest arises.

Treating Patients: When to Intervene and to What End

One of the most controversial bioethical topics of recent years centers around withholding or withdrawing what is considered to be medically futile care. Decisions about withholding or withdrawing medical treatment are generally made by physicians in consultation with patients and family members. Approaches to dealing with these decisions reflect varying attitudes and concerns and may be confusing for all involved. A brief look at history sheds light on current attitudes regarding dealing with contemporary medical treatment. Questions related to the ethical limitations of medical care date back to the time of Hippocrates when physicians were taught that the goal of medicine was to relieve suffering and reduce the effects of disease by lending support to natural processes. Medicine was not intended for situations in which the body was overpowered by disease, since interventions might merely prolong the suffering. The accepted ethical stance recognized the limitations of medicine and withheld treatments that held little potential for healing (Jecker, 1995).

The scientific era that began emerging in the seventeenth century fostered a change in this ethical stance. Rather than revering and working with natural processes, conquering and dominating nature became the goal of science. In the nineteenth century, as medicine began to align more with science and biologic causes for diseases were discovered, the goal of medicine became the conquest of disease by exercising power over nature. Jecker (1995) notes that ethical problems involving aggressive medical treatments where there is little likelihood of success or poor quality of expected outcomes "are the outgrowth of a scientific tradition whose mission is to control and dominate, whose proving ground is nature, and whose means is an unfailing faith in the scientific method" (p. 144). Within this narrow focus of curing disease, ethical issues of personal quality of life and dimensions of suffering are often unrecognized and neglected. With their attention to healing and caring, nurses play an important role in calling attention to concerns that go beyond the narrow focus of curing.

Issues of Life, Death, and Dying

Ethical dilemmas faced in health care settings often relate to issues of and attitudes toward living and dying. Important questions that are deliberated by those involved include "When does life begin?," "When does life end?," "How can we be sure that someone has died?," and "Who decides?" Technology has stretched the boundaries and clouded the waters surrounding life's beginning and ending. Perspectives vary from the belief that life begins at conception to the view that it begins when an infant can survive outside the womb. Technology makes this discussion even more complex and raises questions such as "What happens when conception cannot occur 'naturally' and artificial processes are employed either in vivo or in vitro?" and "Is the laboratory embryo a life?"

Today many low birth weight infants and those with certain birth defects, who would not have survived in prior eras, survive with the support of machines, medications, and surgical procedures. In the process, however, some babies are kept alive only to die after months of expensive treatment. Others survive to face chronic health problems with their associated financial, emotional, and physical strains on families and the health care system. There is no definitive way to predict which infants will have problems as they grow and develop. Dilemmas arise regarding how much effort to invest in "saving" a few infants who have a high probability of living only a short time or with significant health problems.

Ask Yourself

When Does Life Begin?

- What are your beliefs about when life begins? What shaped these beliefs?

- Consider that you are a member of a special task force called together by your hospital to establish guidelines for allocating dwindling funds for support of low birth weight infants in the neonatal intensive care unit. What criteria would you use to determine which of the infants who cannot survive without technology at birth receive such interventions?

- If an infant will die without technology and the technology is withdrawn, do you consider that a natural or unnatural end of life? Why?

In our society death has become an unnatural event frequently associated with hospitals and other institutions, surrounded by tubes, machinery, and heroic efforts. Determining when life ends has become a critical issue related to use of technology, prompting the involvement of courts in decision making. The general attitude, especially among health care providers, is that death is the enemy to be overcome or kept at bay for as long as possible, regardless of the age or health condition of the person. Since death is often viewed as a failure on the part of the health provider, it is understandable that many health care providers have difficulty dealing with death as a possible outcome for patients, thus finding it a difficult topic to discuss. Another reason that the topic of death may be avoided is that discussing death requires health care providers to face issues of meaning in life and anxieties and fears regarding their own mortality. However, lack of discussion of death as a possible outcome may lead families and patients to have unreasonable expectations and false hopes of what the system can offer. Demands for inappropriate interventions or accusations that not enough was done may arise from such situations. Patients and families need support in recognizing and honoring their responses, beliefs, and fears regarding death. By facing their own issues about death, nurses are better able to facilitate this process with patients.

In many cultures death is viewed as part of one's life cycle which comes in its own time. Health care focused on curing is provided when there is reasonable hope of benefit, but one recognizes when it is time for care to mean letting go and facilitating the transition through the dying process. This often occurs at home, surrounded by family and friends.

Ask Yourself

What Are Your Views of Death and Dying?

What many people fear most regarding death is suffering and dying alone.

- How does technology contribute to this concern or attitude?

- What has your experience been related to death, what has shaped your attitudes regarding death, and what are your fears related to death?

- How can nurses minimize or deal with the effects of technology on patients in the dying process?

- How can nurses support patients and families in recognizing and honoring their own responses and beliefs regarding death?

- If machines and medication are keeping a body functioning even if the person is apparently unaware, is that person still alive? Discuss your response.

- Do you think that brain wave activity in the midst of severe deterioration of major systems constitutes living? Discuss your response.

Because attitudes prompt different expectations and scenarios, when faced with decisions about heroic efforts and life sustaining technologies, nurses must be aware of their own attitudes concerning living and dying, as well as the beliefs and expectations of patients, families, and other health care providers. Such awareness alerts the nurse to situations in which there are differing attitudes among the parties involved and provides an opportunity for opening lines of communication before a serious dilemma arises. Consider, for example, the patient who tells the nurse that he feels that his body is just giving up in spite of all the medications and treatments he is receiving and he would like to go home to die peacefully, yet the physician is considering another surgery that is helpful about thirty percent of the time. In such a situation it would be important for the nurse to further explore this area with the patient and either communicate his wishes to the physician or facilitate the patient's talking with the physician about his wishes.

CASE PRESENTATION

A Child with Leukemia

Lucia, a twelve-year-old child with leukemia, has relapsed in spite of routine chemotherapeutic interventions. This child has suffered the side effects of the treatment, including nausea, hair loss, and frequent hospitalizations with infections, and is deteriorating physically. She says she feels as if she is being tortured with all the needles, spinal taps, and bone marrow samples; that she has no friends; and that this kind of life is not worth living. A bone marrow transplant (the only hope for a cure at this point) would mean subjecting her to intensive chemotherapy, total body irradiation, and weeks in isolation following the transplant. The family is told that there is a forty percent chance that the transplant will be effective. The procedure is very expensive, and the family has already had to obtain a second mortgage for their home because their insurance has not covered many of the expenses to date.

Think About It

Factors Influencing Choices Regarding Medical Technology

- What factors do you think need to be considered in making the decision about having the bone marrow transplant?
- How do percentages of risk and benefit affect your decision making?
- In this situation do you think a forty percent chance of success is enough to go ahead with the transplant? What if it were sixty percent? What about twenty percent?
- How can you help patients and families use statistical information in deliberating their decisions?
- Who should be involved in making this decision?

It is important to remember that dying is more than a medical occurrence; it is a spiritual process touching the individual, family, and community. Although medical interventions can assist and support those in the dying process, current technologies can prolong suffering by prolonging the dying process, and separate people from their families by actual physical barriers and institutionalization. Relieving suffering and supporting a dignified death are important elements of the nursing role. Addressing patient needs may require nurses to make decisions to go against institutional policy regarding such things as visitors and visiting hours in order to ensure that the patient is not alone, or to risk confrontations with physicians over pain management or other aspects of care.

Medical Futility

Ethical and legal arguments for initiating or discontinuing life sustaining treatments are based primarily on the relative benefits and burdens for the patient. "Although many health care professionals feel reluctant to discontinue life-sustaining treatments, most philosophical and legal commentators find no important ethical or legal distinction between not instituting a treatment and discontinuing treatment already initiated" (Rushton, 1994, p. 517). Withholding or removing life sustaining treatments in situations in which the burden or harm has been determined to outweigh the benefits is, in essence, allowing the person to die. This is different from **euthanasia,** which is causing the painless death of a person in order to end or prevent suffering. Curtin (1996) suggests that it is not reasonable to say that removal of artificial interventions cause death; rather, it is the condition (such as disease or accident) that prompted the artificial interventions that causes death.

In deliberations regarding withholding, initiating, or withdrawing life sustaining interventions, **medical futility** related to the patient's situation is a major factor. Medical futility refers to situations in which interventions are judged to have no medical benefit or in which the chance for success is low. Futility is often discussed in relation to cardiopulmonary resuscitation (CPR), but it relates as well to interventions that preserve patients in persistent vegetative states or dependent on the technology of tertiary care settings. One difficulty associated with medical futility is that there is no set definition of the concept, only suggested parameters that vary greatly in guiding health care providers. Lo (1995) suggests that there are *strict* definitions of futility that would justify unilateral decisions by physicians to withhold or withdraw interventions, and *loose*, value laden definitions of the concept that do not justify such unilateral decisions. Strict definitions of futility include interventions that have no pathophysiologic rationale, have already failed in the patient, will not achieve the goal of care, and situations where maximal treatment is failing. Determination of futility in these situations "is based on objective data and judgments within the expertise of the physician. Physicians have no ethical duty to provide interventions that are futile in such strict senses; indeed, they generally have an ethical obligation not to provide them even if they are requested" (Lo, 1995, pp. 74–75).

Loose definitions of futility include situations that prompt variable interpretations and thus are more confusing, for example, situations in which the likelihood of success is very small, no worthwhile goals of care can be achieved, patient quality of life is unacceptable, and prospective benefit is not worth the resources required. In these situations the meaning of futility must consider perceptions of the patient and family and judgments of the health care team. In the absence of clear external guidelines, these less clear situations require more skillful nursing care as persons draw on their own understandings and resources shaped by personal beliefs and cultural values.

Ask Yourself

What Constitutes Medical Futility?

- What do you think about these definitions of futility? Where would you envision potential problems or dilemmas based on these definitions?
- Would you consider an expensive treatment that works twenty percent of the time to be futile? What if it only works five percent of the time? Explain.
- Should medical futility be an issue when treatments are not expensive? Explain.
- Do you think a decision about futile treatment should be different with children and younger adults than with the elderly? Discuss your response.
- How would you see a patient's inability to pay for treatment affecting decisions about futility?

Because personal values affect the determination of futility, health care providers, patients, and families may have differing views of what is a benefit or burden, particularly when using looser definitions of futility. For example, a patient or family may find hope and be willing to consider a treatment that has a five percent likelihood of success, while the health care providers see this as a futile effort. When considering quality of life, the perspective of the patient and family is essential in any determination of futility. Deciding when it is not worth continuing life sustaining treatment is another circumstance in which the views of the parties involved may differ. Consider, for example, a seventy-two-year-old quadriplegic patient on a ventilator at home who has been deteriorating and having frequent infections. She had to be resuscitated when recently hospitalized for severe respiratory infection. The physician discussed the futility of the situation with the patient and the family and suggested a **do not resuscitate (DNR) order,** which is a written directive placed in the patient's medical chart indicating that cardiopulmonary resuscitation is to be avoided. (See further discussion of DNR orders later in this chapter.) Even though the patient and most family members indicated agreement, the daughter who is the caregiver said she wants every effort made to keep her mother alive, saying that God will take her mother when He is ready. In another situation health care providers might view continuing treatments that prolong a patient's life a few more days to be causing unnecessary suffering, while for the patient and family this is important "saying goodbye" time.

 CASE PRESENTATION

Mr. Mason and His Son

Mr. Mason is a seventy-eight-year-old retired, widowed ironworker. He has been estranged from his adult son, an only child, for many years. Recently he was diagnosed with advanced lung cancer. He recognized that he needed to make some plans for his immediate future, so he contacted his son and allowed him power of attorney. Mr. Mason is admitted to your unit in severe pain. He is somewhat confused, and you are unable to elicit information from him about his wishes regarding life sustaining measures. You carefully begin discussing this difficult subject with his son, as it is your hospital's policy that everyone admitted to your oncology unit be informed about advance directives. Following are three possible twists this case could take, each of which is based on a real-life situation.

Ending 1. Mr. Mason's son begins to sob uncontrollably, saying, "I was never a very good son. I left home when I was barely nineteen and didn't even write or call for many years. I am just getting to know my dad, and now this happens. I want as much time with him as possible. He told me a few days ago that he was ready to die and didn't want to be kept alive on machines. But it is so unfair to me. I want him alive and more time with him. Please, do everything you can to keep him alive. I need some more time with him. I need for him to forgive me."

Ending 2. Mr. Mason's son seems impatient, continually looking at his watch as you talk to him. Finally, seeming exasperated, he says, "Look, he's going to die anyway, right? Two things: first, I'm a busy man, and the quicker we get this over with the better. Second, I have an appointment in twenty minutes with a real estate agent, and later with Dad's stockbroker. I'd really like to start arranging to sell his house and cash in some of his stocks. My son starts college in two months, and we could use the money. I suppose you think this is cruel, but realistically, would Dad rather we spend the money he worked so hard for on keeping him alive, when he's bound to die anyway, or on his grandson's education? It's pretty clear to me. I say, just let Dad go, that would be the best for everyone concerned."

Ending 3. The son quickly acknowledges that he understands the question. Without hesitation he says, "Do all you can to keep him alive. The tyrant was mean to me all of my life. I hate him. I want him to suffer as long as possible."

Think About It

Family Reactions to Medically Futile Situations

- What is your response to the son's statement in each of these scenarios? Include both your thinking response and your feeling response.
- How would your feelings lead you to advise one option over another?
- How do you think the nurse should react to each response?
- What values and dilemmas are evident in each scenario?
- Identify your personal and professional values related to each scenario.
- Who should make the decision? Do you feel conflicting loyalties?

Economics and Medical Futility. Cost of health care, particularly in relation to technology, has brought economic factors into discussions of futility. Some suggest that the principle of justice indicates that if a particular intervention is judged to be of limited or no benefit for one person, it should be discontinued so it is available for another patient who can make better use of the scarce resource. Lantos (1994) notes that political and economic developments in medicine in recent years, particularly prospective payment, have prompted physicians and hospitals to look more closely at futile treatments. Under prospective payment systems physicians and institutions lose money if patients are maintained on particular treatments beyond a predetermined length of time. Lantos argues that the development of prospective payment systems delegated the responsibility to limit excessive treatments to physicians as a kind of social mandate. He further suggests that it is ethical and justifiable for physicians to limit access to treatments that are expensive while offering limited benefits, and that, given limited health care resources, such decisions are socially responsible. Such an argument is consistent with utilitarian ethics, a perspective often used by government agencies when deciding about distribution of goods and services.

Ask Yourself

How Are Economics and Decisions About Medical Futility Related?

- Under what circumstances do you feel physicians or institutions should be able to limit a patient's access to expensive treatments?
- How do you think economics affects decisions about medical futility?
- How might patient care be affected by these decisions?

Do Not Resuscitate Orders

Cardiopulmonary resuscitation (CPR) is an area in which nurses have an active role in initiating or withholding life-sustaining treatment. Considering whether to initiate CPR with a patient requires attention to professional, ethical, legal, and institutional considerations. Principles utilized to justify decisions regarding resuscitation include autonomy, self-determination, nonmaleficence, and respect for persons.

The general practice regarding CPR is that it must be initiated unless: (1) it would clearly be futile to do so, or (2) the practitioner has specific instructions not to do so. As noted previously, do not resuscitate (DNR) orders are written directives placed in a patient's medical record indicating that the use of cardiopulmonary resuscitation is to be avoided. In situations of the strict definitions of medical futility noted above, Lo (1995) suggests that decisions to withhold or stop CPR are appropriately made by physicians and that, in such situations, resuscitation need not be offered as an option for patients. It has been suggested that nurses are as well qualified as physicians to write DNR orders. "Perhaps the most compelling reason for nurses to be involved in DNR and withdrawal of treatment decisions is that the nurse is the one professional who is in close and continuous contact with the patient, and, thus, is better able to help the patient articulate his or her views or to speak on behalf of the incapacitated person" (Martin & Redland, 1988, p. 6). Communication is key in dealing with DNR decisions with patients and their families or other appropriate surrogates.

Tomlinson and Brody (1988) note that the relevance of considering the patient's or family's values in justifying DNR orders may vary depending on the rationale given for the decision. In situations in which there would be no medical benefits, patient autonomy and consent are considered less relevant. However, when rationale for the decision is based on the patient's quality of life, either after or before CPR, determination of whether the benefit of continued life outweighs the risk of harmful consequences, such as debility or suffering, must flow from the values of the patient or patient's surrogate. Competent patients have the right to refuse CPR and may request DNR orders after they have been informed of the risks and benefits involved. Communication is a key factor in assuring that any DNR decision is acceptable to all parties involved.

CASE PRESENTATION

Mistaken Resuscitation

Jacob has had a chronic lung condition for the past ten of his thirty-two years. The condition causes some restrictions on his life, but he has kept up with a regular job and is very involved in his church. He is currently hospitalized with a severe respiratory infection. Although his condition did not seem to be that serious, when he was admitted he made sure that there was a DNR order in his chart, noting that he has a firm religious conviction that the Creator, and not the doctor, is to decide when it is time for him to die. Because of a staff shortage, Lashanda, a registered nurse who usually works on another unit, has been assigned to Jacob's unit. Although she has been working on the other side of the unit, she is presently covering the whole unit while other staff are at lunch. As she answers a call light from Jacob's roommate, she notices that Jacob is not breathing and has no pulse. Since she is unfamiliar with Jacob's DNR request, she immediately calls a "code" and initiates CPR, figuring that there would be no question that this would be the appropriate action for someone this age. Although Jacob is successfully resuscitated with no serious sequelae, he is intensely angry, saying that it was an interference in the Creator's plan.

Think About It

Decisions Regarding Resuscitation

- What do you think about Jacob's request for a DNR order? What ethical principles are involved in his choice?
- What do you think about Lashanda's response in the situation? Do you think she acted appropriately under the circumstances?
- How do you think you might respond in a similar situation? What principles would guide your actions?
- Describe potential legal ramifications in this situation.

It is very important to understand that DNR orders apply only to resuscitation. The fact that CPR might be considered futile does not imply that other life-sustaining interventions are futile. Health care providers often fail to make this distinction, thus causing confusion for patients as well. Many institutions are beginning to require more specific instructions regarding what is and is not to be done for a patient. These interventions might include treatment of physiological abnormalities like fever or cardiac arrhythmias, nutrition, or use of mechanical ventilation and CPR. Plans for and parameters of DNR orders need to be discussed with all members of the health care team so that the goal of care is clear. The presence of DNR orders requires nurses to become even more focused on providing supportive and comfort interventions and to ensure that there is no reduction in the level of care for the patient and family. A DNR order means only that in the event of cardiac or respiratory arrest there are to be no attempts to resuscitate. The patient may recover from the problem necessitating hospitalization and return home.

At a more philosophical level, Scofield (1995) suggests that decisions to not resuscitate ask us "individually and collectively, to arrive at a consensus on how to integrate death and decisions about it into the legitimating values of our moral universe. Deciding what kind of life we want involves deciding what kind of death we can face" (p. 184). He notes that death, which was once considered fate, is now often a matter of a choice which we do not want to have to make. This is the dilemma that faces those involved in DNR decisions.

Nursing Considerations Related to DNR Orders. Although it is generally considered the domain of the physician to write a DNR order, nurses need to be aware of parameters surrounding such orders. Nurses need to know which patients under their care have DNR orders, and these orders need to be documented clearly in a patient's chart, and perhaps at the bedside, and reviewed periodically as the patient's condition changes. If a patient or appropriate surrogate indicates to the nurse the desire not to be resuscitated and there is no order in the chart, the nurse should record the request and bring this to the immediate attention of the physician. The nurse may wish to explore the request with the patient or surrogate and may need to facilitate discussion of the issue between patient and physician. Orders should specify which interventions are to be withheld and considerations regarding circumstances in which they are to be withheld. All persons involved in care of the patient need to know of the orders. Since attitudes affect one's approach to others, nurses need to reflect on their own attitudes toward decisions regarding withholding of interventions, both in general and in particular patient situations.

Artificial Sources of Nutrition

Maintaining nutrition is a natural life-sustaining measure and a common part of the nursing role. Once a person has difficulty with functions associated with nutrition such as chewing or swallowing, or is not conscious enough to participate in these activities, decisions about artificial sources of nutrition must be made. Ethical dilemmas arise concerning whether to classify such interventions as feeding or medical treatments, as ordinary or extraordinary measures.

Utilizing artificial sources of nutrition may present dilemmas in situations involving persons in persistent vegetative states or end-stage dying processes for whom this intervention is maintaining physical life. We know that withholding food will eventually lead to starvation and death and, under most circumstances, is not considered an ethical action. However, it is considered appropriate to withhold or discontinue life-sustaining medical interventions in the event of medical futility. There are fewer complexities surrounding decisions to withhold artificial sources of nutrition than there are regarding decisions to withdraw medical interventions.

As with any such decision, it is important to consider the wishes of the patient or surrogate. Quality of life is an important factor, and if interventions contribute to, more than relieve, a patient's suffering, the principle of nonmaleficence may sway one toward a decision of not implementing or of discontinuing such therapies. Curtin (1996) reflects that if a person is willing and able to eat and drink, even when death is imminent and the patient is suffering, attempts to quicken death by withholding ordinary nourishment is morally repugnant. However, "in situations in which death is inevitable and the conditions of living intolerable (involve extensive technological isolation from human touch, futile pain and pointless extensions of dying), highly sophisticated means of feeding are not in a patient's best interests and may be withheld or withdrawn" (p. 82). Once artificial measures have been implemented, it is psychologically more difficult to decide on their removal. Curtin suggests that unless a rational adult refuses them, such measures should be continued as long as sentient life is a reasonable expectation, but that they may be terminated when there is a reliable prediction of permanent unconsciousness. A key consideration with any technological intervention is whether its use is prolonging living or prolonging dying. Involved parties may view the use of such interventions from different perspectives.

Legal Issues Related to Technology

As noted in Chapter 7, what is considered an ethical decision by some may not be upheld as a legal action. In the area of health care technology, the courts have intervened in some decisions related to withholding or withdrawing life-sustaining treatments when there has been disagreement among the involved parties. Legal precedents regarding issues such as what constitutes clear evidence of a person's wishes related to these treatments and what is considered standard practice have been set in the process. Examples of two such cases are presented here. When one looks at dilemmas faced by families, health care providers, institutions, and the legal system in situations such as these, the importance of having advance directives becomes evident. **Advance directives** are instructions indicating one's wishes regarding health care interventions or designating someone to act as a surrogate in making such decisions in the event that one loses decision making capacity. These directives are discussed in Chapter 11.

 CASE PRESENTATION

Karen Quinlan

The well known case of Karen Quinlan (Devettere, 1995; Pence, 1995) is a story of a twenty-one-year-old woman who, in 1975, was found to have suffered cardiopulmonary arrest at home alone after having been drinking at a local bar. After the ambulance crew restored heartbeat through CPR, she was admitted to the local hospital and placed on a ventilator. Within a few days she was transferred to a larger hospital where she was kept alive with the assistance of a respirator and feeding tube. Over months she lost weight, developed contractures, and was given no hope of regaining awareness. After much deliberation, the family asked that the respirator be discontinued, but the hospital indicated that it could not grant the request unless the father was named as her guardian. When the father asked the court to appoint him guardian with authority to make decisions to discontinue extraordinary interventions, the court appointed him guardian of her property, but not of her person, and appointed a **guardian *ad litem*** to represent Karen. The guardian *ad litem* felt responsible for preserving Karen's life and opposed removing the respirator. The physician's lawyer argued that removing a respirator from a living person was not standard medical procedure, and the judge sided with this view. When the family appealed the ruling to the New Jersey Supreme Court, the decision of the lower court was reversed and the father was appointed as her guardian. When the father requested that the respirator be removed, the physicians initiated a process of weaning her from it, resulting in her being able to breathe without the machine. Totally unconscious with severe contractures, she was transferred to a nursing home, where she died ten years later.

 CASE PRESENTATION

Nancy Cruzan

In another well known case, Nancy Cruzan (Angell, 1990; Annas, 1990; Pence, 1995) was found unconscious and not breathing after her car went into a ditch in the winter of 1983. Although emergency personnel restored her breathing, she never regained consciousness. After a year of being sustained through the use of a gastrostomy tube for artificial nutrition, it was determined that she was in a persistent vegetative state. When her parents, acting as her guardians, asked that the artificial feeding be discontinued because she had indicated previously that she would not want to be kept alive in this condition, the physicians and hospital refused. When the case went to court, the evidence supporting discontinuing the feeding was based primarily on a statement she had made to a roommate that she would not want to live if she were a vegetable. The judge ruled that the medical nutrition could be removed, but that decision was appealed to the Missouri State Supreme Court by a guardian *ad litem*. The Missouri court reversed the previous decision, claiming that there was no clear and convincing evidence that this would be her wish, that she was not terminally ill or suffering, and that there was no reason to act contrary to the state's interest in preserving life regardless of how minimal that life had become. An appeal to the United States Supreme Court upheld the decision that medical nutrition could not be withdrawn because of the lack of clear and convincing evidence. In 1990, almost eight years after her accident, Nancy's parents appealed again to the local court with the evidence of three of her friends who stated that she had told them that she would not want to live in a vegetative state. At that time, the physician agreed that it was no longer in her best interests to be medically nourished, and the judge agreed that there was now clear and convincing evidence indicating that it was in her best interests to terminate artificial nutrition.

Think About It

When the Courts Intervene

- As you reflect on these two cases, which position do you support, that of the family or that of the guardian *ad litem*?

- Which court decisions do you think are more valid? Defend your position.

- Describe ethical dilemmas and principles involved in these situations.

- If one of your family members was in a similar situation, how do you think you would respond? Would you expect solidarity or disagreement with this position from other members of your family?

- Consider that you are a nurse caring for Karen or Nancy at various stages in her situation. How would you respond to the various parties involved as decisions about her care are being discussed?

- What do you think about the role of the legal system in decisions regarding use of technology?

Examples of Potential Dilemmas with Other Technology

In addition to life-sustaining interventions, advances in technology affect nursing and health care in other arenas as well. Examples of a few such technologies are briefly presented here. Nurses who work with patients whose care involves such technologies need to be aware of potential ethical issues associated with their use, as well as the benefits of such interventions. The intention here is to alert the student to some of the questions and dilemmas that may be associated with these technologies. The student is encouraged to further explore these areas, reflecting on personal values related to each technology.

Reproductive Technology. Because the inability to conceive and bear children can be a very distressing experience for a couple, any technology that can facilitate the process may well be viewed as a life-affirming gift. Such technologies include artificial insemination by donor, in vitro fertilization, and surrogate embryo transfer. While scientists develop and refine these technologies to benefit people, ethicists and others raise questions related to moral implications of their use. Some questions focus on the potential for changing society's concept of family and parenthood. For example, in the case of surrogacy, is the mother of the baby the woman whose ovum is joined with her husband's sperm or the woman who donates her body for the baby's development and birth? One must consider whether the use of such technologies might relegate childbearing into little more than the production of a product. Other ethical questions arise regarding who has custody of frozen embryos and whether these embryos have rights. A related consideration is the potential that women may become more exploited than liberated by the use of these technologies. Because these interventions are expensive, questions arise regarding who should pay for them and for whom they should be made available.

Genetic Diagnosis, Engineering, and Screening. **Genetic diagnosis,** which is usually done within an in vitro fertilization program, involves a process of biopsy of embryos to determine the presence of genetic flaws and gender prior to implantation. At present, such diagnosis is aimed at couples who have a high risk of conceiving a child with a serious genetic disorder, with the intent that only embryos that are free of genetic flaws would be implanted. **Genetic engineering** is the ability to genetically alter organisms for a variety of purposes, such as developing more disease resistant fruits and vegetables, or eventually being able to genetically alter embryos so that the fetus and baby will be healthier. Through **genetic screening** it is possible to determine if persons are predisposed to certain diseases and whether couples have the possibility of giving birth to a genetically impaired infant. The implications of having such technologies available include the potential for correcting some genetic defects in embryo, eliminating some very serious genetic diseases, and producing food that is more nourishing and resilient. Concerns related to these technologies are as varied as their potential benefits, particularly the recognition that relaxing criteria related to a person's value or rights in one arena may lead to abuses or exploitation in other circumstances. Ethicists often speak of these concerns in terms of a *slippery slope* where, for example, one decision based on relaxing criteria supporting the value of human life makes it easy to slide into acceptance of lower standards as ethical guides. For example, one concern is that genetic engineering might produce organisms that could be harmful to humans; another is that employers or insurers might use information gained from genetic screening to exclude people with particular traits from certain jobs or from being insured. Might genetic screening and diagnosis lead to abuses such as forbidding people with certain traits to have children, insurers refusing to cover expenses if insured mothers give birth to genetically impaired infants, or prohibiting the birth of babies with particular genetic features deemed undesirable by those in power in a society? These areas include other broad societal implications such as who pays for the procedures, who determines guidelines for their use, and to whom they are made available.

Organ and Tissue Procurement and Transplantation. Organ transplantation is no longer considered as extraordinary or uncommon a health care event as it was in the not too distant past. As techniques become more refined, the possibility of a transplant becomes a hope for more and more people afflicted with failure of one or another vital organ. Because the demand for organs is great and the supply limited, dilemmas related to allocation of scarce resources emerge. Questions arise regarding eligibility of recipients for organ transplant. Should these determinations be made based on a potential recipient's expectation of survival posttransplant, or ability to pay for the procedure, or power and prestige, or some combination of these and other factors? Transplantation may involve organs from dead or living human donors, animals, or artificial appliances, and there are dilemmas associated with each. This discussion focuses on human donor issues.

Because transplantation requires well nourished organs, procurement must occur as soon after death as possible. Thus, having criteria for determining when death occurs is imperative. Irreversible cessation of cardiopulmonary functioning is one such criterion. However, until CPR has been attempted, how is one to know if the cessation is irreversible? If CPR is initiated, organs to be donated may be damaged, raising an issue of how to deal with a person's desire to be an organ donor with a consideration for CPR. Questions regarding when and how intensively to initiate CPR become important issues regarding organ donation. If a person has been maintained on life support technology, brain death is the most likely criteria to be used, which leads to issues regarding what constitutes brain death. Some suggest that current criteria for brain death which indicate that all functions of the entire brain must cease are more stringent than necessary, and that irreversible cessation of higher brain functions would be sufficient criteria. Such a change in brain death criteria would open the possibility of harvesting organs from people in persistent vegetative states or in permanent comas, and with this would come questions about the ethics of doing so.

The scarcity of available organs and the long waiting lists of potential recipients raise the possibility that people may be declared dead prematurely. This scarcity of organs also affects organ procurement from living human beings. With living donors, issues related to voluntary informed consent and the buying and selling of organs are of concern. There are places in the world where organs are taken from poor people or prisoners without their knowledge or against their will and sold to procurement centers in more affluent countries. Desperate straits have prompted some individuals to sell an organ to raise money for personal or family needs, raising a question about whether there can be true voluntary informed consent under such circumstances.

In cases of sudden accidental death, family members may be asked to consider donation of viable organs. Consider whether there can be true voluntary consent when the family is in the midst of crisis and shock. With the urgency for a decision due to time factors for harvesting organs, coercion could be a factor. In some settings nurses are asked to approach patients or families about considering organ donation. In such situations nurses need to be clear about their own feelings regarding organ procurement and transplantation and remember that attention to family needs takes precedence over time constraints of organ harvesting.

NURSING PRACTICE IN THE MIDST OF TECHNOLOGY

Nursing practice continues to evolve with expanding knowledge and scientific advances in many arenas. As technology has been developed and refined, related nursing responsibilities have expanded. In the midst of these changes, the essence of nursing remains the human focus of caring for patients and families—being attentive to the needs of persons whose lives are affected by the technology. Integrating caring and technology and juggling the demands of each present challenges for nurses in any area of practice. As new technologies become available, they will bring with them associated issues of concern. Regardless of the technology, important considerations for nursing relate to attitudes and values, communication, and maintaining the human focus of care.

Attitudes and Values

The importance of self-awareness related to values, beliefs, and reactions is especially significant when dealing with issues related to technology. The process of being more attentive to personal perspectives regarding such issues as quality of life, living, dying, medical futility, and allocation of scarce resources may be facilitated by pondering questions such as those posed throughout this chapter. Such awareness enables the nurse to differentiate personal values from those of patients and others involved in the situation. Principles of self-determination and autonomy counsel the nurse to understand that individuals may judge benefits of an intervention from varying perspectives. Recognizing where one's values may be different enables nurses to be more attentive to fostering good communication, encouraging others to make their own decisions, avoiding judgment about the rightness or wrongness of the decision based on personal values, and accepting those decisions even if they are different from what the nurse would do.

As the various examples presented in this chapter suggest, many dilemmas that emerge surrounding technology relate to differing values among the parties involved. Facilitating discussion of values among patients and families may help them to clarify their own perspectives. Nurses also need to be alert to situations in which there may be differences in values among the patient, family, and physician. Encouraging timely communication may avert a major dilemma or facilitate more effective resolution of the concern. Nurses who cannot reconcile their values with a particular situation need to take the necessary steps to remove themselves from that situation so as to not compromise patient care or personal integrity. In so doing it is essential to avoid abandoning the patient by assuring that there are others who will provide the needed care for the patient.

The Importance of Communication—Who Decides?

As has been noted, there are many factors involved in making decisions about withholding or withdrawing life sustaining treatments and utilizing other technologies. From the nursing perspective it is important to determine who is involved in making the decision and how the nurse fits into the scenario. Utilizing the decision making process described in Chapter 4 may assist in this process. Nurses need to be aware of institutional policies and protocols regarding various technologies. Such policies should include approaches to reaching decisions about particular patients, ways of dealing with conflicts that may arise, protection of patient rights, description of roles of those involved in the decision making process, and directions for documenting the decision in the patient chart. In most situations the patient or the patient's surrogate has the ultimate authority to decide which interventions to use or withhold.

Since nurses are in close and continual contact with patients, they are often perceived as more available and more approachable than physicians. Patients or family members may more readily discuss their concerns about interventions with the nurse, seeking information or advice. It is important to know what they have been told by the physician and to determine the patient's and family's level of understanding about the situation and whether they have the necessary information to make an informed decision. If information is needed in such areas as risks, discomforts, side effects, potential benefits, likelihood of success, treatment alternatives, or estimated costs, advocating for the patient in this regard is an appropriate nursing response. Nurses are in a key position to utilize conversations with patients and families to discover areas of confusion and to elicit information about the patient's wishes regarding interventions.

Sometimes people just need to talk out their concerns and sort through sometimes conflicting messages coming from the head and the heart. Providing a listening presence can help people vent emotions, speak their fears, and clarify their concerns. At times the concern may be such that the nurse must advocate for the patient by facilitating communication with the physician, support people such as family or pastor, or other appropriate persons such as a patient representative or member of the ethics committee. Collaboration among all involved is important to ensure an informed choice. It is useful to remember that effective communication can be facilitated by providing an environment that is not rushed, using terms and language that are understood by the other person, allowing time for and encouraging questions, practicing attentive listening, and offering a caring presence.

Caring—The Human Focus

In the context of expanding scientific and technological knowledge, nurses have the responsibility for helping patients and families benefit from what technology offers, while remembering always the human focus of care. Davis (1991) suggests that when medical treatment is deemed futile, nursing care in its fullest meaning is most essential. "In fact, one can argue that the concept of futility has little or no place in nursing" (Davis, 1991, p. 414). However alert, and in whatever stage of living and dying, an individual has a life story that continues to unfold, a story that continues to intertwine with lives of others. In the midst of the technology, nurses can encourage family and loved ones to talk with, touch, and be in touch with the patient. In this way nurses acknowledge the primary importance of relationships, even in a health care setting filled with machines, noises, and other evidences of advanced technology.

Attention to the human focus includes helping patients and families become more comfortable with the sometimes formidable array of machines and equipment and make sense of the large amounts of clinical data that are generated. Incorporating family members in caring for the patient provides time for connecting and observing the patient in both good and bad moments and engenders a more realistic view of the patient's condition. Rather than engendering anxiety and mistrust by shutting family out of the patient's life and experiences at critical moments, nurses should encourage them to share directly in the patient's journey. This provides families more experiences upon which to base hard decisions.

The nursing role of providing care and comfort is paramount in any health care setting and has many facets. It may take the shape of explaining, as often as necessary, the purpose and problems related to interventions. Caring requires that the nurse see the experience from another's point of view so that questions, fears, concerns, and frustrations may be addressed appropriately. Providing care and comfort also requires that the nurse support and encourage behaviors that enable patients and families to choose in accordance with their own beliefs and values. Being proficient in technical skills with the intent of doing what is best for the patient is part of human care, as is the ability to be with and wait with persons as they struggle through difficult situations.

SUMMARY

Many of the major ethical dilemmas encountered by nurses and other health care providers today are associated with advances in scientific knowledge and technology. In order to recognize and to deal with such dilemmas, nurses need to clarify their own values and to appreciate differences in values among the various people involved in making patient care decisions. The potential of technology has raised very deep questions about life and death that must be addressed on individual, professional, and societal levels. Issues of quality of life, relief of suffering, and futility of interventions are some facets of these questions. Decisions about when to intervene and reasonable goals of interventions are made more difficult because of varying perceptions of the value of such interventions, nondefinitive outcomes, and issues related to availability of interventions. Principles of beneficence, nonmaleficence, justice, and autonomy provide the basis for arguments on different sides of issues related to technology. Nurses must take into account their responsibilities to patients and the profession, as well as personal integrity, when dealing with ethical dilemmas engendered by technology. It is of prime importance that nurses remember that, in the midst of the technology with its associated dilemmas, there are persons who need the human focus of care that is basic to nursing practice.

CHAPTER HIGHLIGHTS

- The use of technology in health care has prompted the need to address important ethical questions regarding life, death, and allocation of resources.
- Utilization of health care technology may give rise to conflicts between the principles of beneficence and nonmaleficence.
- Appropriate utilization of health care technologies requires that health care providers, patients, and families understand the purposes, benefits, and limitations of specific technologies.
- Attitudes and beliefs concerning life and death affect how health care providers, patients, families, and the legal system approach issues related to health care technology. Ethical dilemmas may arise when there are differing opinions related to the use of technology among the parties involved.
- Determination of medical futility is an important consideration in decisions to withhold or withdraw life sustaining interventions. Ethical decisions regarding these measures require consideration of whether they are prolonging living or prolonging dying.
- Economics may factor into decisions related to medical futility, availability of technology, and accessibility to many interventions.

- Withholding or withdrawing life sustaining treatments in situations in which the burden or harm has been determined to outweigh the benefits constitutes allowing a person to die and is not euthanasia. Dilemmas may arise regarding whether to classify the use of specific interventions as ordinary or extraordinary measures. The courts have sometimes been involved in making this determination.

- Patient self-determination and distributive justice must be considered in decisions regarding technology; and vigilance is required to assure that people are not harmed, exploited, controlled, discriminated against, or excluded from care by the use of health care technologies.

- Nurses are in a key position to help patients and families articulate their preferences regarding technological interventions and to facilitate communication with other health team members in this regard. This role requires familiarity with patient and family decisions and institutional policies regarding life sustaining interventions, and awareness that when medical care is deemed futile, nursing care in its fullest meaning is most essential.

DISCUSSION QUESTIONS AND ACTIVITIES

1. Develop advance directives for yourself considering interventions you would choose and parameters regarding these choices. Discuss and compare your directives with classmates.

2. Discuss your beliefs regarding determinants of the beginning and end of life.

3. Describe quality of life as it relates to health care decisions.

4. Discuss potential *slippery slope* elements related to reproductive and genetic technologies, and organ procurement and transplantation.

5. Plan and engage in a debate in your class focused on economic and justice issues related to health care technologies.

6. Observe several patients who are receiving technological interventions, and note how the technology is affecting them and their families, issues surrounding its use, the focus of nursing care, and your reaction to the situation. Describe strengths of the nursing care you observe, and aspects you might do differently if you were providing care. Talk to nurses and patients regarding the impact of technology on their health and care.

7. Discuss your view about nurses writing DNR orders.

8. How would you handle a situation where you feel the physician's decision regarding life sustaining interventions is inappropriate for your patient?

REFERENCES

Angell, M. (1990). Prisoners of technology: The case of Nancy Cruzan. *New England Journal of Medicine, 322,* 1226–1228.

Annas, G. J. (1990). Nancy Cruzan and the right to die. *New England Journal of Medicine, 323,* 670–672.

Curtin, L. (1996). *Nursing: Into the 21st century.* Springhouse, PA: Springhouse.

Davis, A. J. (1991). Ethical issues in nursing research: My own experience. *Western Journal of Nursing Research, 13,* 414–415.

Devettere, R. J. (1995). *Practical decision making in health care ethics: Cases and concepts.* Washington, DC: Georgetown University Press.

Farquhar, M. (1995). Definitions of quality of life: A taxonomy. *Journal of Advanced Nursing, 22,* 502–508.

Jecker, N. S. (1995). Knowing when to stop: The limits of medicine. In J. H. Howell & W. F. Sale (Eds.), *Life choices: A Hastings Center introduction to bioethics* (pp. 139–148). Washington, DC: Georgetown University Press.

Lantos, J. D. (1994). Futility assessments and the doctor-patient relationship. *JAGS, 42,* 868–870.

Lo, B. (1995). *Resolving ethical dilemmas: A guide for clinicians.* Baltimore: Williams & Wilkins.

Martin, D. A., & Redland, A. R. (1988). Legal and ethical issues in resuscitation and withholding of treatment. *Critical Care Nurse, 10,* pp. 1–8.

Pence, G. E. (1995). *Classic cases in medical ethics.* New York: McGraw-Hill.

Rushton, C. H. (1994). Guidelines on forgoing life-sustaining medical treatment. *Pediatric Nursing, 20,* pp. 517–521.

Scofield, G. R. (1995). Is consent useful when resuscitation isn't? In J. H. Howell & W. F. Sale (Eds.), *Life choices: A Hastings Center introduction to bioethics* (pp. 172–187). Washington, DC: Georgetown University Press.

Tomlinson, T., & Brody, H. (1988). Ethics and communication in do-not-resuscitate orders. *New England Journal of Medicine, 318,* pp. 43–46.

SUGGESTED READINGS

Devettere, R. J. (1995). *Practical decision making in health care ethics: Cases and concepts.* Washington, DC: Georgetown University Press.

Howell, J. H., & Sale, W. F. (1995). *Life choices: A Hastings Center introduction to bioethics.* Washington, DC: Georgetown University Press.

Pence, G. E. (1995). *Classic cases in medical ethics.* New York: McGraw-Hill.

CHAPTER 11

Practice Issues Related to Patient Self-Determination

The task set before us is to find the golden mean between moral autonomy and the cooperative action necessary to contemporary life.

(Curtin, 1982)

OBJECTIVES

After completing this chapter, the reader should be able to:

1. Discuss autonomy and paternalism as they relate to patient self-determination.
2. Describe factors that may threaten autonomy in health care settings and situations in which autonomy may be limited.
3. Examine the interaction of justice and autonomy.
4. Discuss informed consent as it relates to patient self-determination.
5. Examine legal and ethical elements of informed consent.
6. Describe the nursing role and responsibilities related to informed consent.
7. Discuss the place of advance directives in health care decisions.
8. Discuss patient autonomy related to choices for life and health.
9. Describe the nursing role and responsibilities related to patient lifestyle and health choices.
10. Discuss the nursing role regarding complementary therapies.
11. Describe confidentiality in relation to health care choices.

INTRODUCTION

The role of the patient and that of the healer, and the implied responsibilities of each, have varied throughout history and in different cultures. In some cultures, decisions regarding "what is best" for the patient are deferred to the healer who is presumed to know what will bring about healing. Indeed, until recent years, the physician was often viewed in this light. Such paternalism has been challenged in recent years, and greater emphasis has been placed on the role and rights of patients in making health care decisions. This chapter focuses on practice issues related to patient self-determination. Discussion of these issues includes both ethical and legal components and is intertwined with issues of technology and economics.

AUTONOMY AND PATERNALISM

Self-determination derives from the principle of autonomy. **Autonomy,** which is discussed in detail in Chapter 3, denotes having the freedom to make choices about issues that affect one's life and to make decisions about personal goals. Autonomy, which means self-governing, implies respect for persons, the ability to determine personal goals and decide on a plan of action, and the freedom to act on the choices made. The value of the primacy of the individual implicit in autonomy is primarily an Anglo concept and may not be fully accepted in other cultures. It has been suggested that the notion of autonomy is more than a sense of an isolated self and must include an appreciation for the self in relation to others, recognizing that choices are made in the context of community (Sherwin, 1992). Implications of this view for health care include viewing patients as members of a social world in which health care decisions affect others and are made in conjunction with trusted persons.

Factors that may threaten autonomy in health care settings include: a prevailing paternalistic attitude that promotes the dependent role of the patient, assumptions that a patient's values and thought processes are the same as those of the health care provider, failure to appreciate a difference in knowledge level regarding health matters, and a focus on technology rather than caring. Persisting paternalistic attitudes have contributed to increased numbers of patients and families struggling with health care providers over control of health care decisions. **Paternalism** "derives from the privileges associated with the patriarchal family, where fathers are granted the right and responsibility to use their supposedly superior knowledge and judgment to make decisions on behalf of other family members" (Sherwin, 1992, p. 138). Paternalism (or parentalism, as discussed in Chapter 3) implies well intended actions of benevolent decision making, leadership, protection, and discipline, which in the health care arena manifest in the making of decisions on behalf of patients without their full consent or knowledge. Although the principle of beneficence suggests that decisions are focused on the patient's well-being, the power inherent in such a hierarchical arrangement can be abused, and decisions made may reflect the interests of the health care provider more than those of the patient. Consider, for example, many elderly patients in nursing homes who are routinely sedated "for their own protection" because of "agitation and confusion." It is worth pondering whether medication used in this way is for the benefit of the patient or to make life easier for the staff.

CASE PRESENTATION

Determining What Is Best for the Patient

Mr. Zumma, a former butcher who is eighty-four years old, has had evidence of memory loss and periodic confusion for about a year and a half. He has been functional at home—able to do personal care, household chores, and shopping—and has been on no medication. One night he came into the bedroom with two straight razors and told his wife to stay still so he could slit her throat. She was able to escape the situation by exiting through a nearby door and running to a neighbor's house. Reluctant to call the police because "he is not a criminal," she called her son who came and calmed him down. At the advice of another family member, she contacted a geriatric psychiatrist who immediately hospitalized Mr. Zumma and started him on Haldol. When he got worse, the physician increased the dose of the medication. Although he was walking and talking when he was admitted, after one day in the hospital the patient became incontinent, could not walk, was drooling, and had to be restrained. The decline in his condition throughout the week in the hospital concerned Mrs. Zumma, and she approached the psychiatrist about taking him on a previously planned vacation. The psychiatrist indicated that this would be impossible and that the patient would need to go to a nursing home. With persistence, however, Mrs. Zumma was able to convince the psychiatrist to discontinue the medications, after which Mr. Zumma's condition improved and he walked out of the hospital and did well on the vacation trip. Although he still gets confused, he remains functional at home without medication, where his wife makes sure that all sharp or dangerous objects are kept hidden.

Think About It

When Interventions Do More Harm than Good

- How did paternalism factor into the case of Mr. Zumma?
- What ethical issues are evident in this case?
- If you were the nurse caring for Mr. Zumma and his wife approached you with her concerns about his condition, how would you respond?
- Describe patient and family values that you believe influenced decisions about Mr. Zumma's care.

Inherent in the authoritarian medical model is the "belief that neither patients nor health care professionals other than physicians possess the appropriate skills and capacities to exercise decision-making power. In particular, patients (and their guardians) are thought to be too uneducated, too emotionally distraught, or too stupid to make adequate decisions in the face of illness" (Sherwin, 1992, p. 145). What this attitude does not address, however, is that decisions about health require more than scientific expertise. Such decisions must take into account factors such as the patient's values, culture, spiritual and other beliefs; evaluation of risks, benefits, and economic considerations; and effects on lifestyle and role. For this to occur patients must be engaged in the decision making process as autonomous agents in relationship with others who may need to be part of the process.

How Far Does Autonomy Go?

Although the principle of autonomy has become a key consideration in health care ethics, it does have limits. Practitioners are not obligated to honor requests from patients or families for interventions that, in the best judgment of the practitioner, are outside accepted standards of care or that are contrary to the practitioner's own ethical views. Autonomy may also be limited by availability of resources and economic circumstances.

In discussions of patient self-determination, the principle of justice needs to be considered along with that of autonomy. **Justice** implies fair, equitable, and appropriate treatment in light of what is due or owed to persons, recognizing that giving to some may deny receipt to others who might otherwise have received these things. In determining who deserves what portion of finite health care resources, autonomy and justice may come into conflict where needs or demands for health care by autonomous patients outweigh available resources. Issues arise regarding the rights of family members and of society in relation to the needs of individuals. Hardwig (1995) suggests that the medical and nonmedical impact of treatment decisions on both the patient and the family needs to be considered. He reflects that patient autonomy implies the responsible use of freedom, which means considering the needs of family and society as well as one's own desires. He raises the question of whether it is legitimate to ask families to make sacrifices of major resources to meet the needs of one member. The limited availability and expense of many medical interventions have brought such questions to the fore. Since people can be maintained on very expensive treatments for prolonged periods of time, justice requires one to ask not only who deserves an intervention but also who is expected to pay for it. Although the moral relevance of considering the interests of the family is generally not addressed in current ethical theory, dilemmas faced by patients, families, and practitioners include these issues; and it is well worth pondering their implications.

Ask Yourself

Should There Be Limits to Patient Autonomy?

- Can you think of health care situations in which the interests of the family should take precedence over those of the patient? Upon what criteria do you base this decision?
- How would you describe nursing's role regarding patient autonomy?

- How have you experienced paternalism in nursing?
- How do you feel about the suggestion that the physician is most qualified to make health care decisions? What have you experienced in this regard?

INFORMED CONSENT

Informed consent provides legal protection of a patient's right to personal autonomy. The concept of informed consent is one that has come to mean that patients are given the opportunity to autonomously choose a course of action in regard to plans for health care. The choice includes the right to refuse interventions or recommendations about care and to choose from available therapeutic alternatives. This is usually discussed in relation to surgery and complex medical procedures but also includes consent to more common interventions that may have undesirable side effects such as immunizations and contraceptives. Exceptions to informed consent include emergencies in which there is no time to disclose the information and waivers by patients who do not want to know their prognosis or risks of treatment.

The emergence of informed consent as we know it has been affected by several factors. One factor has been the institutionalization of health care in hospitals with their associated technologies and life prolonging techniques over which people have little control and limited understanding. When health providers visited in the home, informed consent was not as necessary because people had more control and better understanding of traditional remedies (Devettere, 1995). The courts, however, have exerted the most significant influence on shaping the doctrine of informed consent.

The history of the concept dates back to at least three landmark legal cases. In *Slater v. Baker & Stapleton* (1767), a decision was made that prohibited "unauthorized touching." This decision held that a person has a right to know what is to be done to his or her body. It did not require any participation in the decision making process. In two similar cases, *Mobe v. Williams* (1905) and *Schloendorff v. The Society of New York Hospital* (1914), separate rulings established the patient's right to know what was to be done and also the right to give or withhold consent. These decisions did not address the patient's right to be informed about risks of treatment or nontreatment or about the existence of alternative therapies. In the case of *Salgo v. Leland Stanford, Jr.* (1957), the California Supreme Court ruled in favor of a patient who had not been informed of the risks of aortography and subsequently became paralyzed. This ruling established a patient's right to be advised of the risks involved in any proposed treatment (Husted & Husted, 1995).

Decision Making Capacity

Informed consent requires that the patient or surrogate have the ability to make a reasonable decision regarding health care concerns. It is presumed that conscious adults have decision making capacity unless there is evidence to the contrary. **Decision making capacity** is a medical determination relating only to the issue at hand, as people may have the ability to make decisions about some areas and not others. For example, a person may be able to make decisions about health while unable to make reasonable decisions about household matters. Persons may have decision making capacity at some times and not others; and in each specific situation, there must be a determination that they have or do not have the capacity. The fact that a person makes a decision that seems unreasonable to the health care provider does not necessarily mean a lack of decision making capacity; it may merely reflect a difference in values. However, if the decision seems unreasonable, it is wise to explore the patient's capacity regarding decision making.

Elements of Decision Making Capacity. When evaluating a patient or surrogate for decision making capacity, several elements must be present. These are listed in Figure 11–1. First, the patient must be able to understand all relevant information, including the nature of the health care problem, the prognosis, treatment options and recommendations, and the risks, benefits, and consequences of each. Second, the patient must be able to communicate this understanding and her or his choices. Third, the patient must possess a set of values and goals that enable evaluation regarding whether this health care decision will be of benefit in terms of personal goals. Fourth, the patient must have the ability to reason and deliberate about available choices, which includes the ability to grasp notions such as risk and percentage, cause and effect, and chance and probability. Although it is not unreasonable to see some indecision or even a change of mind once a choice has been made, a great deal of vacillation between choices would suggest the need to re-evaluate decision making capacity. Nurses are in a key position to observe patients and families for the presence of these elements of decision making capacity. As patient advocates, nurses need to assess, document, and communicate to appropriate members of the health care team any concerns in this regard.

Figure 11–1 **Elements of Decision Making Capacity**

The patient must:
- have the ability to understand all information.
- have the ability to communicate understanding and choices.
- have personal values and goals that guide the decision.
- have the ability to reason and deliberate.

Physicians usually have legal authority and responsibility to determine decision making capacity. This is best done in consultation with family or others who have the patient's best interest in mind. It is important to make a distinction here between decision making capacity and competence. Decisions about **competence,** which is the ability to make meaningful life decisions, require a legal action. Legally, persons are considered competent unless there is a ruling by a judge that they cannot make meaningful life decisions. Legal declarations of incompetence generally stay in effect for the remainder of the person's life and include a court appointed guardian to be the surrogate decision maker for the person.

When a patient lacks decision making capacity, someone else must be identified as a surrogate to make decisions for the patient. In the case of children, the surrogate is usually a parent or legal guardian. With adults the surrogate may be a spouse, parent, adult children, other relatives, or other person named as surrogate in the patient's advance directives.

Ethical and Legal Elements of Informed Consent

It is important to remember that although the informed consent doctrine has foundations in law, it is essentially an ethical imperative. "Ethically valid consent is a process of shared decision-making based upon mutual respect and participation, not a ritual to be equated with reciting the contents of a form that details the risks of particular treatments" (President's Commission, 1983, p. 2). The two major legal elements of informed consent that are inherent in the ethical imperative are *information* and *consent*.

Information.   The information component of informed consent includes both disclosure and understanding of the essential information. Figure 11–2 lists the information that must be included in an informed consent. People need access to sufficient information to help them understand their health concerns and make decisions regarding treatment. The information provided need not be "textbook" detail but does need to offer enough explanation for the person to have a clear picture of the situation, what is being offered, the alternatives and their risks, benefits, and consequences. Determining the adequacy of information disclosed in an informed consent is based on one or more standards: (1) the *professional practice standard*—the disclosure is consistent with the standards of the profession; (2) the *reasonable person standard*—the disclosure is what a reasonable person in similar circumstances would need in order to make an informed decision; (3) the *subjective standard*—the disclosure is what the particular person wants or needs to know. Informed consent implies that the person has received the information and understands what is provided. Verification of understanding can be accomplished through discussion in which patients have an opportunity to ask questions and are asked to describe their understanding of the nature of the intervention, alternatives, risks, and benefits.

Figure 11–2 **Content of Informed Consent**

- The nature of the health concern and prognosis if nothing is done.
- Description of all treatment options, even those that the health care provider does not favor or cannot provide.
- The benefits, risks, and consequences of the various treatment alternatives, including nonintervention.

Consent.   Consent to something implies the freedom to accept or reject it. This means that consent to health care interventions must be voluntary, without coercion, force, or manipulation from health care providers or family. Force entails making someone do something against his or her will. Coercion and manipulation may be overt or subtle and may include threats, rewards, deception, or inducing excessive fear. The voluntary nature of consent does not prohibit health care providers from making recommendations or attempting to persuade patients to accept their suggestions. However, it is important to be alert to situations in which persuasion takes on qualities of coercion or manipulation.

 CASE PRESENTATION

Language and Informed Consent

Mohano is a sixty-seven-year-old deaf man who was admitted to the hospital with atrial fibrillation. The nurse notes that he is alert, apparently oriented, and able to follow simple directions that she acts out, although he does look apprehensive as she cares for him. Mohano's social history indicates that he was brought into the hospital by a community worker who looks in on him because he is deaf and illiterate and has no family in the area. She had indicated that he came to the area as a migrant worker a number of years ago, along with a brother who died the previous year. She had also noted that two of his five siblings were also deaf, and they had developed a type of sign language that was understood only by family members. At the interdisciplinary care conference the medical resident who is in charge of his case voices frustration because of the need to get the patient's permission to do a stress test and to talk to him about medications and risk for stroke. He suggests that they should just get the patient to make an X on the form so they can go ahead with the treatment protocol because it is in the patient's best interest to do so. The social worker suggests that they get an interpreter for the deaf to come in and try to talk to him through sign language, although she is not sure he will understand.

 Think About It

Obtaining Informed Consent When There Is No Common Language

- What ethical dilemmas are evident in this case?
- What do you think about Mohano's decision making capacity?
- Do you think it is possible to obtain an informed consent from Mohano? Support your position with discussion of elements of informed consent and decision making capacity.
- In a situation such as this it is evident that the patient has a language, although it is not understood by the health care providers, and that he has been able to care for himself with some assistance. How would these factors enter into determination of his decision making capacity?

- How does the inability of the health care provider to communicate with a patient affect determination of the patient's decision making capacity?
- What are the implications of denying Mohano important services because of lack of common language and subsequent inability to ensure informed consent?

Nursing Role and Responsibilities

While the practice of documenting informed consent for a procedure usually ends with the signing of a consent form, the process is much more complex. Following the rules laid out previously, informed consent must include explicit verification that the patient is aware of all options, the possible outcomes of each option, and the likely outcome with nontreatment. The patient must also recognize the implications each option will have upon his or her lifestyle. The nurse must be sensitive to the fact that the very act of asking a patient to sign a form giving permission for a particular treatment may constitute a form of coercion. It is the nurse's responsibility as advocate for the patient to ensure that all criteria for autonomous decision making are met. If the nurse believes that the patient does not understand the implications of any part of the process, including nontreatment and alternative options, or that the patient is unable to deliberate and reason on the various choices, it is the responsibility of the nurse to intervene. Legally the nurse must act if it becomes apparent that the patient is not informed; however, no ruling has been made to describe precisely what the nurse must do when it is clear that the patient is not informed (Kapp, 1990). Actions may include notifying the physician and requesting further information for the patient or stopping the process until it is ensured that the decision can be made autonomously. Though the mechanics of the process usually require the nurse to obtain the patient's signature on a consent form, the primary concern of the nurse is to ensure that all criteria for autonomous decision making are met.

Nurses in advanced practice roles are accountable for providing information and obtaining informed consent for interventions that they initiate under their scope of practice. The question of the nurse's right to inform a patient of the risks inherent in a certain procedure or alternative courses of action in other settings is not as clear. In 1977 Jolene Tuma, a nursing instructor, in the course of initiating chemotherapy, answered an elderly patient's questions about cancer treatment alternatives. The patient indicated that she did not want to question the physician because he was not open to considering other therapies. Tuma was also asked to describe the therapies to the patient's son, who was upset by this. Although the patient decided to continue chemotherapy, she died two weeks later. After the patient's death, the son told the physician of Tuma's action. The physician subsequently brought charges against Ms. Tuma for disrupting the physician-patient relationship. She was fired from her job and lost her nursing license as a result. Ms. Tuma pursued an appeal of the decision. In 1979 the Idaho Supreme Court ruled that she could not lose her license for "unprofessional behavior" because there was no statutory description of this offense. The court did not address, however, the nurse's right to inform the patient (Husted & Husted, 1995).

Unfortunately, this leaves the nurse in a sort of limbo in regard to ensuring informed consent. Although the nurse is legally required to act on behalf of the patient to guarantee true informed consent, there is no clear course of action when it is believed that the patient has not been informed or does not understand the information and the physician is uncooperative in remedying the situation. Institutional and legal constraints may impede the nurse from following the ethically correct course of action.

Ask Yourself

What Is Nurse's Responsibility Regarding Informed Consent?

- In the case described above, do you feel that Jolene Tuma's actions were appropriate? Support your position.
- What ethical issues are considerations in situations such as this?
- How does the nurse-patient relationship factor into such a situation?

Advance Directives

Given the dilemmas that can arise regarding the use of technology, it is important that people make known their wishes concerning the use of such interventions. For those who are mentally alert and capable of making decisions, informed consent is needed prior to initiating any life sustaining interventions. To ensure that one's wishes regarding treatment are followed in the event that one has lost decision making capacity, advance directives are needed. **Advance directives** are instructions that indicate health care interventions to initiate or withhold or that designate someone who will act as a surrogate in making such decisions in the event that one loses decision making capacity. Such directives can be considered as a kind of informed consent for future interventions.

Advance directives include living wills and durable powers of attorney. **Living wills** are legal documents giving directions to health care providers related to withholding or withdrawing life support if certain conditions exist. Statutes regulating living wills vary from state to state, so it is important that nurses be familiar with their own state laws. Living wills guide decisions by indicating a person's desires relative to life sustaining interventions; however, they also raise issues of concern. Directives in living wills may be vague and can address only the interventions a person does not want. In many states only persons who are terminally ill or whose death is imminent are allowed to make living wills. Particularly in emergency situations, there is often a concern that a document that may have been developed when a person was in good health may not reflect the patient's current desires.

Durable power of attorney allows a competent person to designate another as a surrogate or proxy to act on her or his behalf in making health care decisions in the event of the loss of decision making capacity. Although there is no particular legal form required, the designation must be in writing and must be signed and dated by the person making the designation and two witnesses other than the designated surrogate. The designating person may revoke the designation at any time by changing the person named as surrogate or by destroying the document. The authority of the surrogate does not become effective until it has been determined that the person has lost decision making capacity. The authority of the surrogate is effective only for the duration of the loss of decision making capacity. For example, in the case of a person who has a temporary loss of consciousness, the surrogate's authority to make decisions would end once the person regained consciousness and the ability to make decisions for self.

It is important that the presence of a living will or durable power of attorney and surrogate designation be documented in a patient's health record. Nurses should routinely ask patients whether they have such documents and be able to discuss the importance of such directives with patients and families. The American Nurses Association (ANA) *Position Statement on Nursing and the Patient Self-Determination Act* recommends including the following questions in nursing admission assessments:

> Do you have basic information about advance care directives including living wills and durable power of attorney? Do you wish to indicate an advance care directive? If you have already prepared an advance care directive, can you provide it now? Have you discussed your end of life choices with your family and/or designated surrogate and health care workers? (ANA, 1991)

It is well known that patients may indicate concerns to nurses that they have not discussed with their physicians. Issues related to advance directives may be one such concern.

Patient Self-Determination Act. The **Patient Self-Determination Act,** which went into effect December 1991, is a federal law requiring institutions such as hospitals, nursing homes, health maintenance organizations, and home care agencies receiving Medicare or Medicaid funds to provide written information to adult patients regarding their rights to make health care decisions. Such decisions include the right to refuse treatments and to write advance directives for guiding decisions should they become incapacitated. The ANA notes that nurses have a responsibility to facilitate informed decision making with patients, particularly regarding end of life care, and that nurses have a critical role in implementing the Patient Self-Determination Act within all health care settings.

> The formation of advance directives is an important decision and will inevitably involve nurses who are the most omnipresent professionals in health care facilities. It is imperative that the decision making that will fall to patients and their families as they make choices about end of life care be facilitated by nurses. (ANA, 1991)

Information concerning advance directives is often provided by a clerical worker on admission to a facility with little explanation or opportunity to ask questions, thus nurses need to explore patient and family understanding of the information given. This gives the nurse an opportunity to stress the importance of having such directives and to advocate for patients who may need assistance in developing advance directives. The law recognizes the need to increase public awareness about advance directives and encourages community education programs to do so. Nursing role in implementation of the Patient Self-Determination Act includes "public education, research, patient care, advocacy, education of the profession and inservice education of other health care providers" (ANA, 1991).

CHOICES CONCERNING LIFE AND HEALTH

Although discussion of patient autonomy frequently centers around issues of informed consent and end of life decisions, issues related to self-determination can arise in any area of nursing practice. In every area of practice nurses must deal with the effects of lifestyle choices on patients' health and healing. Many people who come into our care are suffering from ill effects of such things as overeating; tobacco, drug, or alcohol use; sexual activity; or work related stress. Our job is to deal with the present health concern while encouraging change toward healthier living. However, patients are often not willing to follow the treatment plan and make the changes needed for healthier living. Dealing with patients whose health problems are clearly related to lifestyle choices, yet who are not willing to change their behaviors, may present dilemmas for nurses. Although it might be acknowledged that the autonomous person has the right to choose healthy or unhealthy behaviors, it may be difficult to be as caring toward those who are perceived to have brought problems on themselves.

This is another area where the principle of justice may temper the bounds of autonomy. In situations where resources are limited, questions arise regarding whether it is ethical to put resources into treatments for people whose health problems are brought on by unhealthy life choices. This is countered by the question of whether it is ethical to refuse treatment or provide a lesser level of care to someone because the provider does not agree with the lifestyle choices.

Ask Yourself

Who Should Pay for Ill Effects of Unhealthy Lifestyles?

It is interesting that in the time of Hippocrates physicians were taught that they should not treat persons whose bodies were overmastered by their disease because it was an inappropriate use of medical resources.

- How do you feel about this?

- Would this same stance be considered ethical today?

- To what extent do personal lifestyle choices impinge on the rights of others if significant health care resources are needed to pay for the ill effects of these choices?

Autonomy implies that persons have the right to make choices about things that affect their lives, whether these choices have a positive or negative effect, unless these choices impinge on the rights of others.

- Is it just to expect society to pay for the health care services required for treating the effects of unhealthy behaviors?
- How would you go about allocating health care resources in relation to unhealthy lifestyle choices?

Choices Regarding Recommended Treatment

What are nurses to do when patients are well informed and apparently able to follow plans of care, yet do not? Certainly one hears of physicians who refuse to continue to care for patients who do not comply with instructions—smoking cessation, for example. In a climate of limited resources this is a question worthy of contemplation. The ANA *Code for Nurses* (1985) states clearly that the nurse must "provide services with respect for human dignity and the uniqueness of the client unrestricted by considerations of social or economic status, personal attributes, or the nature of health problems" (p. 2). Further, the nurse must not be affected by the patients' individual differences in background, customs, attitudes, and beliefs. Health care practices are an integral part of patients' backgrounds, customs, and beliefs. Therefore, it is clear that refusal to participate in a plan of care, regardless of the outcome, is the prerogative of the patient and must not affect the caring attitude of the nurse. Unhealthy life practices are part of the whole person and should be taken into consideration when revising plans of care.

 CASE PRESENTATION

A Challenging Patient

Rochelle, a thirty-six-year-old woman who is a known cocaine addict, presented to the emergency room (ER) with severe left leg pain and swelling. The triage nurse reviewed her chart and presenting problem, noting that she had been seen two days prior for chest pain and left leg pain. Assuming these complaints were evaluated then, the nurse sent her to the "fast track" area to be seen by the Nurse Practitioner (NP). The NP noted that her chart was flagged regarding her cocaine addiction and that the physician who had seen her at the previous visit, after doing an EKG, CBC, electrolytes (which were normal), and a urine drug screen (which was positive for cocaine), discharged her with diagnoses of chest pain and illicit drug use. The NP's assessment revealed no shortness of breath, cough, or chest pain; severe swelling and skin tightness of the left leg, with exquisite tenderness and positive Homan's sign, were suggestive of deep vein thrombosis. When the NP went to the ER physician saying that the patient needed to be evaluated by him, she was told to keep the patient over there and do the work-up because he had a patient with a similar problem in the ER.

When the ultrasound confirmed extensive deep vein thrombosis, the NP told the patient the situation and that she needed to be hospitalized. The patient immediately said that she could not stay because she had no one to watch her nine-year-old-daughter, and she began to put on her shoes to leave. The NP told her that she could choose to leave but that the reason she (the NP) wanted her to stay was that this was a very serious problem from which she could die. Rochelle's response was to start crying, saying that she thought she would go home anyway because she had nothing to live for since her husband had died, so she would go home to die. When the NP called Rochelle's primary physician to alert him to the situation, he responded that he would come in to see her only if Rochelle agreed to stay, otherwise it would be a waste of his time. After considerable effort, the NP contacted Rochelle's mother who reluctantly agreed to keep her granddaughter when the NP explained the situation, and Rochelle agreed to stay.

Think About It

Dealing with Patients Who Make Apparently Unhealthy Choices

- What issues of patient self-determination are evident in this case?

- How do you see lifestyle choices affecting Rochelle's care? What ethical issues must be considered here?

- Take an honest look at how you think you might react to Rochelle, knowing that she frequently shows up in the ER and is a cocaine addict?

- As the nurse in this situation, how would you deal with the patient's saying she could not stay? What do you think of the way the NP handled it?

- Evaluate ethical issues involved in the responses of the various health care practitioners in this case.

- Interestingly, Rochelle was indigent, African-American, and without health insurance, and the woman in the ER with similar complaints was middle-class, Caucasian, and had health insurance. Discuss the implications of these factors in this case.

Ultimately, choices about health care practices belong to patients. If allowed to choose, patients should not be labeled in a negative way for choices with which nurses do not agree. It is not appropriate for professionals who express the belief that all competent patients have the right to autonomous choice, to then make value judgments about the choices made, and subsequently label patients as noncompliant. In fact, it is worth pondering whether the term *noncompliant* even belongs in nursing vocabulary. The notion of compliance relates to a paternalistic view that health care providers know what is best for patients and that, providing patients follow these directions, they will get well. It might be better to speak in terms of motivation to follow a mutually agreed upon plan of care that incorporates patient and family values and beliefs. It is important to remember that patients have a right to refuse interventions, and they have a right to seek therapies other than those offered by conventional Western medicine.

Complementary Therapies. Many people utilize therapies that may be termed complementary, alternative, or unconventional in regard to Western allopathic medicine (Eisenberg, Kessler, Foster, Norlock, Calkins, & Delbanco, 1993). Examples of **complementary therapies** include acupuncture, herbal and nutritional interventions, healing touch, massage, and guided imagery. Most people tend to use such therapies along with conventional modalities, but some will choose to use them in lieu of what is offered by medical practitioners. Most people do not inform their medical practitioner that they are using these therapies.

Several issues regarding the use of complementary therapies need to be considered. First, people have a right to utilize modalities other than conventional medicine to address their health care needs. Second, nurses and other health care practitioners need to develop at least a talking knowledge, and better yet a working knowledge, of such therapies in order to be better able to discuss their use with patients. Many therapies work as an adjunct to medical interventions, some may interact in unhealthy ways, and the efficacy of many modalities is not yet known. Nurses need not be practitioners of other modalities in order to discuss them with patients any more than they need to be able to do surgery in order to discuss it. It is important to create an atmosphere that encourages nonjudgmental discussion of all modalities being considered or employed, with a goal of using whatever is beneficial for the particular patient. Transcultural considerations (which are discussed in Chapter 18) may influence a person's choice of treatment modalities. Third, complementary modalities should not be discounted merely because they are not understood within the Western medical framework; however, it is also important to counsel patients to explore the validity of claims made about a particular therapy. Fourth, as research continues and expands in the area of complementary therapies, the question of whether informed consent will need to at least acknowledge these therapies as treatment options must be addressed. Fifth, nurses who are skilled in one or more complementary therapies need to be clear about what is within their scope of practice according to their state's nurse practice act. The ethical stance with complementary therapies, as with other interventions, requires offering an explanation of the intervention and receiving permission from the patient or family prior to initiating the therapy. Because these therapies can affect conventional interventions, practitioners should apprise other health team members of their use and document both treatments and their effects.

Controversial Choices

The value of patient self-determination has been used to support two decisions that have been the focus of much controversy in this country for many years: abortion and active euthanasia. Both of these choices are surrounded by ethical and religious opinion and debate. Abortion in particular is an example of an issue in which legal answers have been sought for ethical dilemmas. The potential for transmission of HIV infections within health care settings raises controversial issues regarding testing and disclosure. This discussion presents some of the arguments on both sides of these issues.

Nurses need to be very clear about their own values regarding each of these issues and find a balance between personal values and professional obligations to patients and families. Nurses must sort out their own beliefs about what is right and wrong so that they can differentiate between tasks and roles that are consistent with their ethical stance and those that are not, and make responsible practice decisions accordingly. It has been suggested that in the process of reasoning through dilemmas such as those involved with these issues, the least that can be expected is that the nurse not abandon the patient. "The most that can be hoped is that each nurse regard the rights of others as precious, as she would want her own regarded, and that within this complex context she view her obligations to self, to the patient, to nursing, and to her place of employment" (Davis & Aroskar, 1991, p. 136).

Abortion.　The abortion debate sparks passionate, emotion laden arguments in political, social, legal, religious, and moral arenas. Issues of self-determination arise regarding the mother's right to control her body and her life (right to choose) in contrast to rights of the unborn fetus to a chance at life (right to life). Those in the right-to-life camp believe that abortion constitutes murder of an unborn person, suggesting that it is a legal as well as an ethical matter. This has raised questions about the role of government in dealing with this ethical concern. Those who hold to the right to choose maintain that the right to privacy regarding health care decisions includes a woman's reproductive choices, implying that governmental regulation is an infringement on this privacy.

Values in relation to life are fundamental considerations in regard to abortion. Such values include beliefs about when life begins, considerations regarding quality of life for children who are unwanted, and concerns about the mother's life and health. Some believe that life starts at conception while others hold that life begins only when a fetus is viable outside the womb. Discussions regarding viability continue to change as technology enables the survival of babies of lower and lower birth weights and results in saving some imperiled newborns of the same gestational age as some aborted fetuses.

Opponents of abortion hold the position that because a fetus possesses humanity, it must be accorded all human rights, including the right to life. Proponents of abortion argue that, based on autonomy, a woman has a right to her own body and that no woman should be forced to bear a child that she does not want. Because abortion is a situation in which two lives are involved, dilemmas arise regarding who has rights, and whose rights take precedence.

> Some take the position that pregnant women, no matter what the circumstances of conception, have obligations toward the life and well-being of the fetus that overshadow any discussion of the woman's rights. . . . So we have a moral argument, where the stakes are high, in which some people support abortion on demand based on the woman's autonomy. At the same time we have people who oppose

> abortion perhaps except to save the life of the mother or not at all, based on the sanctity of life principle and the personhood of the fetus. To think in a simple way about this ethical dilemma, on the one hand the fetus is viewed as an object or thing while on the other, the woman is viewed as an object or thing. (Davis & Aroskar, 1991, pp. 130–131)

From either perspective, the consideration of abortion presents a dilemma for those involved.

There is no agreement about the morality of abortion in our society. It is a complex issue with many facets to consider. Although debate generally focuses on areas related to rights of the woman or the fetus, Mahowald (1995) suggests that it is also important to consider the morality of circumstances that provide fertile ground for abortion. She notes that immoral conditions that sometimes occasion abortion include: poverty, lack of social and medical supports for pregnancy and parenthood, stereotypic views of sex roles and biological parenthood, and a eugenic mentality that welcomes only "premium babies," those babies that meet the parents' desired specifications (p. 107). She stresses the need for society to direct more effort into rectifying these conditions.

Active Euthanasia. As noted in Chapter 10, technology has caused death to become an unnatural event in the lives of many people. Lo (1995) notes that active euthanasia is currently illegal in all states, and assisted suicide is explicitly prohibited in two-thirds of states. However, public dissatisfaction with end of life care has prompted efforts to legalize these acts. Because of the concern that health care providers will not adhere to personal wishes regarding end of life issues, fears about prolonged suffering resulting from prolongation of dying, and the lack of control that each of these engenders, many people consider the possibility of active euthanasia or assisted suicide. **Active voluntary euthanasia** is an act in which the physician both provides the means of death and administers it, such as a lethal dose of medication. With **assisted suicide** the patients receive the means of death from someone, such as a physician, but activate the process themselves. Justification offered by proponents of these acts include respect for the person's autonomy in choosing to end his or her life if it is deemed intolerable due to conditions of a lingering terminal illness, and compassion exhibited in relief of the patient's suffering. Opponents argue from a stance of the sanctity of life, saying that any such act violates the prohibition against killing human beings. They hold that suffering can almost always be relieved, and they voice concerns about potential abuses, such as involuntary euthanasia to contain health care costs, if such acts were permitted (Lo, 1995).

It is particularly important to consider the reason for a patient's requesting assisted suicide or euthanasia. When the patient indicates that life has become intolerable, it is important to determine why this is so. Often inadequate pain management and depression are factors that enter into this perception, which, when treated appropriately, can change the patient's perspective. Attentiveness to the nature and cause of a person's suffering and provision of comfort care throughout the dying process are important components of the nursing role that may influence choices regarding active voluntary euthanasia or assisted suicide.

Issues Related to HIV/AIDS. It is well known that human immunodeficiency virus and acquired immunodeficiency syndrome (HIV/AIDS) is a major worldwide health concern and that the virus is generally contracted through sexual contact. Although most cases of HIV/AIDS have resulted from a choice to have unprotected sexual relations, it is important to remember that not all HIV/AIDS results from lifestyle choices. The ANA *Code for Nurses* directs nurses to care for patients regardless of their values or lifestyle; thus, nurses need to be aware of potential judgmental attitudes toward persons with HIV/AIDS and be alert to how these attitudes may affect the quality of their care.

Because of the risk of exposure to HIV in health care settings, questions arise regarding issues of autonomy and confidentiality in relation to HIV testing and status. One issue relates to whether patients can be required to submit to HIV testing in situations of potential or actual percutaneous exposure of health care workers to their blood. In order to protect persons from potential discrimination, confidentiality of HIV testing and status is generally assured by law; thus, it is generally illegal to perform HIV testing without a person's written consent. "Ethically speaking, HIV testing over the patient's objections violates the patient's autonomy and privacy as well as the spirit of informed consent . . . consent for HIV testing is important because stigma and discrimination may occur if other people know that the patient is seropositive" (Lo, 1995, p. 332).

Because of concerns about potential stigma in work or home settings related to having a documented HIV test, regardless of its result, patients may refuse a test even if they are sure it will be negative. In order to ensure confidentiality and to encourage patient agreement to testing in the event of exposure of a health care worker to a patient's blood, Lo (1995) suggests an approach of anonymous testing of the patient. Such an approach would necessitate paying for the test by a source other than the patient's insurer (such as an employee health fund), recording the results in a location other than the patient's medical record (such as a special occupational health file), and labeling the blood sample with a code rather than the patient's name. In this way the health care worker could know if he or she is at risk while protecting the patient from potential stigma resulting from the test.

Another issue that has become a public concern relates to potential exposure of patients to the blood of a seropositive health care worker. Questions arise whether HIV testing among health care workers, or at least those involved in certain invasive procedures, should be mandatory; whether seropositive health care workers should have restrictions on their practice; and whether the HIV status of health care workers should be made known to patients. Some argue that if it becomes mandatory for health care workers to be tested, then it should be mandatory for all patients as well. Principles of autonomy, confidentiality, and nonmaleficence become part of this discussion. Health care workers, as well as patients, have a right to autonomy and confidentiality regarding health matters, particularly where discrimination could result from disclosure. At the same time, nonmaleficence directs them to do no harm to patients, and the doctrine of informed consent requires advising patients of potential risks related to interventions being considered. Economic factors enter into the discussion as well. At the present time, presuming health care workers follow universal infection control precautions, the risk of a patient's contracting HIV from a seroposi-tive health care worker is low, in contrast to the high cost of mandatory testing. Requiring such testing could well divert money from other more effective areas of health promotion and protection.

Current issues related to HIV/AIDS may become less of a concern as technology ad-vances toward more effective prevention and treatment of the disease. However, ethi-cal concerns surrounding these issues apply to other health problems of similar nature. Nurses and other health care workers must be aware of any factors in their own health that might put their patients at risk and take necessary precautions to protect patients from harm. It is also essential that nurses follow universal precautions aimed at pro-tecting them and others from harm. If behaviors on the part of health care workers are observed that might put patients at risk, the imperatives of beneficence and nonmalef-icence direct nurses to do what is necessary to protect the patient. Actions may include approaching the person involved, reporting the situation to appropriate persons within the agency, and working with groups to institute changes to prevent similar situations from occurring.

Although cases of HIV/AIDS must be reported, as with other infectious diseases, caregivers cannot disclose a person's HIV status without consent. The legal and ethical right to confidentiality regarding HIV/AIDS raises an ethical issue related to protection of others when the infected individual continues behaviors that may expose others to the infection. In some circumstances physicians are allowed limited disclosure without consent, such as to the patient's spouse. In such situations the imperative of confiden-tiality must be weighed against the duty to warn others in order to protect them from potential harm. At the present time there are no clear directives in this area for health care providers.

Confidentiality

The imperative of **confidentiality** in health care, which is discussed in Chapter 3, can be traced at least as far back as the Hippocratic vow not to reveal secrets. In order to care for people with health concerns, nurses must be privy to very personal, and sometimes secret, information. Without assurance of confidentiality, many people would not disclose information that is important in diagnosis and treatment of, and car-ing for, health concerns. This is especially true in situations where there is stigma at-tached to, or other risks for social repercussions from, the information disclosed. Nurses need to remember that a patient's trust is sacred, and any breach of confiden-tiality, no matter how small it might seem to the nurse, is a violation of this trust. As with so many other areas, there are situations where other factors override confiden-tiality. In circumstances such as court cases, the law might require disclosure. In situa-tions where secrets entrusted to the nurse suggest potential harm for the patient or others, the duty to warn may take precedence over confidentiality. For example, if a patient tells a nurse about suicide plans that the nurse believes are genuine, and the patient is not willing to be hospitalized, protection of the patient may require the nurse to initiate the process of involuntary hospitalization.

SUMMARY

This chapter discussed considerations for nursing practice related to patient self-determination. The concept of self-determination derives from the principle of autonomy and denotes the right and freedom to make choices about issues that affect one's life. Principles of justice, beneficence, and nonmaleficence may temper the bounds of autonomy in some circumstances. The doctrine of informed consent, which has developed as both a legal and ethical imperative for protecting a person's right to self-determination in health care decisions, implies the right to accept or reject recommended treatment plans. In their role as patient advocates, nurses need to be alert for situations in which patient autonomy may be limited or in which there is a lack of sufficient information for the patient or family to make informed decisions. Nurses have a particular responsibility for facilitating informed decision making regarding patient choices for end of life care. Nursing's professional code directs nurses to provide services with respect for the rights and dignity of the patient regardless of a person's background or the nature of the health concern. If professional responsibilities expected of a nurse in a patient care situation are inconsistent with the nurse's ethical stance, integrity and accountability counsel her to remove herself from that situation after ensuring that there are others to assume care for the patient. A nurse's attention to the many faceted issues surrounding patient self-determination may be the factor that ensures the patient's involvement in important health care decisions.

CHAPTER HIGHLIGHTS

- Self-determination derives from the principle of autonomy and implies having freedom to make choices about issues affecting one's life, an ability to make decisions about personal goals, and an appreciation for self in relation to others.

- Autonomy may be threatened by factors such as paternalism; presumptions that a patient's values, knowledge level, and ways of dealing with issues are consistent with those of health care providers; and greater attention to technology than caring. In some situations, principles such as justice or nonmaleficence may temper the bounds of autonomy.

- Decisions about health care require attention to patient values, culture, and beliefs; effects of lifestyle and role; others who are affected by a patient's choices; and evaluation of risks, benefits, and economic considerations.

- Practitioners are not required to honor requests for interventions that are outside accepted standards of care or contrary to the practitioner's ethical views.

- Informed consent provides legal and ethical protection of a patient's right to personal autonomy regarding plans for health care, including the right to refuse interventions and to choose from available alternatives. Information necessary in an informed consent includes: the nature of the concern and prognosis if nothing is done; description of treatment options; and benefits, risks, and consequences of treatment options or nonintervention.

- Decision making capacity, which is a medical determination and essential for informed consent, includes evidence of the ability to understand information, to communicate understanding and choices, to evaluate decisions in relation to personal values and goals, and to reason and deliberate. It is presumed that conscious adults have decision making capacity unless there is evidence to the contrary.

- Nursing responsibility regarding informed consent includes verifying that the patient is aware of options and the implications of each and advocating for patients to ensure that criteria for autonomous decision making are met in situations where the physician has not attended to these criteria. Nurses in advanced practice must obtain informed consent for interventions that they initiate within their scope of practice.

- Advance directives, which include living wills and durable powers of attorney, provide instructions regarding health care interventions in the event that one loses decision making capacity. The Patient Self-Determination Act provides legal support for ensuring that patients are informed of their rights regarding health care decisions.

- In dealing with patient lifestyle choices, nurses must remember the instructions in the ANA *Code for Nurses* to provide services with respect for human dignity and to avoid value judgments related to differences in background, customs, attitudes, and beliefs.

- Nurses need to be aware of their own values and beliefs regarding various lifestyle and health care choices and know how these affect their care with patients.

- Nurses must recognize the patient's right to use complementary therapies, become more knowledgeable about other modalities, and create an atmosphere encouraging of nonjudgmental discussion of such interventions.

- Ethical codes direct nurses to maintain confidentiality regarding patient health status and choices, except in special circumstances in which the "secrets" revealed suggest potential harm for the patient or another.

DISCUSSION QUESTIONS AND ACTIVITIES

1. Discuss your understanding of patient self-determination, including its ethical and legal basis, and nursing practice considerations.

2. Describe dilemmas that may arise for nurses related to patient self-determination and suggest approaches for dealing with such dilemmas.

3. Explore how practicing nurses in your institution perceive their role regarding informed consent. What dilemmas related to consent have they encountered and how did they deal with these issues?

4. Analyze your own values regarding abortion and active voluntary euthanasia. How would you respond to a patient under your care who was deliberating such a choice?

5. Explore your state's statutes regarding advance directives, HIV testing and disclosure, euthanasia, assisted suicide, and abortion. What are the implications of these regulations for nursing practice in your state?

6. What are your views on mandatory HIV testing for health care professionals? What about limiting the practice of seropositive health care workers? Review current literature to determine recommendations by professional organizations concerning these issues.

7. Determine how your institution meets requirements of the Patient Self-Determination Act. Discuss the adequacy of the process and nursing's involvement.

REFERENCES

American Nurses Association. (1985). *Code for nurses with interpretive statements.* Washington, DC: Author.

American Nurses Association. (1991). *Position statement on nursing and the Patient Self-Determination Act.* Kansas City, MO: Author.

Curtin, L. (1982). Autonomy, accountability, and nursing practice. *Topics in Clinical Nursing, 4,* 7–14.

Davis, A. J. & Aroskar, M. A. (1991). *Ethical dilemmas and nursing practice* (3rd ed.). Norwalk, CT: Appleton & Lange.

Devettere, R. J. (1995). *Practical decision making in health care ethics: Cases and concepts.* Washington, DC: Georgetown University Press.

Eisenberg, D. M., Kessler, R. C., Foster, C., Norlock, F. E., Calkins, D. R., & Delbanco, T. L. (1993). Unconventional medicine in the United States. *New England Journal of Medicine, 328,* 246–252.

Hardwig, J. (1995). What About the Family? In J. H. Howell & W. F. Sale (Eds.), *Life choices: A Hastings Center introduction to bioethics* (pp. 53–67). Washington, DC: Georgetown University Press.

Husted, G., & Husted, J. (1995). *Ethical decision making in nursing* (2nd ed.). St. Louis, MO: Mosby.

Kapp, M. B. (1990). Informed, assisted, delegated consent for elderly patients. *AORN, 52,* 857–860.

Lo, B. (1995). *Resolving ethical dilemmas: A guide for clinicians.* Baltimore: Williams & Wilkins.

Mahowald, M. B. (1995). Is there life after Roe v. Wade? In J. H. Howell & W. F. Sale (Eds.), *Life choices: A Hastings Center introduction to bioethics* (pp. 96–110). Washington, DC: Georgetown University Press.

President's Commission for the Study of Ethical Problems in Medicine and Biomedical and Behavioral Research. (1983). *Making health care decisions,* pp. 1–6, Washington, DC: U.S. Government Printing Office.

Sherwin, W. (1992). Paternalism. In *No longer patient: Feminist ethics and health care* (pp. 137–157). Philadelphia: Temple University Press.

CHAPTER 12

Scholarship Issues

My experience tells me that people instinctively trust those whose personality is founded upon correct principles.

(Covey, 1992, p. 18)

OBJECTIVES

After completing this chapter, the reader should be able to:

1. Describe scholarship issues encountered by nurses in academic and clinical settings.
2. Discuss principles basic to academic honesty and the ethical treatment of research data.
3. Describe principles and nursing standards undergirding the protection of human rights in research.
4. Explain why informed consent is mandated for research involving human subjects, and describe the elements required for this consent.
5. Discuss the nursing role regarding protection of human rights in research.
6. Describe principles guiding personal response to dilemmas regarding nursing scholarship.

INTRODUCTION

Scholarship issues face students, teachers, researchers, and clinicians from the moment a person enters a nursing program and throughout that person's professional career. This chapter discusses principles that undergird ethical behavior in academic matters, in conducting research, and in the treatment of data both during the research process and in presentations or publication. Respect for all persons, including oneself, is basic to ethical behavior regarding scholarship. Personal values affect how one approaches situations that present ethical dilemmas; thus, it is essential that nurses be knowledgeable about principles guiding ethical conduct, whether dealing with academic assignments, research data, or research with human subjects.

ACADEMIC HONESTY

Integrity in upholding the principles of veracity and fidelity is expected of nurses in any setting and is at the core of academic honesty. Veracity refers to truth telling, which is an essential ingredient for trust among humans. Husted and Husted (1995) suggest that true interaction and communication cannot occur where there is no trust. These authors describe fidelity as promise keeping, suggesting that it is the form that truth takes in an agreement between persons such as nurse-patient, researcher-participant, or student-teacher. Integrity implies respect for self and others, and a personal commitment to principled behavior over time in one's personal and professional life. When integrity is present, there is no need for monitoring a person's behavior; rather, there is an implicit trust that one represents oneself in a truthful way. Honesty and integrity are key considerations in both academic and clinical situations. Personal values such as honesty serve as the basis for professional integrity.

Students at all levels face many stresses in regard to academic performance, and nursing students are no exception. Pressures may come from many areas, such as family expectations, personal goals of being accepted into graduate school, needing a certain grade to receive tuition reimbursement, or self-expectations that say "I always get good grades." When pressures become intense, values such as honesty and integrity may become challenged.

Issues of academic honesty include plagiarism, cheating, and forgery. **Plagiarism** is taking another's ideas or work and presenting them as one's own. Examples include submitting written, oral, or visual materials—such as a paper, report, speech, or thesis—that have been knowingly copied or obtained, in whole or in part, from another's work without appropriate acknowledgment. **Cheating** refers to dishonesty and deception regarding examinations, projects, or papers. Examples include receiving help from or giving help to another student during an exam, allowing another to copy one's work, or doing work for another student that is to be submitted by that student. **Forgery** includes fraud or intentional misrepresentation, for example, altering or causing a grade to be altered in an academic record or presenting false data on admission records (West Virginia University, 1995–1997).

Ask Yourself

What Are Your Perspectives on Academic Honesty?

- One of your closest friends is in a different section of the same course, and his section meets two days after yours. You know he has been very stressed because of his mother's illness and that he needs good grades to keep his scholarship. You have just taken the mid-term exam, and he asks you to give him an idea of the topics covered so he can focus his studying. What would you do? How do you feel in this situation? What principles would guide your decisions?

- During an exam you notice two students passing what appears to be notes between them. You are fairly sure that the instructor has not seen this. How do you feel in response to this? What would you do, and why?

- You are struggling with an assignment that is due in just a few days. A classmate says she has a paper that her cousin did for this same course three years ago that she is using as a guide, changing the text so that it seems like her writing. She offers to let you see her cousin's paper to do the same. What do you think about her plan? How would you respond? What would guide your decision?

Implicit in academic honesty is a trust that work submitted by a student, whether papers, projects, or exams, is indeed the work of that student. When material from other sources are included in papers, students must utilize appropriate referencing so as to avoid plagiarizing. One university catalog suggests that academic dishonesty indicates an "inability to meet and face issues . . . creating an atmosphere of mistrust, disrespect, and insecurity" (West Virginia University, 1995–1997, p. 35). The breach of trust and potential consequences within a student-teacher relationship that academic dishonesty engenders are self-evident. Litigation is another potential consequence in severe situations. Because of the value of honesty, academic institutions frequently have written policies that may carry consequences as serious as the student's being suspended or expelled for dishonest practices.

 ## CASE PRESENTATION

Suspicions of Dishonesty

Sabrina and Jude have been close friends and study partners throughout their nursing program. They discuss their readings and class notes and frequently choose the same topic, sharing articles between them when writing papers. After a recent submission of papers, the instructor called them in and noted that their papers were almost identical, including mistakes in grammar, and said that it appeared that one had copied the other's paper. They each denied copying from the other.

Think About It

Considering Consequences for Academic Dishonesty

- What ethical issues are involved in this situation?
- How do you feel about incidences of academic dishonesty?
- How do you think this situation should be handled? What consequences would you consider?
- In light of the standards that guide nursing practice, what is your position on allowing a student who has violated academic honesty through plagiarism, cheating, or forgery to continue in a nursing program?

RESEARCH ISSUES AND ETHICS

As nursing continues to seek to enhance its professional image and develop a unique body of scientific knowledge, research becomes a more prominent issue for the discipline. Nurses are being called to greater accountability for the quality of care delivered and to document the efficacy of their practice of nursing. The scientific knowledge base, which is expanded through research, provides an organizing framework for clinical practice.

Participating in research can be exciting and encourage professional growth. It can also present some dilemmas for the nurse and nurse researcher in the academic and clinical realms. Seeking new knowledge and understanding is the expected motivation for conducting research. However, personal or institutional gains related to rewards like grant monies, prestige, the need to succeed, or promoting a product can be other motivating factors that may challenge principled behavior in regard to research.

A nurse who works in clinical areas where research is being conducted must be aware of principles for the conduct of research, regardless of whether the nurse has an active role with the research project. In this regard, guidelines from the American Nurses Association (ANA) state:

> A relationship of trust between nurse and patient has always been an essential element of the professional code of ethics. In research, a relationship of trust between subject and investigator requires that the investigator assume special obligations to safeguard the subject. . . . The individual has the right of self-determination concerning what will be done to his person. Each practitioner of nursing has an obligation to endorse and support self-determination as a moral and legal right of the individual. The responsibilities of safeguarding the rights of others must be fully accepted by nurses whether their roles are as practitioners, educators, or researchers. (ANA, 1985, p. 3)

Ethical Issues in Research

Discussions of ethical issues in research found in research texts focus a good deal on protection of human rights. This emphasis is understandable because of violations that have occurred in the past. The most often cited violations of human rights in research are those that were perpetrated by the Nazis during World War II and that came to public awareness during the Nuremberg trials. International efforts to provide guidelines for protection of human rights have been documented in the **Nuremberg Code,** which was developed as a set of principles for the ethical conduct of research against which the experiments in the concentration camps could be judged, and the **Declaration of Helsinki,** issued by the World Medical Assembly in 1964 and revised in 1975, to guide clinical research. Included in the **Belmont Report,** the principles set forth in these codes serve as the basis for policies developed by the United States National Commission for the Protection of Human Subjects of Biomedical and Behavioral Research (1978).

Principles underlying the ethical conduct of research noted in the *Belmont Report* (1978) and echoed in the American Nurses Association Human Rights Guidelines for Nurses in Clinical and Other Research (1985) are beneficence, respect for human dignity, and justice. The principle of **beneficence** implies the right to protection from harm and discomfort, including a balance between the benefits and risks of a study. The principle of **respect for human dignity** implies the rights to full disclosure and self-determination or autonomy. The principle of **justice** implies the rights of fair treatment and privacy, including anonymity and confidentiality. A brief discussion of each principle follows. The ANA guidelines for the protection of human rights are summarized in Figure 12–1.

Figure 12–1 **Protection of Human Rights**

Right to Freedom from Intrinsic Risk of Injury

- When an individual participating in research is exposed to increased risk for social, emotional, or physical injury, the investigator must specify the degree of risk and estimate how the risk to the individual compares to the benefit to humanity through knowledge gained.

- All relevant information concerning activities that go beyond established and accepted procedures for meeting personal needs must be given to a prospective participant prior to that person's participation in the study.

- Nurses must be vigilant in their concern for persons who are unable to effectively protect themselves from harm or injury due to illness or other condition and be aware of potentials for exploiting captive populations, such as persons in institutions, students, or prisoners.

Right to Privacy

- Since an investigator cannot decide for another what is considered an invasion of privacy for that person, all proposals, protocols, investigative instruments, and procedures to be used in research activities must be specified and discussed with the prospective participant.

- The above must be discussed as well with any workers who are expected to take part in the research as data gatherers or research participants.

Right to Anonymity

- There must be safeguards against unanticipated physical, psychological, or social disadvantages occurring to participants because of their role in the research, either during the study or from dissemination of findings.

- Assurance that a participant's anonymity will be protected must be provided when the participant agrees to share personal information that might not be divulged to others in another context.

- When collected data is not to remain under the control of the investigator, mechanisms for protecting the identity of the participant and safeguarding confidentiality must be established.

- When the plan of the study or the report of the findings will sacrifice the participant's anonymity or confidentiality, specific prior consent must be obtained.

- Potential violations of human dignity from demeaning or dehumanizing situations in the research protocol require special consideration, recognizing that such violations can have long-range repercussions when significant values of the individual are involved.

Adapted from American Nurses Association (1985). *Human rights guidelines for nurses in clinical and other research* (p. 67). Kansas City, MO: Author.

Beneficence. This principle derives from the maxim that says "above all, do no harm." In research situations this means that researchers need to design and conduct studies so as to protect the participants from physical, mental, emotional, spiritual, economic, and social harm. Discomfort can range from no anticipated effects to certainty of permanent damage and include such things as fatigue, physical pain, anxiety, embarrassment, confronting meaning and purpose in life, threats to self-esteem or to values, lost earnings for time given to participate in research, and social stigma (Burns & Groves, 1993; Harrison, 1993; Wilson, 1993). If discomfort is anticipated as part of the research protocol, the participant must be willing to experience the discomfort after being given all relevant information, and the risk for harm must be balanced with anticipated benefits. In general, a minimal risk is that which is no more than would be expected within the context of routine life activities. When risks are greater than minimal, the researcher's aim must be to minimize risks while maximizing the benefits to participants. "By virtue of their calling, practitioners in the health professions seek to protect individuals under their care from unnecessary physical or mental suffering" (ANA, 1985, p. 6). If the risks outweigh the benefits, the study should be redesigned or discontinued.

Respect for Human Dignity. Implicit in this principle is the right to self-determination, which acknowledges the autonomy of the potential participant in research. This means that persons have the right to choose whether or not they wish to participate in the research, that is, participation is voluntary and free from coercion of any type. **Coercion** includes threat of harm or penalty for not participating in the research, or offering excessive rewards for participation. The right of self-determination means that the person has the right to withdraw from participating in the study at any time without imposed consequences such as denial of health care or benefits. Voluntary participation requires **full disclosure,** that is, that the potential participant be fully informed of the nature of the study, the anticipated risks and benefits, time commitment, what is expected of the participant and the researcher, and the right to refuse to participate. This is addressed through the process of informed consent, which is discussed below.

Justice. Included under the principle of justice are the rights to privacy and to fair treatment. The nature of research is to gather information about that which is being studied. When persons are the focus of study, the **right to privacy** is a critical issue. Attentiveness to privacy means the participant determines when, where, and what kind of information is shared, with an assurance that information, attitudes, behaviors, records, opinions, and the like that are observed or collected will be treated with respect and kept in strict confidence. Anonymity, confidentiality, and informed consent are processes by which privacy is maintained. If even the researcher cannot link information with a particular participant, then **anonymity** exists. **Confidentiality** refers to the researcher's assurance to participants that information provided will not be made public or available to anyone other than those involved in the research process without the participant's consent. Confidentiality is maintained by using codes rather than personal identification on data collection forms and restricting access to raw data to those on the research team who need to use the data.

The **right to fair treatment** is related to the right to self-determination. Equitable treatment of participants in the selection process, during the study, and after the completion of the study is at the basis of this right. Factors to consider in fair treatment include: selecting participants based on the research needs, not on the convenience or compromised position of a group of people; equitably distributing the risks and benefits of the research among participants regardless of age, gender, socioeconomic status, race, or ethnic background; honoring any agreements made or benefits promised; treating participants with respect, providing access to research personnel or other professionals as needed; treating persons who decline to participate or withdraw from the study without prejudice; and debriefing as needed to clarify issues or when information had been withheld prior to the study.

CASE PRESENTATION

Protecting Patients Who Are Research Subjects

Annissa, a nurse in a primary care clinic, talked with her coworker Bill about his non-nursing graduate program. Bill said he has decided to study emotional attitudes of patients using a standardized instrument for his required research project. When Annissa asked about recruiting participants, he said he will have all his patients complete the instrument when he sees them for routine visits over the next few weeks. In response to Annissa's questions about the possibility of patients not wanting to participate, Bill said that he'll just tell them it's for a student project, and he's sure they'll fill out the form to help him out and keep on his good side. Annissa asked which Institutional Review Board (IRB) reviewed his proposal, and Bill replied that his school does not have an IRB so only his advisor had to give approval.

Think About It

What Principles Guide Ethical Conduct of Clinical Research?

- What principles are involved in this situation?
- What dilemmas may arise with Bill's research project?
- What are Annissa's ethical responsibilities in this situation?
- What is the responsibility of the primary care agency related to research conducted within the agency?

Informed Consent. As noted above, voluntary participation in a research study requires full disclosure. Informing potential participants of the research purpose, expected commitment, risks and benefits, any invasion of privacy, and ways that anonymity and confidentiality will be addressed are included in the process of **informed consent.** It is important that there is evidence that the person who is agreeing to participate in the study comprehends the information included in the consent and has a chance to receive clarifications and additional information when needed. Written consent forms should be developed using common language and avoiding jargon. The literacy level of the person signing the informed consent should be determined and recorded, and the person agreeing to participate in the research must be mentally and emotionally competent to make the decision.

Munhall (1993) suggests that the process of informed consent provides a way of including the person as a collaborator in the research rather than as a mere "subject." It is important, however, to guard against the element of coercion. When the nurse who cares for the patient is on the research team and the one obtaining the informed consent, determining whether the patient is giving consent to the "nurse" or to the "researcher" can be somewhat tricky. The nurse-researcher must determine whether the patient truly feels the freedom to refuse to participate.

The *Code of Federal Regulations* (1981) lists basic elements that need to be included in informed consent:

1. A statement that the study involves research, an explanation of the purpose of the research and the expected duration of the subject's participation, a

description of the procedures to be followed, and identification of any procedures that are experimental.

2. A description of any reasonably foreseeable risks or discomforts to the participant.

3. A description of any benefits to the participant or to others that may reasonably be expected from the research.

4. A disclosure of appropriate alternative procedures or courses of treatment, if any, that might be advantageous to the subject.

5. A statement describing the extent, if any, to which confidentiality of records identifying the subject will be maintained.

6. For research involving more than minimal risk, an explanation as to whether any compensation and an explanation as to whether medical treatments are available if injury occurs and, if so, what they consist of, or where further information may be obtained.

7. An explanation of whom to contact for answers to pertinent questions about the research and research subjects' rights, and whom to contact in the event of a research-related injury to the subject.

8. A statement that participation is voluntary, that refusal to participate will involve no penalty or loss of benefits to which the subject is otherwise entitled, and the subject may discontinue participation at any time without penalty or loss of benefits to which the subject is otherwise entitled.

Nurses who are assisting with research or who work on units where research is being conducted must be familiar with these elements of informed consent. If consent forms do not contain these elements, nurses should bring this to the attention of the investigators or the institution ethics committee.

 CASE PRESENTATION

Nurses, Research, and Informed Consent

Juan, a registered nurse, works in a small rural hospital clinic that has a strong commitment to the underserved population in its area, yet has been struggling financially because of the large number of indigent patients. There has been talk of possibly eliminating some positions because of the financial crisis. In a recent staff meeting he learned that a pharmaceutical company has negotiated an agreement with the physicians to use a new medication with their hypertensive patients and gather data about side effects of this medication. A sizable financial reimbursement for the hospital is part of the agreement. As the RN, Juan will be responsible for checking patients' blood pressures and completing the side effect surveys. Juan asks about informed consent and is told that the pharmaceutical company said it is not needed because this medication has been through the clinical trials already. Juan does not feel comfortable about participating in the project but recognizes that the money is needed by the hospital and, in fact, may make the difference in avoiding elimination of staff positions.

Think About It

Decisions About Participating in Research

- What issues do you identify in this case situation?
- What ethical principles are being violated or potentially violated?
- What ethical dilemmas do you think Juan is experiencing?
- What do you think Juan should do, and why?
- How might potential consequences affect the decision making process?

Special Considerations: Vulnerable Populations

A vulnerability or diminished autonomy exists among certain populations that requires the nurse to be more attentive to protection of rights to self-determination regarding research in clinical situations. These populations include physically, mentally, or emotionally disabled or challenged persons; children or elderly persons; those who are dying, sedated, or unconscious; persons who are institutionalized or incarcerated; pregnant women; and fetuses. Because people in these populations are vulnerable to deception and coercion and may have decreased ability to give informed consent, advocates or guardians who have the person's best interest in mind need to be involved in decisions regarding their participation in research. "The fundamental rule here is that the less able a subject is to give informed consent, the greater the burden on the investigator to protect the subject's rights" (Wilson, 1993). Nurses who work with these populations need to be especially cognizant of their roles as advocates, particularly when research is proposed or being conducted in their settings.

More than Protection of Human Rights

Protection of human subjects is a very important consideration when looking at ethical issues in nursing research. However, there are other issues equally important to consider. Wilson (1993) discusses characteristics of ethical research that go beyond the protection of human rights. These include:

Scientific objectivity—reporting all data, both supportive and unsupportive of hypotheses, and not engaging in misconduct, fraud, or acts of bad faith;

Cooperation—submitting proposals to and following recommendations of those authorized to review the research for protection of human rights;

Nobility—working actively to ensure protection of participants from harm, deceit, coercion, and invasions of privacy, even when this may inconvenience the study;

Integrity and Truthfulness—honestly describing the research process, including the purpose, procedures, methods, risks, discomforts, benefits, and findings;

Impeccability—ensuring anonymity and confidentiality of data and using discretion with information learned about people;

Illumination—publishing and presenting research findings in order to enhance nursing's body of scientific knowledge;

Equitability—noting contributions of others in publications and presentations;

Forthrightness—disclosing funding sources and sponsorship in publication and presentation of research findings; and

Courage—publicly clarifying any distortions of research findings made by others.

When nurses are working in agencies or institutions where research is being conducted, whether or not they are directly involved in the research, they must be aware of standards for ethical research so as to guard against violations of these standards.

Nurses who participate in conducting research may at times experience role conflict. A nurse is held to standards of professional practice that delineate the nurse's concern as safeguarding the health and well being of the patient. A researcher is focused on processes and outcomes of a study in which patients may be used as sources of data. A responsible researcher is guided by humanistic values of moral concern in decisions regarding research participants (Fry, 1981). Thus, when there is a question of potential harm to a patient involved in a research study, the advocacy role of the nurse and the therapeutic imperative takes precedence over integrity of the research protocol (Fowler, 1988a; Munhall, 1993; Namei, King, Byrne, & Proffitt, 1993). Ignorance of ethical and legal guidelines related to research is no excuse for a nurse failing to be a patient advocate in research situations. Although research is necessary for development of scientific and therapeutic knowledge, a balance between principles guiding scientific inquiry and those guiding nursing practice must be maintained.

When nurses are employed, particularly in institutions that are research focused, they need to clarify what is expected of them in regard to research. Nurses should know prior to accepting a position whether they will be required to gather data or administer treatments as part of research protocols, and whether such treatments may have potential risks to patients. Nurses in such settings need to know whether their positions will be jeopardized if they refuse to participate as part of a research team. When participation in research is expected as part of a nurse's job, it is imperative that the nurse know the protocol, whether it has been approved by the institutional review board, and who to consult with any concerns about the research process and effect on patients.

Ask Yourself

What Takes Precedence—Research or Nursing Care?

Fowler (1988b, p. 354) poses some questions that are worth pondering.

- Is the good of the patient ever subservient to the acquisition of nursing knowledge?

- Does the therapeutic imperative of clinical care and the good of the patient always preempt the mandate to enlarge the nursing profession's body of knowledge?

- At what point must a nurse stop a specific nursing research project?
- When must a nurse intervene to halt a specific medical research project?
- Are there conditions under which a nurse should not include a specific subject in a study, even though consent has been secured?

ETHICAL TREATMENT OF DATA

Scholarship issues regarding data include how the data is handled during the collection and analysis process and how the data is reported. **Ethical treatment of data** implies integrity of research protocols and honesty in reporting findings. The honesty and integrity of the researcher are of utmost importance in the ethical treatment of data. Taking care to ensure that only those who are involved in the research process have access to the data and to maintain confidentiality were mentioned previously. Munhall (1993) notes that "the most critical, ethical obligation that qualitative nurse researchers have is to describe the experiences of others in the most faithful way possible. The ethical obligation is to describe and report in the most authentic manner possible the experience that unfolds even if contrary to your aims" (p. 399). The ethical obligation to report the findings as accurately as possible is imperative in quantitative studies as well.

 CASE PRESENTATION

Ethical Issues in Handling Research Data

A classmate and good friend is in the process of doing a research project required for graduation. You know she is frustrated because the surveys she sent out are not being returned and the project needs to be completed soon if she is to graduate on time. She also needs to do well on this project in order to graduate with honors. In order to have a large enough sample, she tells you that she is going to fill in several forms herself and asks if you will do some for her too, noting that several other friends have already completed forms. She says that, after all, the object of the assignment is to see if one can collect and analyze the data. You are also aware that the best studies will be published in the student nursing newsletter.

 Think About It

Honesty in Nursing Research

- What is your reaction to her plan and request?
- Discuss the ethical issues involved in this scenario.
- Describe the appropriate ethical stance in this situation. What factors would enable or mitigate against your taking this stance?

- What would you do with this information and what principles would guide your actions?

Nurses involved in research are accountable to professional standards for reporting findings. Principles that guide academic honesty apply as well to nurse researchers in reporting outcomes of studies. It is dishonest to exaggerate results or adjust facts of a study in order to maximize or minimize particular outcomes or hypotheses. When information from someone else is included in a report without appropriate referencing, this is plagiarism. In recent years, scientific misconduct has become a concern within the scientific community. Articles have been published in professional journals reporting studies that were never conducted, findings that were fabricated, or findings that were intentionally distorted by researchers (Burns & Groves, 1993; Chop & Silva, 1991; Friedman, 1990; Hawley & Jeffers, 1992). Although these reports have related more to biomedical studies than to nursing research, such reports present problems to disciplines whose clinical practice may be changed based on research findings. They also serve as a reminder to nurses to be vigilant regarding ethical reporting of research findings.

Ask Yourself

Consequences of Reporting Fraudulent Research

Pause and think about the havoc rendered by publication of fraudulent research.

- How might this affect how others view the integrity of the profession?
- How might this affect a reader's response to other research published in the same journal?
- How would this affect your ability as a nurse to determine whether you should adjust your practice based on reported research?
- Imagine that you have just read the report of a research project for which you gathered data and discovered that the process described was quite a bit different from what you had done, making the results take on a different meaning. How would you react and what would you do?

SUMMARY

Nurses are expected to exhibit principled behavior in all situations. This chapter has focused on principles related to scholarship issues that may be encountered by nurses. Decisions related to academic honesty face nursing students before they ever encounter a patient. Since personal values affect professional behavior, choices made in the academic arena concerning actions such as plagiarism, cheating, or forgery may foreshadow values used to guide future professional decisions. Nurses must be familiar with principles guiding ethical practices in research and reporting of research findings in order to make sound judgments regarding research in which they may be involved, and to guide decisions related to advocacy for patients regarding research issues. Ethical practices regarding scholarship are essential to the integrity of both the professional and the profession.

CHAPTER HIGHLIGHTS

- Principles of veracity and integrity are core to academic honesty and to ethical treatment of research data.

- Nursing research and researchers must adhere to nursing standards regarding the ethical conduct of research that affirm a participant's right to freedom from intrinsic risk of injury, right to privacy, and right to anonymity.

- Protection of human rights, a prime focus of research ethics, is based on principles of beneficence, respect for human dignity, and justice. These principles imply protection from physical, emotional, spiritual, economic, and social harm; voluntary participation in research; and assurance of privacy and equitable treatment of all research participants.

- Informed consent for research studies, which helps to ensure that a participant's rights are protected, must include the elements promulgated in the *Code of Federal Regulations*.

- When there is a question of potential harm to a patient involved in a research study, the nurse's advocacy role and therapeutic imperative takes precedence over the integrity of the research protocol. Nurses need to be especially attentive to protection of rights of vulnerable groups in clinical and research settings.

- When considering employment, nurses should clarify expectations regarding potential participation in research.

DISCUSSION QUESTIONS AND ACTIVITIES

1. Review your school's policy regarding academic honesty and discuss ethical principles that are violated in cases of academic dishonesty.

2. What factors should be taken into consideration by persons reviewing cases of academic dishonesty?

3. How did protection of human rights come to be required for research involving human subjects?

4. What guidance do nursing standards offer nurses who are participating in or conducting research? What principles underlie the ethical conduct of research? Discuss nursing roles related to these principles and standards.

5. Interview a nurse-researcher regarding how human rights are protected in the study. Have all the required elements been included in the informed consent?

6. Give examples of situations in which the nursing roles of patient advocate and researcher might be in conflict. Which role takes precedence and why?

7. Discuss potential effects of unethical treatment of data on patient care.

REFERENCES

American Nurses Association. (1985). *Human rights guidelines for nurses in clinical and other research*. Kansas City, MO: Author.

Burns, N., & Groves, S. K. (1993). *The practice of nursing research* (2nd ed.). Philadelphia: Saunders.

Chop, R., & Silva, M. C. (1991). Scientific fraud: Definitions, policies, and implications for nursing research. *Journal of Professional Nursing, 7,* 166–171.

Code of Federal Regulations. (1981, January 26). Title 45, part 46. Washington, DC.

Covey, S. R. (1992). *Principle-centered leadership*. New York: A Fireside Book.

Fowler, M. D. M. (1988a). Ethical issues in nursing research: Issues in qualitative research. *Western Journal of Nursing Research, 10,* 109–111.

Fowler, M. D. M. (1988b). Ethical issues in nursing research: A call for an international code of ethics for nursing. *Western Journal of Nursing Research, 10,* 352–355.

Friedman, P. J. (1990). Correcting the literature following fraudulent publication. *Journal of the American Medical Association, 263,* 1416–1419.

Fry, S. T. (1981). Accountability in research: The relationship of scientific and humanistic values. *Advances in Nursing Science, 4,* 1–13.

Harrison, L. (1993). Issues related to the protection of human research participants. *Journal of Neuroscience Nursing, 25,* 187–193.

Hawley, D. J., & Jeffers, J. M. (1992). Scientific misconduct as a dilemma for nursing. *Image, 24,* 51–55.

Husted, G. L., & Husted J. H. (1995). *Ethical decision making in nursing* (2nd ed.). St. Louis, MO: Mosby.

Munhall, P. L., & Boyd, C. O. (1993). *Nursing research: A qualitative perspective*. New York: National League of Nursing Press.

Namei, S. K., King, M. O., Byrne, M., & Proffitt, C. (1993). The ethics of role conflict. *Journal of Neuroscience Nursing, 25,* 326–330.

United States National Commission for the Protection of Human Subjects of Biomedical and Behavioral Research. (1978). *The Belmont report: Ethical principles and guidelines for the protection of human subjects of research* (DHEW Publication No. (OS)78-0012). Washington, DC: U.S. Government Printing Office.

West Virginia University. (1995–1997). *Robert C. Byrd Health Sciences Center Catalogue*. Morgantown, WV: Author.

Wilson, H. S. (1993). *Introducing research in nursing* (2nd ed.). Redwood City, CA: Addison-Wesley.

GLOBAL ISSUES THAT IMPINGE ON NURSING PRACTICE

Part IV recognizes each person as part of an interrelated global population affected by various forces. Focusing on nursing, this part begins by addressing challenges and changes in health care delivery and moves to examination of local, national, and global issues. Nurses are encouraged to be responsible professionals and citizens in acknowledging and participating in decisions related to various political, economic, social, gender, transcultural, and spirituality issues.

CHAPTER 13

Health Care Changes and Challenges

By Barbara Kupchak

What we remember, we can change; what we forget we always are.

(Tafoya, 1996)

OBJECTIVES

After completing this chapter, the reader should be able to:

1. Identify patterns of health care delivery from ancient times to the present.
2. Discuss historical events that have helped to shape the current system of health care delivery in the United States.
3. Examine trends in health care delivery and financing that have emerged in recent history.
4. Describe challenges facing health care delivery systems around the globe.
5. Discuss factors prompting a renewed interest in traditional healing systems worldwide.
6. Briefly describe factors affecting health care delivery for rural and urban aggregates.

INTRODUCTION

The health care delivery system and the way it is financed define the parameters within which nurses and other health care personnel function. Issues of health care delivery and the function of the health care delivery system are of worldwide concern. In the United States and most of the Western world, delivery of health care is much like a runaway train of high technology—there is a proliferation of markets for new medications and expensive treatments. Further, the system is challenged to provide for an ever increasing global population with decreasing resources. At the basis of this global concern is the ever increasing cost of health care and the issue of its sustainability. Developing countries are recognizing that current and future health care systems have at their foundation expensive medicines and technologies that are imported from more developed regions of the globe. Questions arise about prioritizing health expenditures. Can countries address the health needs of their people without relying on expensive medications and treatments? Can local, existing systems of health care be utilized to provide basic health services to rural and urban poor communities? In developing countries, can traditional methods and systems of health care be utilized to promote health care and prevent disease, thus reducing the burden on the system? Has modern Western health care practice been lax in preserving and utilizing the traditional methods in favor of technology, and at what cost?

In order to gain an understanding of the changes and challenges that must be addressed by health care systems worldwide if they are to survive into the twenty-first century and beyond, one needs to explore the history of health care systems and financing that are presently in use as well as traditional methods of health care. In addition, one must look at rural and urban at-risk communities and factors that impede the delivery of health care in an overburdened system.

Ask Yourself

What Cultural Influences Affect Your Health Care Practices?

All persons have roots in beliefs and cultural heritage from their family of origin and place of birth.

- What do you know about the health care practices of your cultural origins?

- Have you or persons you know ever utilized any healing modalities that are not part of what would be deemed *modern health care?*

A BRIEF HISTORY OF HEALTH CARE DELIVERY: THE EURO-AMERICAN EXPERIENCE

From the earliest civilizations there is evidence of some type of health care. The methods of health care were often a mixture of religious, civil, and mythological belief that combined to keep away disease, prevent wars, and ensure survival of populations in order to keep the various empires strong. In every culture there have been individuals designated to provide care to the sick. Some were formally trained as nurses and physicians, while others seemed to have a natural gift for the art of healing. Eastern and Middle Eastern peoples such as the Mesopotamians, Babylonians, Hebrews, Persians, Hindus, and Chinese have recorded some type of system for the delivery of health care. In all of these cultures, religious or civil laws enforced systems of disease prevention in matters of hygiene and diet, some of which were connected to the various religious practices of the ancient civilizations.

Early Eras of Health Care Delivery

Achterberg (1990) notes that "the Sumerians, and not the ancient Greeks and Romans, are the parents of Western healing systems" (p. 14). Archeological findings in the area of ancient Sumer, which is located in the vicinity of modern Iraq, include numerous prescriptions and two tablets that are considered to be the oldest medical text in existence (Achterberg, 1990). Sumerian knowledge of healing and theories of disease were dispersed to other areas through trade with the Phoenicians, Greeks, and Egyptians.

The ancient Greek civilization represents a major force in the systematic organization of education, both in secular and scientific fields. The most well known name in ancient Greek medicine and health care is Hippocrates, known as the Father of Medicine. His approach of separating medicine and health care from religion, magic, and myth was considered purely scientific for his time. He diagnosed from observed symptoms with emphasis on treating the whole patient, and he promoted continuous bedside care. His method of systematic record keeping of the patient's appearance, vital signs, and general bodily functioning became a standard for health care. Hippocrates approached medicine and health care from the highest ethical standard, believing medicine to be the noblest of arts. In addition, he believed that the physician's conduct should be of the highest quality and above reproach. Hippocrates gave the health care system organized writings of medical books that include detailed descriptive case histories, technical practices, and reports of research on various disease treatments, including treatments that worked and those that did not, so as to avoid repeating errors in care (Kelly, 1985).

As nations and populations expanded, knowledge was disseminated from culture to culture, constantly redefining the approach to health care, research, and practice. Alexander the Great, who conquered Greece in about 339 B.C.E., spread what he learned in Greece throughout the entire world. He established medical schools in Egypt that included clinics, laboratories, and libraries. Physicians were supported by the government and could devote their time to practice and research. Gradually, through various wars and assimilation of culture, Greek medicine supplemented or replaced practices throughout the known Western world.

The empire of Rome replaced methods of health care that were based on folklore and magic with a knowledge base developed in Greece. Within this developing culture, medicine and health care soon became a part of the necessary education of upper-class men, and women's health issues and childbearing practices regained importance. Midwives became key figures in the care of women (Kelly, 1985). Important contributions to health care delivery of the Roman Empire include public health sanitation and public health law. The Romans instituted city planning that provided for development of sewage systems, aqueducts, and baths. In addition, they can be credited for the development of hospitals with male and female attendants to care for the sick.

A new era in the care of the sick occurred after Christianity became the official religion of Rome. The Christian attitude of care for persons based on a strong belief in the sanctity of human life was derived from Hebrew tradition as well as the teachings of Christ. Bishops assigned individuals to care for widows, orphans, the sick, and the poor. Hospitals to care for the sick and institutions to care for the poor offered combinations of outpatient and welfare services. Monastic orders of monks and nuns, who were generally better educated than the ordinary person, controlled the health care institutions and kept writings of the care given to the sick and techniques used, which provide early records of diseases, practices, and research for cure and care (Bullough & Bullough, 1978).

Changes Through the Middle Ages and Reformation

During the thirteenth and fourteenth centuries, the organization and founding of medical schools and universities and the advent of book binding all worked to promote a better educated health care provider. Nurses, who were not as fully established as physicians, functioned as attendants who made beds and gave baths to the sick.

As noted in Chapter 1, amidst the religious revolution that had taken place against the church of Rome (known as the Reformation) in the early sixteenth to seventeenth century, the disbanding of convents and monasteries led to severe impediments in the care of the sick. During this time some progress was made in midwifery, medicine, and nursing. However, it was not until the mid-nineteenth century and the Industrial Revolution, when the demand for intellectual freedom brought about educational institutions for men, that the health care system as we know it began to emerge. During the nineteenth century, Florence Nightingale's leadership influenced nursing education, nursing care, and ultimately, because of organized nursing, the health care of the world (Bullough & Bullough, 1978; Nightingale, 1990).

Ask Yourself

How Have Things Changed?

- Consider the discussion of the early era of the health care delivery system and identify problems in early civilization that might still be seen in today's world.

Changes Influencing Development of Modern Health Care in the United States

Health services in the United States developed from health care models in European countries. These systems share the products of medical innovations that took place from the late nineteenth century to the time of World War I, a time when major nations were changing from agricultural to industrial economies. Such innovations as the use of anesthesia in surgery and the recognition of bacteria as a causative factor in many widespread diseases provided the impetus that led to the development of the modern hospital as it stands today. The dissemination and incorporation of this knowledge among the large number of practicing physicians took at least a generation to accomplish; consequently, the importance of the place of the modern hospital in society was not felt until the late nineteenth century and into the early twentieth century. At the time of this revolution of knowledge, physicians, who were the primary health care practitioners, engaged primarily in a private practice, fee-for-service system.

Physicians and Hospitals. In the United States, hospitals were generally privately funded, while European nations had both tax supported charity hospitals and private hospitals for those patients who had the ability to pay for their own health care (Anderson, 1963). The primary purpose for hospitals built in Europe was ministry to the low-income or charity patient, while in the United States, hospitals that were built by private funding were open to charity patients as well as private pay patients.

The development of hospitals affected European physicians by creating a class of specialists who operated in the general hospital and also had the option of treating private pay patients. These specialists often created their own cottage hospitals where they could treat their private pay patients. All other physicians in that system were excluded from practicing in a hospital. In the United States, on the other hand, practitioners sought out appointments to the hospital system in order to be able to admit patients, while at the same time maintaining private offices in which to see their patients. This began a new approach to the use of the hospital system in which resources were used more extravagantly and the system was more democratic in its care of patients than the European system. The United States health care system became immersed in greater use of technology, industrial and management skills, and scientific methods, creating by some estimates the best health care system in the world, and the most expensive (Anderson, 1963).

As an outgrowth of the development of hospitals, a greater awareness of public health problems arose. Prevention programs for the public, such as sanitation, environmental issues, control of communicable diseases, and maternity and infant care, developed. Curative programs, which were generally hospital based, were supported by private and public funding. Hospital clinics that provided outpatient services became the primary site of health care for low-income and indigent patients. At that time in history, physicians provided these outpatient services free of charge and, in return, were able to participate in the hospital system where the latest in knowledge and technologies was being introduced. This information could then be applied to the care of large numbers of both private and charity patients. Hospitals provided physicians an opportunity to develop their skills and to provide service to the public, thus fulfilling the physician's commitment to the public interest (Anderson, 1963).

Twentieth Century Changes and Challenges. The United States health care delivery system in the latter nineteenth century was affected by sources of funding (private or public), the ability of the patient to pay, and the type of control exercised by independent practitioners, which now included physicians, pharmacists, and dentists. The development of an industrialized society in the United States, the growth of the economy, and the increased capability of a growing health care system produced a healthier and more aware population. (See Figure 13–1.) However, twentieth century changes created new challenges for the health care system.

Figure 13–1 **Selected Significant Events in Health Care History**

Date	Event
1862	William Rathbone opened a nurse training school, the Liverpool Royal Infirmary, in consultation with Florence Nightingale.
1869	The first Board of Health was established in Massachusetts.
1872	The American Public Health Association was established.
1886	The Visiting Nurse Society of Philadelphia was established.
1893	The Henry Street Settlement, under the direction of Lillian Wald, was founded to provide health promotion, disease prevention, case finding, and follow-up care. Out of this system came the first school nurse, Lina Rogers, who was assigned to the public school system.
1896	The Nurses Associated Alumnae of the United States was established, later to become the American Nurses Association.
1901	The Army Nurse Corp was established by an act of Congress.
1910	The Flexner Report exposed abuses in medical education and proposed reforms.
1916	The Pure Food and Drug Act was enacted.
1918	An influenza epidemic produced 500,000 deaths in the United States.
1918	The Chamberlain-Kahn Act established the Venereal Disease Division of the United States Public Health Service.
1921	The Sheppard-Towner Act was passed, providing grants-in-aid to enable states to create their own bureaus of Maternal and Child Health.
1923	The Goldmark Report was published, entitled *Nursing and Nursing Education in the United States.*
1946	The Hospital Survey and Construction Act, known as the Hill-Burton Act, provided for matching funds for the building of hospitals to state and local communities.
1948	The Brown Report, *Nursing for the Future,* was published by Esther Lucille Brown, emphasizing higher education for nurses.

1948	Eli Ginzberg's report, *A Program for the Nursing Profession,* recommended two levels of nursing: professional and practical.
1956	The Health Amendments Act was passed to provide traineeships for public health personnel. It gave nurses an opportunity for advanced preparation for positions in teaching, administration, and supervision.
1965	The American Nurses Association published its "Position Paper."
1965	The Social Security Act was amended to provide funds for the health care of the elderly (Medicare–Title XVIII) and the health care of the medically indigent (Medicaid–Title XIX).
1978	Louise Brown, the first test tube baby, was born in England.
1981	AIDS was identified in the United States.
1983	A prospective payment system based on Diagnosis Related Groups (DRGs) was created under Medicare.
1989	The Omnibus Budget Reconciliation Act (OBRA '89) phased in new Medicare payment scales for physicians. It mandated direct Medicaid reimbursement for pediatric and family nurse practitioners.
1990	The Patient Self-Determination Act and the Americans with Disabilities Act were enacted.
1993	The Omnibus Budget Reconciliation Act (OBRA '93) established an all-time record cut in Medicare funding and contained the Comprehensive Childhood Immunization Act to provide vaccines for Medicaid eligible and Native American children.
1994	President Clinton's health reform proposal, the American Health Security Act, failed.

Ask Yourself

How Do Nineteenth Century Concepts Affect Twentieth Century Health Care?

- What concepts or practices regarding health care from the late 1800s and early 1900s still affect a patient's access to health care today?

- How is the health care delivery system that we know different from the system at the turn of the century?

In the early part of the twentieth century, a growing nation experienced population increases and a greater influx of immigrants, over one million immigrants from southern and eastern Europe in 1905 alone. The need for health care and related services warranted attention. Medical schools and nursing schools expanded to provide personnel to meet the demand. Science, technology, public health services, and medicine progressed at an increased rate. Physicians and scientists began to use such diagnostic tools as x-rays, to make strides toward reduction of infectious organisms through the use of rubber gloves, and to research the causes and cures of diseases such as yellow fever and typhoid and the use of radiation to treat breast cancer. Amidst such major advances as the discovery of penicillin, the proliferation of science and technology, the advancement of the professions of nursing and medicine, and the changing conceptualization about disease, a phenomenon unique to the United States emerged: the American hospital system, which has colored the health care system in the twentieth century and possibly into the twenty-first century (Stevens, 1989).

The later part of the nineteenth century and the first two decades of the twentieth century saw the transformation of hospitals from asylums for the poor to modern institutions dedicated to science and improved patient care. Physicians expanded surgical interventions such as tonsillectomies, removal of tumors, and many gynecological operations. Nurses began to take a more active role in managing the hospital environment to control infection and began to have more responsibility for technical management of patient care through duties such as taking the patient's pulse, temperature, and blood pressure (Stevens, 1989). Patterns that developed in the health care delivery system in the early part of the century can still be seen today. Physicians gained a new and strong identity and prestige, and the American Medical Association became a powerful force. Physicians gained increased authority in the routine workings of hospital systems, shifting the balance of power from boards of trustees to the medical decision makers (Stevens, 1989).

As a result of battlefield experiences in World War I, nurses, physicians, and other health care workers designed and set up streamlined, technically proficient, and very efficient specialized hospitals for the acutely ill or injured patient. On the home front, in response to ever increasing numbers of immigrants, models of health care with emphasis on prevention and community interaction were developed. Prior to the war, the elite area of nursing was public health, with nurses at the forefront of campaigns for infant care and welfare, tuberculosis, and infectious disease. The war, however, emphasized the glamour of hospitals, and by 1920, more than half of the general hospitals in this country had schools of nursing attached to them. Student nurses staffed hospitals and were socialized into the hospital system. Like physicians, nurses became caught up in the culture of the acute health care environment and reluctant to expand their professional interests into public health and the social aspect of health care (Stevens, 1989).

After World War I, the idea of group practices for physicians began to take hold, and the movement for health insurance began to develop. With the encouragement of President Theodore Roosevelt, workers' compensation was the first form of social insurance to become prominent in this country. Thirty-seven states passed laws that sanctioned workers' compensation by 1919. Through this movement, the cost of injury and damage to workers because of job related hazards was passed on to industry. The health insurance movement entered a fast track, supported by the American Medical Association and various physicians' groups around the country. During this time, the struggle for access to care and control of fees and services escalated (Stevens, 1989).

The ten years after 1920 were years of growth and expansion of the health care industry. Consumerism flowered in direct relationship to the growth of the health care industry. As the public became aware of the availability of modern techniques, they wanted the best available. The health care delivery system developed into a middle-class entity in which many advances were taking place in private care while the poor were increasingly underserved. By the end of this ten-year period, there was increasing criticism of the cost and financing of the health care system, and the question of equal care for all income levels was raised. The rich and middle class were accused of having the best available to them while the poor were viewed as manipulative of the very system that wanted to provide *charity* care to them.

During the Great Depression, government and charity hospitals were overrun with patients unable to afford health care, causing health care institutions to lose income and question their survival. The various health care professions pulled together to care for the sick, and a renewed sense of dedication kept a strained system afloat. Continually rising costs of health care led to development of plans for health insurance for everyone in the 1930s. The original Blue Cross plans were an outgrowth of the need for payment for continued growth of hospital and health care technologies. Thus, a prepayment insurance plan was born, and the health care delivery system grew by leaps and bounds. During the ensuing years major federal grant programs such as the Hill-Burton Act of 1946 funded the construction of health care facilities, and the science of medicine expanded through laboratory and clinical research. World War II prompted advances in health services that included therapy for prevention and treatment of shock, better blood replacement techniques, and research on gamma globulin, steroids, and other drugs, all of which increased the possibilities for successful treatment in surgery and internal medicine (Stevens, 1989). Expansion in the health care industry continued in the postwar years.

Think About It

How Do World Events Affect Health Care Delivery?

In reviewing history it is evident that seemingly nonrelated events can steer the course of other events, as has been noted in the development of the health care delivery system.

- How have major world events of your lifetime affected the course of health care delivery?

Between the passing of the Hill-Burton Act in 1946 and the advent of Medicare legislation in 1965, the United States health care delivery system hit a new wave of expansion. The most widely known image of expansion in hospitals was the intensive care unit, with the greatest expansion between 1950 and 1965. In the early 1960s, coronary care units began to flourish, and by the mid 1960s premature nurseries, respiratory units, physical therapy units, and units dealing specifically with postoperative surgeries and neurosurgery were functioning in every fully operational hospital. Because of technological expansion, the cost of health care increased rapidly.

Expanding Health Insurance Coverage. Seeing a need and opportunity, the insurance industry began to compete with Blue Cross plans to provide third party coverage for health care. These insurance plans removed the anxiety related to paying large hospital and health care bills and also removed incentives from health care institutions to keep their costs down. Hospitals passed down increased costs to insurance companies who in turn passed the cost on to the individual insurance subscriber. Because individual citizens had insurance, they demanded more and better service, and the system drove itself through the supply and demand cycle (Califano, 1986).

Medicare Parts A and B, which was passed in 1965 and enacted in 1966, essentially gave hospitals and other health care institutions a license to spend, and bigger and better were the watch words. The health care delivery system was caught up in a whirlwind that has escalated to the point where the system is facing the need for serious change and the possibility of rationing in this last decade of the twentieth century. Spiraling costs have prompted development of cost containment mechanisms such as Diagnostic Related Grouping, case management, and managed care systems, which affect current health care delivery. Standardization is more and more defining the care that patients receive in the present health care delivery system. Many people have no insurance for health care, and health care institutions have reverted to the charity care that existed in the first part of the twentieth century. The future of the system is uncertain and continues to be influenced by political structures, economic constraints, and worldwide societal needs and demands.

HEALTH CARE PERSPECTIVES—A GLOBAL CONCERN

The challenge to provide health care for populations across the globe requires increasing effort and creativity. Many variables play a part in this challenge, including economics, cultural factors, epidemics, environment, war, and national crises. The problems are further compounded by the relationship or lack of relationship between modern medicine and traditional healing systems, national versus private health insurance, and preventive methods of health promotion contrasted with curative methods of treating illness. These factors all affect the functioning of health systems in various countries around the world (Bodeker, 1996).

All industrialized nations, with the exception of the United States and South Africa, have comprehensive national health care programs. The countries that operate with a nationalized system include: Australia, Austria, Belgium, Bulgaria, Canada, Czechoslovakia, Denmark, Finland, France, Germany, Great Britain, Greece, Hungary, Ireland, Italy, Japan, The Netherlands, New Zealand, Norway, Poland, Portugal, Romania, Russia, Spain, Sweden, and Switzerland. However, even with health care programs in place, all are not equal and do not function as smoothly as one would hope (Shikles, 1991).

Russia, for example, is suffering from a health care system that is at grave risk. There is a shortage of essential drugs, basic sterile equipment such as syringes, antibiotics, x-ray equipment, and basic medical supplies. Hospitals are dark and dirty, personnel are overworked, and there is a neglect of sanitation procedures. Rural areas in the former Soviet Union fare much worse. Problems occur in situations where some rural clinics have nonfunctioning or nonexistent sewage systems. Some clinics lack piped in water, or if water is piped in there is no system for heating it safely. Many of the hospital personnel such as physicians, nurses, and technicians have gone on strike because of poor working conditions and poor rewards for service. In this system, a physician may be paid less than a bus driver and a nurse less than a housemaid (Erlanger, 1992).

South Africa, while technically an industrialized nation with many natural resources, is plagued with health care problems similar to those occurring in many developing countries. The government of South Africa has as its long-term goal affordable and accessible health care for all its citizens. This goal is far from being realized, however, because the rise in urbanization and the proliferation of Third World illness is causing a deterioration in the process of setting up health care for all. In their present system, physicians and nurses are overworked, hospitals are overcrowded, and much of the equipment is nonfunctioning or outdated (Randolph, 1991).

In pro-Castro Cuba, the health care system is said to be one of the most glorious accomplishments of the revolution. Both the World Health Organization (WHO) and the United Nations agencies laud the Cuban system as a major achievement for the citizens. This system provides services from primary care to the most sophisticated procedures available, free to urban and rural citizens alike. It has been upheld as a model for other developing nations. Available data document that there are more than thirty-nine thousand practicing physicians. Infant mortality rates have declined to less than eleven deaths per one thousand live births. Communicable diseases such as diphtheria, malaria, polio, and whooping cough are on the verge of being eliminated. Primary care clinics abound in rural areas and are open around the clock. Nurses and physicians make house calls to older or very ill residents. Continuing education offerings are readily available. Research and development in heart disease and cancer therapy is occurring (Shikles, 1991).

As was mentioned earlier, most industrialized nations have some type of universal health coverage. These systems vary in regard to the amount of government and private pay insurance, and some countries have a combination of several methods.

Germany, France, and Japan have systems of health care coverage that are mandated benefits coverage, the cost of which is shared by employees, employers, and government taxed revenues. The health care delivery system shares three traits with the system in the United States. Medical care is offered through private physicians and through private and public hospitals. Patients may choose their providers. Most people in these countries have health insurance coverage through their place of employment. Health insurance is offered to the citizens of these countries through multiple third party insurance agencies.

In all three of the above mentioned countries, reimbursement rates are standardized for physicians and hospitals through a negotiation system between hospitals, physicians, third party payers, and the government. Similar problems to those existing in the United States are present, such as high cost and increased spending for technology. However, every citizen has some type of health care coverage. In an attempt to hold down rising health care spending, all have instituted direct controls on the price of health care. The controls apply to all of the health care systems in the respective countries, and policies are strictly enforced to comply with the set limit on health care spending (Shikles, 1991).

Canada and Great Britain have developed national health care systems that provide health care for their citizens. The government-run plans provide cradle-to-grave services that are financed through taxes. These plans enable patients to receive services free and to choose their own hospitals and physicians. The plans pay salaries to physicians and operate their own hospitals.

There are both champions and critics of the national health insurance systems in Canada and Britain. Some say the systems are sound while others says they are flawed. In Canada, for example, on the positive side, citizens of these countries can go to physicians or hospitals of their choice when they need care. Physicians bill the province for patient care. Patients do not pay for services, nor are they required to fill out endless forms. Negotiations for fees, cost containment measures, and salaries take place between the provinces and the health care system.

Citizens of Canada and Great Britain consider health care to be one of their basic rights, and they value and respect their health care systems. Major political parties in these countries support the systems, and physicians and hospitals seem generally satisfied as well since they receive a guaranteed payment. Businesses applaud the programs because payment is spread across society and they do not have to carry a large part of the payment burden for employees (Beatty, 1991).

The national health insurance system in these countries have their critics. Some say the system is flawed and that being insured in this way sets up a system of rationing because of insufficient funds for specialized health care. It has been said that waiting for care in these systems sometimes means death. Access to certain procedures and technologies is limited. Waiting lists are getting longer. Critics say that there is an unequal access to health care from province to province, depending on the affluence of the province. Some Canadian citizens who can afford to pay out of pocket come to the United States for specialized care and surgeries. In all instances, the high cost of technologies and research is having an impact on these systems in much the same ways as it is across the globe (Walker, 1992).

Ask Yourself

Access to Health Care—Rights and Responsibilities

Much of the discussion regarding the health care delivery systems of the United States as well as those of many countries in the world is a commentary on access to what is termed *modern medical care.*

- How does access to health care affect an individual's participation in the health care system?

- What is our individual responsibility in the big picture of these vast health care systems?

- Do you consider health care a basic right? If it is a right, what are our individual responsibilities in ensuring this right for all citizens?

ALTERNATIVE TRADITIONS OF HEALTH CARE

Indigenous populations in cultures throughout the world have traditional forms of health care that view humanity as connected to the wider dimensions of the earth and nature. In developing countries, these forms of traditional healing systems provide comprehensive approaches to prevention of illness and promotion of health that go beyond the scope of modern medical care. The World Health Organization (WHO) refers to these systems as holistic, that is, viewing a person in totality within a vast ecological spectrum and emphasizing the notion that illness or disease occurs as a result of an imbalance between the person and his or her ecological systems (WHO, 1978).

An important component of traditional systems of health care is their basis in models that take into account mental, spiritual, physical, and ecological factors in assessing health and well being. A basic concept of all traditional health care systems is that of balance between mind and body, function and need, and individual, community, and environment. Illness or disease is thought to be a breakdown in the balance in one or more of these areas. Treatments are designed to restore health and balance between the individual and his or her internal and external environments. While these models of traditional health care systems have been considered primitive and unsophisticated by modern practitioners, an increasing number of developing countries are showing a new interest in program development toward revitalizing these traditional systems. There are several factors at work in promoting this resurgence of interest.

Many, if not the majority, of rural populations of developing countries cannot afford Western types of medical health care. Rural people have to travel many days to reach the larger health care centers, resulting in loss of wages in addition to money spent for travel and medicines. In Asia, the traditional systems are being incorporated into other more formal health care systems to provide for care and ease the burden of cost. India has over two hundred thousand traditional practitioners. In Thailand, the ministry of health promotes the use of traditional medicinal plants in primary health care, state run hospitals, and health service centers. In Korea, twenty percent of the national health care budget is directed to traditional health care services. Health insurance coverage is available for Oriental medical treatments and traditional health care methods (Bodeker, 1996).

In Africa, the governments are facing huge bills for the AIDS crisis that continues to grow. These governments are exploring their traditional indigenous medicinal treatments for inexpensive and effective ways to relieve the suffering of AIDS patients. Health care providers in Uganda have been active in promoting research into traditional medicine for treating people with AIDS.

China has had a policy of integrating traditional health care into the national health care policy for over forty years. The Chinese are trying to combine the modern and the traditional as formal components of health care provision. In China, the traditional health care providers perform the majority of care to the poor and rural communities. The country physicians are educated in a three year program that includes a combination of traditional medicine and modern medicine. Modern Western medicine is being strongly pursued at great financial cost to the government. But at the same time hospitals and health care systems offer a choice to patients. Persons who take advantage of these choices are often the older and the less affluent. As the country is opening up to capitalist beliefs and free enterprise, some Chinese citizens, who now have the financial means to make different choices, are choosing Western methods of treatments and often ignoring the tried and true Oriental methods for status reasons. The younger generation of Chinese seem to believe that what is Western is always better. In observing some of the health care delivery in China, there is evidence that the government, while allowing the practice of the ancient Oriental medicine, is putting a strong emphasis on a belief that technology is the answer to health care in this vastly populated country. This is especially disconcerting in view of the fact that Oriental medicine and the tradition of health care with alternative choices have been functioning well for two thousand years, and Western health care providers are beginning to research and utilize these traditional systems of care in order to offer them to their patients.

Ask Yourself

What Do You Know About Traditional Healing?

Traditional methods of healing and health care have kept indigenous populations healthy and functioning for thousands of years. Many countries are trying to reinstate these practices to promote health and reduce the cost of health care and health care delivery.

- How do you think traditional and modern healing systems should relate to each other?

- What traditional methods of health care are available in your community or nearby area?

- With what traditional or *folk* health practices are you familiar? Have you or persons you know utilized these practices?

CHALLENGES FOR RURAL AND URBAN AGGREGATES

Problems in the delivery of health care to populations around the world occur not only because of expensive technology or lack of money to pay for insurance but also because of geographic barriers. Rural populations in the United States and abroad often have to do without services because of lack of providers and facilities within a reasonable distance from their homes. Health care for persons in these populations requires a day off of work for travel and waiting in crowded waiting rooms. Many rural areas lack health care personnel, and emergency care is often nonexistent. In one mid-Atlantic state, all counties boast of an access to a 911 emergency number, but for some, the switchboard and EMT vehicle is three counties away and travel is over narrow mountain roads. Patients often delay treatment or do not become involved with prevention or health education plans because they require so much effort to accomplish. In addition, many rural citizens tend to be older persons for whom travel and finances are a great consideration in health care services.

The urban poor face similar access problems, not because care is geographically distant, but because access requires trips to places they cannot afford or free clinics where lines are long and workers are few. Individuals are often required to take time from work, like their rural counterparts, in order to see a provider. Medications may be unaffordable. Large immigrant populations live in overcrowded situations in the urban setting. In addition to financial constraints, there may be language and cultural barriers and lack of knowledge about how to access the system.

 Think About It

Health Care Changes and Challenges

The challenges and changes in health care can seem insurmountable and over-whelming. It seems as though only the very wealthy will be able to have health care services. Some sociologists say that the middle class is disappearing and that this country, as well as other world countries, will have only the rich and the poor. Health care costs are rising, and there seems to be no end to it.

- How should these issues be addressed? How should nurses respond to these issues?
- What issues have you encountered in accessing health care providers for you and your family?
- Are you able to afford a comprehensive health plan? If not, what do you do when you become ill?

SUMMARY

Historical awareness enables one to have a more informed view of circumstances in the present. Contemporary issues and concerns regarding health care delivery and financing are related to the historical interplay of advances in scientific and medical knowledge, social and political climate, and waxing and waning of economic and other resources. Current parameters in which health care providers function are changing. Acute care hospitals are changing the focus of, and in some cases limit-ing, services; and many people are looking to the traditional healing systems of var-ious cultures to provide needed health care services. Although some countries ensure access to basic health care services for their citizens, many individuals throughout the world community have limited or no access to basic health care. Questions regarding access to and availability of resources are not new, but they must be addressed anew in light of the various currents within contemporary soci-ety. The future of the system is uncertain, and one must consider whether issues of the past are destined to repeat themselves. Perhaps we can take what is positive from the past and blend this with both traditional and modern healing approaches in order to rescue a flawed health care system in this country and around the world.

CHAPTER HIGHLIGHTS

- Systems of health care, which have existed to address societal needs for healing from early civilization to the present, have been influenced by cultural, political, economic, religious, and scientific factors throughout history.

- Scientific and medical innovations coinciding with the shift in Western nations from agricultural to industrial economics in the latter nineteenth and early twentieth centuries provided a basis for modern day health care. Societal changes such as wars, women working more outside the home, and the influx of immigrants have raised new issues and concerns for health care delivery at various times in United States history.

- Skyrocketing health care costs can be traced to the advent of health insurance (1930s and forward) and the enactment of Medicare and Medicaid (1960s), which removed incentives from health care institutions and physicians to keep costs down, and to public awareness of the availability of medical interventions, which prompted consumers to demand the best care and services available.

- Expansion of hospital and other health care services has reached a point of crisis in which out of control health care costs have prompted imposition of external controls on institutions and health care providers. Many people have no means of paying for expensive services.

- Some nations provide basic health care services for their citizens, while people in many areas suffer from limited access to or availability of such services. People in both developing and industrialized countries are exploring ways to incorporate traditional and modern healing practices into contemporary health care systems in an effort to utilize the benefits of both systems in meeting the health care needs of society.

- Problems of access to and payment for health care services are of special concern among rural populations and the urban poor.

DISCUSSION QUESTIONS AND ACTIVITIES

1. Interview a person who worked as a nurse during or within the decade following World War II and discuss nursing roles and duties, types of health concerns for which patients were hospitalized, and what was considered new therapies at the time. Compare the information you obtain to your experience of health care today.

2. Review nursing and medical journals and texts from the earlier part of this century regarding issues of concern in practice and to the profession. Compare and contrast these issues to issues of current concern.

3. Imagine that it is the year 2035 and you are being interviewed by a nursing student about factors that affected health care delivery and financing in your early days in nursing. What would you say?

4. Discuss global issues related to health care delivery. Which of these issues would have the greatest impact on your nursing practice and why?

5. Describe the impact of health delivery and financing on patient care and outcomes. Identify potential ethical dilemmas related to current systems of delivery or financing.

6. How should traditional and modern healing practices and practitioners relate to each other?

REFERENCES

Achterberg. J. (1990). *Woman as healer.* Boston: Shambhala.

Anderson, O. W. (1963). Medical care: Its social and organizational aspects. Health services systems in the United States and other countries—critical comparisons. *The New England Journal of Medicine, 269,* 839–843.

Beatty, P. (1991). Canada's health care system is sound. In G. McCuen (Ed.), *Health care and human values* (pp. 162–176). Hudson, WI: GEM Publications.

Bodeker, G. C. (1996). Global health traditions. In M. S. Micozzi (Ed.), *Fundamentals of complementary and alternative medicine* (pp. 279–290). New York: Churchill Livingstone.

Brown, P. (1989). *Perspectives in medical sociology.* Belmont, CA: Wadsworth.

Bullough, B., & Bullough, V. (1978). *The care of the sick: The emergence of modern nursing.* New York: Prodist.

Califano, J. A., Jr. (1986). *America's health care revolution: Who lives? Who dies? Who pays?* New York: Random House.

Erlanger, S. (1992, May). Cuts gut Russian health care. *The New York Times.*

Kelly, L. Y. (1985). *Dimensions of professional nursing* (5th ed.). New York: Macmillan.

Nightingale, F. (1990). *Notes on nursing: What it is and what it is not* (Commemorative ed.). Philadelphia: Lippincott.

Randolph, E. (1991, November). Soviet hospitals besieged by filth, shortage of drugs. *Washington Post.*

Shikles, J. L. (1991, November). Health care spending: The experience of France, Germany and Japan. *U.S. General Accounting Office Report.*

Stevens, R. (1989). *In sickness and in wealth.* New York: Basic Books.

Tafoya, T. (1996, May). *Embracing the shadow: Mending the sacred hoop.* Paper presented at the South Texas AIDS Training (STAT) for Mental Health Providers: The Human, Transcultural, and Spiritual Dimensions of HIV/AIDS, San Antonio, TX.

Walker, M. (1992). How they don't do it in Canada. *Reason, 35–42.*

WHO (1978). *Traditional medicine.* Geneva: WHO Publications.

SUGGESTED READINGS

Bullough, B., & Bullough, V. (1994). *Nursing issues.* New York: Springer.

Castro, J. (1994). *The American way of health.* Boston: Little, Brown.

Dauner, C. D. (1994). *The health care solution.* Sacramento, CA: Vision.

Kalisch, P., & Kalisch, B. (1989). *The advance of American nursing* (2nd ed.) Boston: Little, Brown.

Knowles, J. H. (Ed.). (1977). *Doing better and feeling worse.* New York: Norton.

Kovner A. (1995). *Health care delivery in the United States* (5th ed.). New York: Springer.

Long, R. E. (Ed.). (1991). *The crisis in health care.* New York: Wilson.

Rosenberg, C. E. (1987). *The care of strangers.* New York: Basic Books.

Wekesser, C. (Ed.). (1994). *Health care in America: Opposing viewpoints.* San Diego, CA: Greenhaven Press.

CHAPTER **14**

Political Issues

To leave the world a bit better,
*   whether by a healthy child, a garden patch*
*   or a redeemed social condition;*
To know even one life has breathed easier
*   because you have lived;*
This is to have succeeded.
*   (Ralph Waldo Emerson, What Is Success?)*

OBJECTIVES

After completing this chapter, the reader should be able to:

1. Describe the process by which issues become "political issues."
2. Distinguish between the terms *political* and *partisan*.
3. Give examples of specific political issues related to health care.
4. Discuss your personal stand on various political issues in relation to ethics.
5. Describe the health policy process.
6. Discuss the role of ethics in policy making.
7. Explain the role of nurses in the policy making process.
8. Describe various methods of influencing public policy.

INTRODUCTION

Health policy and politics are viewed in a number of different ways. There are those who perceive health policy as a political process strongly influenced by ideology and party politics. Others see the health policy making process as a thoughtful one by which decisions are based on data and the rational analysis of needs, outcomes, and costs (Donley, 1996). In reality the health policy process is a combination of both informed rational judgments and ideological partisan politics.

Both individual nurses and the profession of nursing have become increasingly involved in the political process, particularly in the realm of health policy. Nurses view health, at least in part, as dependent upon various environmental factors that can be altered by health policy decisions. Recognizing their role as advocates for patients' health, and acknowledging the importance of being involved in regulatory processes, nurses are assuming more responsibility in the political arena. This chapter features examples of selected political issues in the discussion of the process of creating health policy and describes specific methods that nurses can utilize to influence policy.

POLITICAL ISSUES

The term **political** relates to the complex process of policy making within the government. Government is an essential element of society, and politics is inherent in government. Political issues are those that are created, affected, or regulated by decisions within either the executive, judicial, or legislative branches of government. **Political parties** are organized groups with distinct ideologies that seek to control government. When political parties take opposing positions on an issue, the different opinions and subsequent decisions are said to be **partisan.** Though individuals may genuinely and independently agree with the position of a particular party, partisanism is sometimes portrayed in a negative light—that is, consisting of blind, prejudiced, and unreasoning allegiance to a party. Because many people think that every problem in society can be solved by passing a law, legislatures make more and more laws to satisfy demands. Depending upon the existence of legitimate need or the interest or whim of either society-at-large, special interest groups, individuals, or government, any issue can become a political one.

Think About It

Abortion—A Moral and Political Issue

Abortion, a moral issue, raises questions about basic beliefs regarding life and death, sanctity of life, the beginning of life, and a woman's individual rights. Over time, abortion has become a political issue. Examples of this change include legal arguments over women's choice versus right to life, as in *Roe v. Wade*; congressional discussions regarding public funding of abortions, including debate related to the level of coverage; and the definition of acceptable circumstances surrounding conception and abortion. Within the last two decades, the two major

United States political parties have polarized on the issue. One party supports freedom of a woman to make her own decision while the opposing party advocates the fetus's right to life. As a result, abortion has become a partisan issue.

- What is your moral stand on abortion?
- How did you develop this stand?
- How is your opinion about abortion related to the position of the political party to which you belong?
- Would you support a particular party based solely upon one issue?
- What is the government's role related to moral issues? Explain your position.
- How does your opinion influence your ability to give quality care?

An issue can become "political" in a number of ways. As discussed in Chapters 7 and 8, the administrative branch of government is involved in the operation of government agencies. State boards of medicine, nursing, and health, for example, are administrative agencies that are charged with regulating the activity of specific groups of professionals or particular aspects of health care delivery with the goal of protecting the public. Rules and regulations promulgated by these groups can have a profound effect upon health care delivery. Because positions on these boards are often granted through the process of political appointment, decisions are occasionally viewed as partisan. Examples of political issues occurring within the administrative branch include prescriptive authority for nurses in advanced practice and implementation of mandatory standards of care.

The judicial branch of government influences health care professions and health care delivery through the common law system. As was noted in Chapter 7, judicial precedents take on the force of the law. Consider, for example, the profound effect on the American health care system of the landmark Supreme Court decision in *Roe v. Wade*. Though the Supreme Court is considered to be a nonpartisan entity, partisan politics plays a tremendous role in judicial appointments. Supreme Court appointments are particularly important to political parties because of the potential to further party ideology through the unusual power granted the Court in the United States by virtue of the common law system, the small number of justices, the durability of Supreme Court decisions, the Court's relative freedom from special interest groups, and the fact that Supreme Court justices are appointed for their lifetime.

Ask Yourself

Is the Supreme Court Partisan?

Supreme Court justices are nominated by the president of the United States and, following long sessions of questioning, are confirmed or rejected by a committee of the Senate. Try to recall the confirmation process of nominees for the Supreme Court within the past fifteen years.

- Were the prospective justices questioned about issues with moral/ethical implications?
- Were they questioned about their position on specific partisan issues?
- Why do you think it is important to political parties that judges with certain beliefs are appointed to the Supreme Court?
- What role does the Supreme Court have in shaping the country's health policy?

Nurses are most familiar with political issues discussed in the legislative arena. These issues are the ones that are decided through the passage of federal or state laws. It is within the legislative forum that nurses can be particularly effective in influencing the outcome of various political issues. Examples of well-publicized legislative issues with health care implications include: Medicare and Medicaid revisions, health insurance reform, and issues related to advanced practice nursing, such as prescriptive authority, scope of practice, and third party reimbursement.

Nurses function in a variety of roles. They are citizens, knowledgeable consumers of health care, professionals whose practice is regulated by government, and advocates for patients. Responsible political involvement is an important function of each of these roles. Because nurses are individuals with a variety of backgrounds, experiences, beliefs, and values, opinions about political issues are diverse. This diversity, when coupled with sensitivity to moral and ethical implications, provides a foundation for productive and fair political discussion.

Political issues of particular interest to nurses fall into four distinct categories: those involving moral values, those involving professional regulation, those involving the health of individuals in society, and those involving distributive justice. Nurses' positions on these issues are based upon personal experience, ethical orientation, religion, cultural bias, and a number of other factors. Naturally, there is a healthy diversity of opinion among nurses on most issues—particularly those involving moral values. Figure 14–1 shows examples of selected political issues of interest to many nurses.

Figure 14–1 **Selected Examples of Political Issues**

Issues Involving Moral Values

Beginning of Life Issues

- Abortion
- Use of Fetal Tissue
- Genetic Testing
- Contraception and Sterilization

Health Care Issues

- Medically-Assisted Pregnancy
- Deciding for Infants and Children

- Distributing Harvested Organs
- Use of Animal Organs for Research and Treatment
- Informed Consent

End of Life Issues
- Active and Passive Euthanasia
- Physician Assisted Suicide
- Patient Self-Determination
- Organ Procurement

Issues Involving Professional Regulation

Nursing Education
- Entry into Practice
- Funding for Nursing Education and Research

Workplace Issues
- Safety
- Americans with Disabilities Act

Advanced Practice Issues
- Third Party Reimbursement
- Prescriptive Authority
- Scope of Practice

Issues Involving the Health of Individuals in Society

Environmental Health
- Clean Indoor Air
- Clean Groundwater
- Air Pollution Control

Public Health
- Treatment and Reporting of STDs
- Family Planning Programs and Regulations
- Tobacco Legislation
- Childhood Immunizations
- Gun Control
- Seatbelt and Helmet Laws
- Food and Product Labeling

Issues Involving Access to Care
- Social Security
- Medicare and Medicaid
- Regulation of Private Insurance
- Managed Care Legislation
- Health Care Reform

HEALTH POLICY

Health plays a critical role in the physical, psychological, and economic condition of individuals and their society. Having the central purpose of enhancing health, health policies are intended to "influence the actions, decisions, and behaviors of people in the domains of the environmental conditions under which people live; their lifestyles and personal behaviors; and through improvements in the availability, accessibility, and quality of their health care services" (Longest, 1995, p. 7). Because health is an integral component of the social and economic lives of citizens, health related issues receive considerable attention from individual citizens as well as public policy makers.

Health is conceptualized differently by different people. The prevailing definition of health determines, in part, the extent to which society is willing to go toward maximizing health among its members. A society that defines health narrowly, in terms of illness, for example, might choose to intervene in illness but avoid the financial support of health promoting behaviors. In contrast, a society that defines health positively, in terms related to wellness, would be more likely to focus on encouraging individuals to seek preventive interventions in the quest for health.

Health policies are formal and authoritative decisions focusing on health that are made in the legislative, executive, or judicial branches of government and are intended to direct or influence the actions, behaviors, or decisions of others. Policy is comprised of a very large set of decisions. Examples of health policy are those codified in the statutory language of specific pieces of legislation, rules and regulations established for the purpose of implementing legislation, rules and regulations established to operate government and its various programs, and judicial decisions related to health. **Statutes** or **laws** are pieces of legislation that have been enacted by legislative bodies and approved by the executive branch of government. **Rules** or **regulations** are policies that are established to guide the implementation of laws and programs. **Judicial decisions** are authoritative court decisions that direct or influence the actions, behaviors, or decisions of others (Longest, 1995). In addition to these different types of policies, there are also two broad categories of health policies.

Although there is significant potential for overlap, health policies fit into two basic categories: allocative and regulatory. **Allocative policies** are those that are "designed to provide net benefits to some distinct group or class of individuals or organizations, at the expense of others, in order to ensure that public objectives are met" (Longest, 1995, p. 6). Allocative policies are essentially economic in nature and are geared toward guaranteeing access to goods and services for the disadvantaged. The most well known examples of allocative health policies are those of Medicare and Medicaid. **Regulatory policies** are those that are "designed to influence the actions, behaviors, and decisions of others through directive techniques" (Longest, 1995, p. 7). Longest (1995) lists five basic classes of regulatory policies:

1. market entry restrictions;

2. rate or price-setting controls on providers;

3. provider quality controls;

4. market-preserving controls; and

5. social regulation (geared toward such socially desired ends as safe workplaces and nondiscriminatory provision of health care).

As with all policies, the purpose of regulatory policy is to ensure that public objectives are met.

The Health Policy Process

Health policies are those that impact health in any way—either directly, as with immunization programs, or indirectly, as with statutes that describe scope of practice of health care providers. The process of health policy includes three distinct phases. These phases are both consecutive and circular. The first phase is that of **policy formulation.** This phase includes such actions as agenda setting and the subsequent development of legislation. The second phase is that of **policy implementation.** This phase follows enactment of legislation and includes taking actions and making additional decisions necessary to implement legislation such as rule making and policy operation. The final stage is **policy modification.** This stage exists to improve or perfect legislation previously enacted. This might entail only minor adjustments made in the implementation phase, or it may involve major changes or the elimination of particular statutes (Longest, 1995).

Policy Formulation.   The first phase of policy making is policy formulation. This phase is divided into two distinct sequentially related sets of activities—agenda setting and legislation development (Longest, 1995). At any point in time, there is a complex mix of three variables: health related problems, possible solutions and alternatives, and diverse political interests. As agenda setting progresses, the emerging issues can proceed to the development of legislation.

Problems.   The existence of real or perceived problems is the impetus for the policy formulation phase of policy making. Problems may become evident in a number of ways. Some problems occur as the result of the interaction of certain variables related to previous policy. For example, it is likely that the predicted shortfall of Social Security is related to a policy that did not take into account inequities between program budget and rapidly escalating expenditures. Other problems may gain attention as they reach unacceptable levels. Growth in the numbers of people with AIDS is an example of this type of problem. Other problems emerge as a result of some specific event that forces public attention. Examples of this type of problem include the discovery of waste products washing up on beaches and the development of a new drug for treating AIDS that is so expensive few people can afford to purchase it (Longest, 1995). Nevertheless, the mere existence of problems is not always sufficient to ensure the formulation of legislation. There must also be feasible solutions to the problems and the political will to enact legislation.

Solutions.   In order to trigger the development of legislation, even serious problems must be coupled with ideas for solving the problems. The process of offering solutions to problems involves generating ideas for solving the problems, refining the ideas, and selecting from among the options (Longest, 1995). *Nursing's Agenda for Health Care*

Reform (American Nurses Association [ANA], 1991) is an example of the profession's attempt to formulate specific solutions to problems in health care delivery.

Political Circumstances. In addition to the existence of particular problems and the potential for feasible solutions, there must also be people in influential policy making positions with the political will and energy to create a particular policy. Factors that influence political will include: public attitudes, concerns, and opinions surrounding an issue; the preferences and relative ability to influence political decisions; the positions of key political leaders on the issue; and the other competing items on the policy agenda. Longest (1995) believes that creating a political thrust forceful enough to cause policy makers to formulate and implement new policy is often the most problematic area. Nurses, as a significant percentage of the voting population, are in a good position to collectively influence political decisions and thus enhance the political will essential to formulate health policy.

Think About It

Failure of the Health Care Reform Initiative

Whatever happened to health care reform? On September 22, 1993, President Bill Clinton introduced the American Health Security Act. Following months of high-level negotiation and planning, this reform package included many of the ideas presented in at least eleven separate proposals made within the preceding five years. Administration officials thought the public and many special interest groups were demanding a radical reform of the health care system. Leah Curtin, nursing leader and ethicist, predicted in May of 1991 that there would be a universal access system within three to eight years (Curtin, 1996, p. 225). Yet Clinton's proposal, along with all of its predecessors, failed. Universal access did not become a reality, and it does not appear that it will happen anytime soon.

- A great deal of time and energy was invested in the policy formulation phase. How effective do you believe leaders were in this phase?
- What was the problem being addressed? How clear was the problem?
- Were the proposed solutions realistic and acceptable? Discuss specific solutions.
- Do you think the political circumstances were favorable for passage of a health care reform proposal? Why or why not?
- Do you think the influence of special interest groups affected the eventual outcome of the proposal? Explain your thinking.
- At what point in the policy making process do you think the proposal failed?

Policy Implementation. Policy implementation immediately follows the enactment of legislation. Because legislation seldom contains explicit language on how it is to be implemented, details are left to the process of rule making. A formal part of the implementation phase, the promulgation of rules, is accomplished by specific implementing organizations. For example, the various states' boards of nursing are the organizations responsible for promulgating rules related to nursing practice. Generally, these organizations accept input from affected groups during the rule making process. Thompson (1991) calls the interaction between the implementing organizations and affected interest groups "strategic interaction." Interest groups routinely seek to influence rule making because they are so often the targets of rules established to implement health policies. Lobbying is one of the major means by which interest groups attempt to influence policy makers. Lobbying is especially intense when various interests groups disagree upon the formulation of a particular policy.

Policy Modification.   As the third phase of the policy making process, policy modification results when the outcomes, perceptions, and consequences of existing policies indicate that either the original problems still exist or new problems have arisen from unforeseen circumstances or from the policy itself. The policy modification phase is intended to spiral backward, with feedback, into the agenda-setting and legislation-development stages of the formulation phase—potentially creating new legislation—and spiral forward into the rule making and policy operation stages of the implementation phase, stimulating changes in rules or operations. Many programs are routinely amended, some of them repeatedly over a period of many years. These modifications may reflect, among other things, the development of new technologies, changing economic conditions, and public demand (Longest, 1995). Newly proposed changes in Medicare and Medicaid programs are examples of the policy modification process.

Ethics in Policy Making

Because policy affects people's lives and relationships and is often part of the distributive justice process, policy making is an inherently ethical endeavor. The outcomes and consequences of most health policy affect large groups of people. There are two equally important functions of ethics in public policy making. In the policy formulation phase, ethics can guide the original development of new policies. Ethics is also useful in the policy modification phase as a means to legitimately criticize policies that are already implemented (Thompson, 1985). However, there is some practical difficulty in adhering strictly to specific ethical principles during the policy making process. Discussing the complexity of policy making in terms of ethics, Beauchamp and Childress (1994) write:

> Policy formation and criticism involve more complex forms of judgment than merely invoking ethical principles and rules. The ethics of public policy must proceed from impure and unsettled cases, in which there are profound social disagreements, uncertainties, different interpretations of history, and imperfect procedures to resolve the disagreements. Obviously, no body of abstract principles and rules can dictate policy, because it cannot contain enough specific information or provide direct and discerning guidance. The specification and

implementation of moral principles and rules must take account of problems of feasibility, efficiency, cultural pluralism, political procedures, uncertainty about risk, noncompliance by patients, and the like. Principles and rules provide background moral considerations for policy evaluation, but a policy must also be shaped by empirical data and by special information available in relevant fields of [nursing], medicine, economics, law, psychology, and so on. In this process, moral principles and various uses of empirical data are often closely connected. (p. 10)

Thus, Beauchamp and Childress suggest that health policy is so complex as to prohibit the strict and exclusive use of specific rules or principles in guiding policy formulation; rather, the authors suggest that ethical considerations must be accompanied by the rational use of empirical data.

Think About It

Ethics and Politics of Tobacco Sales

The sale and distribution of tobacco products has become a highly publicized political issue. The tobacco industry is increasingly affected by legislative and judicial decisions regarding the health effects of tobacco.

- What are the ethical issues of which the policy makers should be aware?
- Can you think of ethical arguments in favor of regulating the production and sale of tobacco products?
- Can you think of ethical arguments in favor of allowing the industry to operate on the free market—unrestricted?
- There are judicial precedents that assign at least some responsibility for the health problems of smokers to the tobacco companies. Is this a legal, ethical, or political issue—or some combination of these?
- Is this an issue in which nurses should be interested? What factors determine whether nurses should be interested in this issue?

Research Data In Policy Making

As a defense against ideological dominance in decision making, it is important that policy makers be furnished with reliable data. Research findings are useful in identifying problems, making comparisons, establishing trends, and developing policy based on evidence (Donley, 1996). Recognizing that time is precious for most policy makers, Pender (1992) observes that officials are generally more interested in research findings that address a particular issue than in unsubstantiated personal opinion. She suggests that nurses who plan to discuss policy with officials carefully review research findings that pertain to the issue and be ready to quote a few statistics that are particularly attention getting, recognizing that the potential for cost savings often gets attention when other facts elicit little response.

The federal government recognizes the importance of health care research in the development of policy. Established by Congress as part of the 1989 Omnibus Budget Reconciliation Act, the Agency for Health Care Policy and Research is one of eight agencies of the United States Public Health Service. Seeking answers to some of the most pressing health concerns facing our population, this agency serves as a bridge between researchers, clinicians, and policy makers (Bavier, 1995).

NURSING, POLICY, AND POLITICS

Not since the days of Lavinia Lloyd Dock have nurses been so actively involved with policy making and politics. It is through the perspective of knowledge, experience, and intimacy with the health care needs of the population that nursing is in the unique position to bring balance to the policy making process (Murphy, 1992). Moreover, the ANA *Code for Nurses* (1985), in identifying the goals and values of the profession, explicitly calls for nurses to be involved in policy formulation. Insofar as this document specifically identifies the community at large as one recipient of nursing care, nurses are called to look beyond immediate problems of individuals to broader political and social dimensions. The following points from the ANA *Code for Nurses* (1985) identify at least four areas of policy making for which nurses are accountable:

Point 8   The nurse participates in the profession's efforts to implement and improve standards of nursing.

Point 9   The nurse participates in the profession's efforts to establish and maintain conditions of employment conducive to high quality nursing care.

Point 10 The nurse participates in the profession's effort to protect the public from misinformation and misrepresentation and to maintain the integrity of nursing.

Point 11 The nurse collaborates with members of the health professions and other citizens in promoting community and national efforts to meet the health needs of the public. (pp. 13–16)

The formulation of health policy requires strong nursing leadership and an understanding of the nature of local and national policy making (Nagelkerk, 1994). Calling for the political empowerment of nurses, Batra (1992) charges that:

> Any serious effort to promote health must include an understanding of the crucial role that public policy plays. For the nursing profession, this new thinking means developing the ability to think, teach, research, and act in ways relevant to policy: awareness of the clinical impact of policies; clinical placements in policy-oriented settings; policy research, especially with short-term, qualitative research methods; and better strategic planning by professional nursing organizations to influence the health relevance of state and national policy agendas. (p. 171)

Recognizing health problems as policy issues allows nurses to move into the realm of policy formulation.

Nursing's Political Strengths.   There are at least two notable strengths with which nursing enters the political arena. First, the most sizable group of health care providers, the nursing profession boasts an extremely large number of political constituents. Acting together, the nation's nurses have the potential to be a formidable political force. In addition, nurses have traditionally been perceived in a favorable light. Nurses are viewed as much less self-interested than any of the other major health related interest groups (Hadley, 1996).

Nursing's Political Weaknesses.   Counterbalancing certain political strengths, nursing also has a number of political weaknesses. First, relatively new to the political arena, many nurses are not astute or comfortable in policy making or lobbyist roles. Second, there has historically been a lack of ideological and political unity within the profession, a weakness Hadley (1996) believes stems from the lack of uniform educational requirements and titles. Third, though nurses comprise the largest number of professionals, there are fewer dollars in nursing coffers specifically earmarked for intense lobbying than in those of many other special interest groups.

Policy Goals for Nursing

How do nurses become aware of the issues that are important and require energy and focus? Each individual has the responsibility to reflect upon problems and potential solutions. In addition, one of the major functions of professional organizations is to provide leadership and assistance to members in political and other matters. Congruent with the *Code for Nurses*, the American Nurses Association has developed a specific agenda for nurses interested in policy making. Nursing's legislative and regulatory agenda, as devised by the American Nurses Association, encompasses four basic goals: (1) to maintain nursing control of nursing practice, (2) to have a positive impact on health care policy, (3) to advocate on behalf of the client, and (4) to institute workplace reforms (deVries & Vanderbilt, 1992).

Think About It

Nurses Take Positions on Political Issues

In 1993 the American Nurses Association published a book outlining the profession's position on a variety of political issues. These positions were derived from the strategic goals of the organization. Altogether there are position statements covering over sixty different issues. Examples of issues include the following: campaign finance reform, child and elder care, civil rights, collective bargaining, domestic violence, drug control policy, family and medical leave, gun control, homelessness, malpractice/liability reform, migrant and seasonal farm worker health issues, pay equity, rural health care, and sexual harassment. These are but a few of the published position statements.

- Why do you think the professional organization published these position statements?

- Why are nurses concerned with issues such as campaign finance reform and gun control?

- What impact do you think the profession could make if each nurse became familiar with all of the issues and promoted them to policy makers?

LOBBYING

Sometimes nurses are privileged to be legitimate members of governmental or institutional policy making bodies. More often, the nurse's role in policy formulation, implementation, and modification is that of lobbyist. "**Lobbying** is the art of persuasion—attempting to convince a legislator, a government official, the head of an agency, or a state official to comply with a request—whether it is convincing them to support your position on an issue or to follow a particular course of action" (deVries & Vanderbilt, 1992, p. 1). Though many special interest groups employ lobbyists, every nurse can be a lobbyist and should lobby on issues of concern. Lobbyists have a powerful voice in determining the policy making process—from agenda setting to policy modification. In fact, some nurses believe it is a nurse's duty to participate in political **activism.** Hagerdorn (1995) defines activism as "a passionate approach to everyday activities that is committed to seeking a more just social order through critical analysis, provocation, transformation, and rebalancing of power" (p. 2). Activism promotes "exposing, provoking, and unbalancing the social power that maintains people in a state of disease, while simultaneously nurturing caring" (p. 2). There are others who believe that constrained, subtle, and persistent political activity is more effective in the long term than overt activism.

To be effective in the political domain, nurses are charged to become politically astute. According to Jennings (1996), "most decisions at the policy table and in the halls of Congress are politically driven. . . . one can have the best policy proposal on the table but if he or she doesn't know how to play the political game, all will be lost. Nurses must be very adept at discerning who has the power in the policy arena and how to link to that source" (p. 4). Knowing the "power players" in the political arena is one of the most important steps in the lobbying process.

Methods of Lobbying

The most familiar type of lobbying is the face-to-face approach. This process involves either meeting directly with a policy maker to request a desired action or testifying at a hearing. When possible, both paid and volunteer lobbyists should utilize the face-to-face method of lobbying. A second form of lobbying is **grassroots lobbying.** Grassroots lobbying involves mobilizing a committed constituency to influence the opinions of policy makers. Different types of grassroots lobbying include organized letter writing and implementing campaigns designed to mobilize public opinion (deVries & Vanderbilt, 1992).

One of the most important facets of lobbying is knowing whom to lobby. In seeking help to promote a particular legislative agenda, nurses want to begin by enlisting policy makers who have the following characteristics: (1) legitimate power, (2) an interest in the problem, (3) an affinity for nursing or for health care issues in general, (4) time and energy to invest in the process, (5) the respect of colleagues, and (6) committee or other positions that are appropriate to the particular legislation. Finding an official with all of these characteristics will greatly enhance the probability of legislative success. Neophyte lobbyists waste a great deal of time and energy lobbying officials who are disinterested, have conflicting loyalty, are powerless, or are not respected by their colleagues. The first step in lobbying is to connect with the appropriate policy makers.

The Lobbying Campaign. Once nurses have identified the appropriate policy making officials and are familiar with the issues and the legislative and regulatory process, the lobbying campaign can begin. There are two basic types of lobbying—direct and indirect. Indirect lobbying strategies are geared toward influencing public opinion, which in turn will influence policy makers. Methods of indirect lobbying include: media broadcasts, newspapers and other written materials, dissemination of the results of opinion polls, paid advertisements, educational campaigns, and organizations' agendas. Direct methods used to influence policy makers include: party platforms, political elections, influence of committees, agency regulations, face-to-face lobbying, letter writing, and contact with policy makers during social events (deVries & Vanderbilt, 1992).

Letter Writing. Handwritten, personal, mass letter writing is a powerful grassroots lobbying technique that has been successfully used by groups of nurses. In order to influence policy makers, there are certain letter writing techniques that have been found to be more effective. Following are some practical tips for letter writing:

- Whenever possible, individualize and legibly handwrite or type letters on personal stationery. Though more effective than no letters at all, form letters are much less likely to be read by officials than individualized letters.
- Write the letter in your own words, using your own thoughts and logic and drawing pertinent inferences.
- Identify yourself as a nurse and state your reason for writing in the first paragraph, including the title and number of the legislation in which you are interested.
- Be specific and include key information and examples supporting your position.
- Be explicit. Tell the official exactly what you want. If you are writing to ask for cosponsorship or a vote for or against a bill, say so.
- Be brief but informative. Keep your letter to a maximum of one to two pages.
- Include only one topic in each letter.
- Never threaten or use hostility. This immediately destroys your chances of developing a cooperative relationship.
- Offer your assistance as a resource.
- Promptly thank the official for favorable votes.

Personal Visits. A personal visit is usually a more powerful lobbying tool than letter writing. Whenever possible, nurses should seize the opportunity to meet with policy makers face to face. Following are a few suggestions for personal visits with policy making officials:

- Be prepared. Develop your plan of action and know what you intend to say.

- Be on time for your appointment, and be patient if the official is late.

- Be courteous and greet the official with a firm handshake, introduce yourself, and present your business card.

- Identify the subject of the meeting and present your facts in an orderly, succinct, and direct fashion.

- Support your position with personal experiences and anecdotes; use valid research and statistics when appropriate.

- Keep your presentation simple. Avoid technical language and professional jargon. Your goal is to inform and influence, not to impress.

- Close the meeting strongly and effectively, asking for the official's support.

- Leave a short fact sheet summarizing the issue and your position. Include the names and telephone numbers of contact people.

- Send a letter within a few days thanking the official for the meeting, restating your position, and including any information requested during the meeting.

Think About It

Be Careful of Your Wording

Nurses must be careful in choosing words to use when lobbying. One nurse relates a story of her first experience testifying before a state legislative committee. Feeling her presentation was well prepared and would be effective, the nurse decided at the last minute to substitute the words *nurse voters* for the word *nurses*. There were many people giving testimony that day. Following the completion of the testimony phase, the legislators were given an opportunity to make comments or ask questions. There were no questions. Every comment was directed toward the nurse, who was surprised to learn that the legislators perceived the term *nurse voters* to indicate a veiled threat. They did not hear the substance of the presentation, but rather the perceived threat; "If you do not support our position, we will vote you out of office." By unintentionally giving this impression, the nurse negatively affected the potential for a productive relationship with these legislators. The legislation that the nurses were supporting failed.

- Why do you think the nurse changed the wording of her presentation in the first place?

- What words would you have used?

- Describe similar circumstances in which you were speaking and the reaction of the listeners was based upon their inferences from your choice of words rather than their intended meaning?
- How can nurses avoid mistakes of this sort?

Political Campaigns

One very effective direct lobbying technique is for nurses to become involved in either supporting candidates or themselves running for elective office. According to Wakefield (1990), nurses are extolled to get involved in lobbying for specific legislation, not realizing that the ability to influence decisions related to the health care system occurs long before the issues are revealed to the public. Wakefield suggests that nurses become involved in campaigns and elections. This can be done in any number of ways. First, nurses should become involved in political party organizations. Political party activity serves as a vehicle for developing important relationships with elected officials. Involvement in a political party is essential to building a political network. Second, nurses can become involved through district and state nurses' associations. These organizations provide an opportunity to meet candidates, form relationships, and offer candidates forums. Forums serve to remind a candidate that nurses are an organized group interested in politics and public policy and to acquaint nurses with the candidate's position on important issues. Third, nurses can become actively involved in campaigning for candidates who support their positions on various health care issues. This may take the form of campaigning door to door, stuffing envelopes, publicly endorsing candidates, and so forth. Actively supporting candidates for public office helps to forge relationships with officials and elect candidates to public office who will sympathize with issues important to nurses. Involvement with political parties and the consequent relationships with public officials can also lead to either nurses' candidacy and election to public office or nurses' appointments to important policy making positions.

SUMMARY

There are many political issues that are important to nurses. Most issues for which nurses are actively concerned are related to health policy: issues of a moral nature, issues related to professional regulation, issues related to public health, and issues related to distributive justice. Fulfilling the role of advocate, nurses are challenged to become politically active: to know and become involved with important issues, to learn the political process, to form relationships with public officials, and to become astute in methods of influencing health policy.

CHAPTER HIGHLIGHTS

- The term *political* relates to the policy making process within the government.
- Political issues are those that are created, affected, or regulated by any of the government branches.

- Political parties are organized groups with distinct ideologies that seek to control government.
- Partisan issues are those issues for which the political parties have distinct ideology.
- Health policies influence the actions, decisions, and behaviors of people in the domain of health.
- Society's definition of health reflects the extent to which society is willing to go toward maximizing the health of citizens.
- Allocative health policies are designed to provide benefits to a distinct group.
- Regulatory policies are designed to influence others through directive techniques.
- The process of health policy includes the phases of policy formulation, policy implementation, and policy modification.
- There are two important functions of ethics in public policy making—guiding the original development of policy and criticizing previously implemented policy.
- Nurses are able to affect health policy through various political means.

DISCUSSION QUESTIONS AND ACTIVITIES

1. Discuss the issues listed in Figure 14–1 in class. How do classmates' positions compare to those of the major political parties? Are each student's opinions politically consistent from issue to issue?

2. Discuss the following question in class: What purpose do political parties serve?

3. Compile a list of political issues and classify them as to the branch of government with which the issue is most closely aligned—administrative, judicial, or legislative.

4. Discuss methods for influencing health policy in the administrative and judicial domains.

5. Compile a list of at least five political issues related to health that have been decided within the judicial domain. How have the judicial decisions affected health care delivery?

6. Compile a list of political issues related to moral values. Discuss the role of the professional organization in guiding members' actions related to these moral issues.

7. Discuss popular definitions of health and determine how each definition, if adopted by government, would affect health care delivery.

8. Discuss the role of ethics in policy making.

REFERENCES

American Nurses Association. (1985). *Code for nurses with interpretive statements*. Washington, DC: Author.

American Nurses Association. (1991). *Nursing's agenda for health care reform*. Kansas City, MO: Author.

Batra, C. (1992). Empowering for professional, political, and health policy involvement. *Nursing Outlook, 40*(4), 170–176.

Bavier, A. (1995). Where research and practice meet: Opportunities at the Agency for Health Care and Policy and Research. *Nursing Policy Forum, 1*(4), 20–38.

Beauchamp, T. L., & Childress, J. F. (1994). *Principles of biomedical ethics* (4th ed.). New York: Oxford University Press.

Curtin, L. (1996). *Nursing into the 21st century: Health care reform, restructuring, practice, leadership.* Springhouse, PA: Springhouse.

deVries, C. M., & Vanderbilt, M. W. (1992). *The grassroots lobbying handbook: Empowering nurses through legislative and political action.* Washington, DC: American Nurses Association.

Donley, R. (1996). Shaping health policy. *Nursing Policy Forum, 2*(1), 12–19.

Emerson, R. (1995). What is success? In W. Bennett (Ed.). *The moral compass: A companion to the book of virtues.* New York: Simon & Schuster.

Hadley, E. (1996). Nursing in the political and economic marketplace: Challenges for the 21st century. *Nursing Outlook 44*(1), 6–10.

Hagerdorn, S. (1995). The politics of caring: The role of activism in primary care. *Advances in Nursing Science, 17*(4), 1–11.

Jennings, C. (1996). Politics and nursing do mix! *Nursing Policy Forum 2*(3), 4.

Longest, B. B., Jr. (1995). *Health policymaking in the United States.* Ann Arbor, MI: AUPHA Press/Health Administration Press.

Murphy, N. (1992). Nursing leadership in health policy decision making. *Nursing Outlook 10*(4), 158–161.

Nagelkerk, J. (1994). Policy making. *JONA 24*(5), 14–15.

Pender, N. (1992). Making a difference in health policy. *Nursing Outlook 40*(3), 104–105.

Roe v. Wade, 410 U.S. 113 (1973).

Thompson, D. (1985). Philosophy and policy. *Philosophy and Public Affairs 14*(2), 205–218.

Thompson, F. J. (1991). The enduring challenge of health policy implementation. In T. J. Litman & L. S. Robins (Eds.), *Health politics and policy* (2nd ed., pp. 148–169). Albany, NY: Delmar.

Wakefield, M. (1990). Political involvement: A nursing necessity. *Nursing Economics 8*(5), 352–353.

CHAPTER 15

Economic Issues

I begin with the assumption that suffering and death from lack of food, shelter, and medical care are bad. I think most people will agree about this....

(Singer, 1972, p. 229)

OBJECTIVES

After completing this chapter, the reader should be able to:

1. Describe the role of economics in health care.
2. Explain the concept of distributive justice.
3. Discuss utilitarian, libertarian, communitarian, and egalitarian theories.
4. Discuss basic questions related to the distribution of health care resources.
5. Describe recent trends in health care economics and the relationship of economic trends to the delivery of health care.
6. Discuss ethics in relation to managed care systems of health care delivery.

INTRODUCTION

Nursing, other health care professions, and the overall health care delivery system exist to deliver health care to society. Over the past several decades, dynamic forces have worked together to create a complex system that has been called the best in the world. From advances in knowledge and technology to changes in health care financing, the system has experienced rapid and drastic changes. It is not unusual to hear the term *crisis* used to describe the state of the current health care system. This "crisis" relates to problems with cost, quality, and access to health care services. Current debates about social justice are fueled by inequalities in access to health care and health insurance combined with dramatic increases in the costs of care (Beauchamp & Childress, 1994). Thoughtful, systematic consideration of ethics is necessary for the process of devising solutions to the current problems. This chapter discusses particular aspects of health care economics, distributive justice, and emerging trends.

OVERVIEW OF TODAY'S HEALTH CARE ECONOMICS

Though given its own twists, the history of economic thought is closely associated with the utilitarian movement in the last century (Honderich, 1995). One of the main assumptions in traditional economics is that it is inappropriate to judge the institutions of a society except by reference to the preferences of the people they affect. There are different ways to judge the total preference of society. One method claims that one arrangement is better than another only if it satisfies the preferences of some and does not frustrate the preferences of any. This idea is at the center of what is known as welfare economics. Another method suggests that one arrangement is better than another only if it would be preferred by people allowed to make a collective choice. Given that institutions are only properly judged according to the preferences of the people they affect, the institution of health care should be judged by the society it serves. Discussion and debate about the current state of health care economics is integral to the process of evaluating the present system and formulating one that is more just.

The current American health care system is the most technologically advanced, and the most expensive, in the world. A legacy of progressively higher standards that require the most and the best care for a large segment of the population regardless of cost, coupled with the irresponsibility that comes from neither providers nor patients required to be stewards of cost, has led to a skewed model that focuses heavily on technology and personal autonomy and ignores basic principles of social responsibility and distributive justice. Except for newer managed care programs, this system features an odd split between those who make the spending decisions (patients and physicians) and those who must actually pay for those decisions (third party payers such as insurance companies, business corporations, or government) (Morreim, 1995). Moreover, there are staggering contrasts within this system. In some instances, hundreds of thousands of dollars are spent on what is recognized as futile care, yet much of the population has no access to even basic health care services.

Within the traditional fee-for-service system, ethics is predominately driven by codes of ethical behavior and patients' rights statements with a strong focus on the principle of autonomy. This model focuses on the individual patient, protects physician autonomy, promotes treatment that offers potential benefit or prolonged life, and assumes unlimited resources. Clearly, there are ethical problems associated with this model, including both overutilization and rationing on the basis of financial means (Biblo, Christopher, Johnson, & Potter, 1995).

Ask Yourself

Paying for Futile Care

One often hears stories about elderly patients with terminal illness, and even "no code" status, who remain in intensive care settings for extended periods of time, often because of family members who insist that everything be done for their loved one.

- Is the expenditure of expensive health care resources appropriate for these types of situations? Explain your position.
- Who should bear the financial burden for futile care?
- What are the ethical principles that conflict in situations of this sort?

In an essay on reforming American health care, deBlois, Norris, and O'Rourke (1994) discuss the problems with today's health care financing system. Though most people agree that modern health care in America is highly sophisticated and technologically advanced, they also recognize that there are many deficiencies in the system. First, health care services and resources are inaccessible to nearly twenty percent of the population. Second, health care costs are accelerating at an unsustainable annual rate, consuming a huge portion of the gross national product. Third, the high cost of health care threatens the competitiveness and profitability of business and industry. Fourth, the benefits to the individual and corporate providers within the system are often pursued at the expense (and sometimes harm) of persons who are in need of health care. DeBlois et al. propose that the real problems with the current system are related to its priorities and the values and commitments that support them, the most significant of which are:

1. an extreme form of individualism that routinely prefers individual interests over concerns about the community of persons;

2. an endorsement of profit making as a primary motive for providing health care services; and

3. an uncritical acceptance of technology as morally neutral and as unambiguously in the service of human goods and goals. (p. 55)

DeBlois et al. charge that the health and well-being of people subjected to a system under the influence of these values are often threatened by the kinds of services offered, the manner in which they are provided, and the priorities that determine both. Further, if improvements in the system are intended to promote health and well-being of people, efforts need to be ethically grounded and challenge the values that drive the present system.

DISTRIBUTIVE JUSTICE

The ethics of **justice** relates to fair, equitable, and appropriate treatment in light of what is due or owed to persons, recognizing that giving to some will deny receipt to others who might otherwise have received these things (Beauchamp & Childress, 1994; Honderich, 1995). The "others" may be those living in a person's community, or those in other communities, or even those yet to live. For example, if Social Security becomes bankrupt through excessive expenditures in the present, "others" who would have received benefits in the future (even if they are not yet born) will be denied these benefits. As mentioned in Chapter 3, the relevant application of the ethical principle of justice within the health care system focuses on the fair distribution of goods and services. This application is called **distributive justice.** Beauchamp and Childress (1994) define distributive justice as fair, equitable, and appropriate distribution of diverse benefits and burdens such as property, resources, taxation, privileges, and opportunities. Because there is a scarcity of resources and competition for resources and services, it is impossible for all people to have everything they might want or need. One of the primary purposes of government is to formulate and enforce policies that deal with distribution of scarce resources.

Three areas of health care are relevant to questions of distributive justice. First, which population groups should be the recipients of health care resources? Second, what percentage of society's resources is it reasonable to spend on health care? Third, recognizing that health care resources are limited, which aspects of health care should receive the most resources? These are important questions, both practical and ethical in nature.

Entitlement

In deciding questions of distributive justice, one must ask, "Who are entitled to these services?" As with all of ethics, there is no universally accepted answer. Distribution of limited resources is the function of various levels of governing bodies. In attempting to fairly distribute limited resources, leaders will seek systematic means of deciding. Historically, these questions have been answered by such **material rules** as: to each person an equal share, to each person according to need, to each person according to merit, to each person according to social contribution, to each according to the person's rights, to each person according to effort, to each person according to ability to pay, or to each person according to the greatest good to the greatest number. Most societies will utilize several of these principles in establishing public policies. We find many of these principles in effect in the United States where, for example, welfare payments and many health care programs are distributed on the basis of need; jobs and promotions in many sectors are awarded on the basis of demonstrated achievement and merit; comparably high incomes of some are awarded on the basis of superior effort, merit, or potential social contribution; and the opportunity for basic education is distributed equally to all citizens (Beauchamp & Childress, 1994).

Ask Yourself

Is Health Care a Right or a Privilege?

- Discuss whether you think health care is a right or a privilege. Explain your thinking.
- Should all people have access to the same health care services regardless of ability to pay? How should ability to pay influence access to health care services?
- If you believe health care is a right, to how much health care is each person entitled?

Right to Health Care.   In examining who should receive care, one hears questions about the basic right to health care. Is health care a right or a privilege? This is a question that is debated fiercely in the media, in the professional and political arenas, and around the dinner table. Is society responsible for providing health care for all citizens, and if so, to what degree? Should each person be eligible for minimum basic health care, or should everyone be allowed to have everything there is to offer—from organ transplants to tummy tucks? Would the public benefit from a strict free market system that would provide health care services only to those who can pay, or should the government be responsible for the health care needs of all citizens? If health care is a right and health care resources are scarce, what resources are allocated to which group of people? These and other questions fuel the debate about the right to health care.

Discussion of health care as a right is not new. On December 10, 1948, the General Assembly of the United Nations adopted the Universal Declaration of Human Rights which identifies medical care as a necessary social service ensuring the right to a standard of living adequate for health and well-being (Giesen, 1994). In 1983 the President's Commission for the Study of Ethical Problems in Medicine and Biomedical and Behavioral Research concluded that society has a moral obligation to ensure that everyone has access to adequate care without being subject to excessive burdens. The commission made a clear distinction between society and government, recognizing that a collective or societal obligation does not imply that government should be the primary institution involved in making health care available but, rather, that government should participate with the private sector.

The issue of health care as a right has some basis in constitutional law. The commission reported that neither the Supreme Court nor any appellate court has found a constitutional right to health care, but many federal and state statutes have been interpreted to provide statutory rights in the form of entitlements to some vulnerable groups. As a consequence, these groups have benefited from many legal decisions. Bandman and

Bandman (1978) argue that the common welfare clause of the Constitution implies the protection of basic needs including a right to the protection of health.

Health care as a right is not a universal belief. There are those who believe that health care is a privilege to be enjoyed by some, but beyond the common advantage of all citizens. The entrepreneurial model of libertarianism declares that health care is not a right but a commodity that must be purchased on the open market like any other service. This model compares the health care professional's right to conduct a practice and charge fees with the baker's and the candlestick maker's right to do likewise. It can be argued that this model provides health care only for those who can pay (or for those who are given health care services as a gift). It is hypothesized that as a result of a free market system of health care delivery, supply-and-demand and pricing competition would result in lower health care costs. This in turn would result in health care services becoming more accessible to a larger portion of the population. Except for the fact that professionals can choose to provide services free of charge, this model makes little allowance for children and the very poor (Bandman & Bandman, 1978; Beauchamp & Childress, 1994).

How Much and to Whom?   If one accepts that health care is a right (albeit limited) or that society has an ethical obligation to provide health care services to vulnerable populations, then one is required to examine the question of how much health care is to be provided and to whom. There are two broad views regarding the right to access to health care: some believe all should have equal access to health care, while others believe the right extends only to a decent minimum of health care. Consider the following case.

CASE PRESENTATION

Should Public Funds Pay for Extraordinary Procedures?

There was a recent court case in which a middle-aged indigent woman, who suffered from insulin dependent diabetes mellitus, demanded that Medicaid pay for a pancreas transplant. This patient was reported to be uncooperative in her previous diabetic regimen and disliked giving herself insulin injections. Even though Medicaid in that state has a fiscal policy that denies payment for this surgery to all program recipients, the state supreme court ruled that this woman had a right to the surgery by virtue of the fact that those with insurance or adequate funds have access to the surgery. The decision was based on the principle of nondiscrimination.

Think About It

Decisions About Entitlements

- Do you think the patient had a "right" to this surgery? Why or why not?
- Should society (through tax) pay for the surgery even though the patient was known to be nonparticipative in her previous regimen? Why or why not?

- Should the government make arbitrary decisions permitting or prohibiting certain therapies? Explain.
- Do you think there were others who might have received benefits but were subsequently denied them because extraordinary funds were used for this patient?
- What are the ethical implications of the court decision?
- What are ethical arguments for and against the court decision?

Fair Distribution

The court's decision to require public payment for the pancreas transplant in the previous case study raises questions about restricting health care services. Few people would argue that there are enough resources to pay for all services. Think about your household budget. If you have only $300 to spend on Christmas gifts for your three sisters and you also need to purchase groceries for the week and antibiotics for yourself, it would be foolish to spend $150 on one gift. By doing that, you would ensure that your sisters would not be treated equitably, that you probably would not be eating very well for the next week, and that you would not feel well anyway, since you could not afford your prescription medication. The same principle applies to health care dollars. The limited public budget must be divided among many interests. In order to maintain a functioning infrastructure, the government must ensure that public schools, highways, police, national defense, social security, and other services in the public domain have a proportionate share of the total budget. Policy makers are charged with the difficult task of making equitable decisions about distribution of resources. These decisions must balance health care spending with other programs and must carefully avoid both extravagant excess spending and frugality that threaten the health of citizens.

Distribution of Resources

Limited health care dollars must be spent wisely. There are several different criteria that have been proposed to make distributive justice decisions. One method involves making judgments about cost in relation to predicted benefit. For example, one could question the practice of allowing patients in the last stages of terminal illness to monopolize limited and expensive intensive care beds, thus utilizing the most expensive kind of health care for the least benefit. Some propose that the best way to avoid making arbitrary decisions in these kinds of situations is to set mandatory guidelines. For example, some suggest that expensive therapies, such as dialysis or organ transplant, be reserved only for those below a certain age. A second method involves making judgments about the utility of given therapies. Immunizations, for example, are very cost effective and are also beneficial to a large percentage of the population. Some would suggest that the most utile therapies (the ones that are less costly and nearly guaranteed to help a large number of people) are the ones that should have priority.

Theories of Justice

There are distinct theories of distributive justice that render these diverse principles coherent. Several theories have been proposed to determine how resources and services should be distributed. Utilitarian, libertarian, communitarian, and egalitarian theories are examples of popular theories of justice. Because of society's fragmented beliefs about social justice, no single theory can be expected to bring coherence to the situation. Beauchamp & Childress (1994) discuss the current system in the United States:

> We seek to provide the best possible health care for all citizens, while promoting the public interest through cost-containment programs. We promote the ideal of equal access to health care for everyone, including care for indigents, while maintaining a free-market competitive environment. These desirable goals of superior care, equality of access, freedom of choice, and social efficiency are difficult to render coherent in a social system. Different conceptions of the just society underlie them, and one goal is likely to diminish another. (p. 335)

Recognizing that no single theory will satisfy society by fulfilling all principles, the authors suggest that several theories of justice attempt to balance competing social goals.

Utilitarian Theories. Based, in general, upon the rule that it is good to maximize the "greatest good for the greatest number," **utilitarian theories** favor social programs that protect public health and distribute basic health care equally to all citizens. This is based on the belief that the outcome of these programs maximizes utility. Though these theories are the basis of many social programs, there are problems in their application. For example, because utilitarianism places aggregate social good before individual rights, it could be determined that social utility is maximized by denying access to health care for some of society's sickest and most vulnerable populations (Beauchamp & Childress, 1994).

Libertarian Theories. **Libertarian theories** propose that the just society protects the rights of property and liberty of each person, allowing citizens to improve their circumstances by their own effort. Privatization in the health care system is a protected value under this conception. Libertarian theory does not classify health care as a right but rather as a commodity that operates on the material principle of ability to pay either directly or indirectly through insurance. Strict libertarians view taxation as an unjust redistribution of private property but do not oppose other methods of distribution if they are freely chosen. Market strategies and managed competition are proposals in the United States that are influenced by libertarianism (Beauchamp & Childress, 1994).

Communitarian Theories. **Communitarianism** places the community, rather than the individual, the state, the nation, or any other entity, at the center of the value system. Less fully developed than utilitarianism or libertarianism, communitarianism emphasizes the value of public goods and maintains that values are rooted in communal practices. Communitarians believe that human life will go better if collective and public values guide peoples' lives. They have a commitment to facilities and practices designed to help members of the community develop their common and hence their personal lives (Honderich, 1995). Modern communitarian writers disagree on the application of these theories to health care access. Some envision a federation of interlinking community health programs that are democratically administered by citizen-members. In this model, each individual program would determine which benefits to provide, which care is most important, and whether expensive services will be included or excluded. Another communitarian theory holds that community tradition includes commitments of equal access to health care and suggests that as long as communal funds are spent, services must be equally available (Beauchamp & Childress, 1994).

Egalitarian Theories. **Egalitarianism** is related to the concept of equality in which people who are similarly situated should be treated similarly, though much depends on what kinds of similarity count as relevant and what constitutes similar treatment (Honderich, 1995). Promoting ideals of equal distribution of social benefits and burdens, egalitarian theories recognize the social obligation to eliminate or reduce barriers that prevent fair equality of opportunity. These theories are cautiously formulated to avoid requiring equal sharing of all possible social benefits. A leading proponent of egalitarianism, John Rawls (1996) suggests that in making decisions of justice, one should examine the situation behind a veil of ignorance. In this hypothetical situation, "no one knows his place in society, his class position or social status, nor does anyone know his fortune in the distribution of natural assets and abilities, his intelligence, strength, and the like" (p. 567). This veil of ignorance ensures that no one is able to design principles to favor his or her particular condition. Supporters of Rawls's theory recognize a positive social obligation to eliminate or reduce barriers that prevent fair equality of opportunity and suggest that health policy formulated according to egalitarian principles would guarantee a safety net or minimum floor below which citizens would not be allowed to fall (Beauchamp & Childress, 1994).

Ask Yourself

Making Fair Decisions

- Which theory of distribution appeals to you as the most fair and equitable? Why?
- Do you think the theory you chose would be fair to all people in all circumstances? Discuss your thinking.
- Could you combine two or more theories to make a system that is fair and equitable?

RECENT TRENDS AND HEALTH ECONOMIC ISSUES

Questions of ethics and distributive justice began to be discussed well before the mid 1990s. Claims that the United States was experiencing a crisis in health care economics reached a crescendo in the 1980s and 1990s. Skyrocketing expenditures and a general tightening of health care dollars resulted in fiscal scarcity. Both government and business responded by attempting to gain control over expenditures. This tightening assumed a variety of forms including managed care systems, prospective payment, and utilization review. Sacrificing, in part, the traditional focus on the welfare of patients, health care corporations began devising ways to cut costs, improve profits, increase efficiency, and branch out into more profitable ventures such as landscaping, catering, and laundry service.

Government was the prime mover of cost containment during the early 1980s. Having experienced virtually no incentives for cost controls up to this point, hospitals in the 1980s were unprepared when the government instituted the payment system based on Diagnosis Related Groups (DRGs). This shift represented the first major change in the way hospitals were paid for Medicare patients and placed the responsibility for efficiency and cost savings on hospitals and physicians. Certificate of Need programs were established to restrain the building or purchasing of unnecessary and expensive technologies and capital construction. Organizations such as Professional Standards Review Organizations (PSROs) and Peer Review Organizations (PROs) were established to require physicians to develop more efficient practice standards (Sherrill, 1995). By the early 1990s the system was in a state of disequilibrium. While large hospital corporations were finding ways to cut costs (utilizing such methods as eliminating support services and reducing nursing staff) and many small rural hospitals were closing as a result of the financial strain, inherent problems were unsolved—care remained excellent, though expensive, for some but inaccessible to many.

Economic influences also arose from outside the health care system. Two of the major outside influences were increased malpractice litigation and employment negotiated health insurance plans. Malpractice litigation resulting in huge awards and the subsequent birth of defensive medicine added to the expense of the system. Califano (1986) attributes this to dynamic forces that included elements from many distinct programs and entities. The system moved from one that traditionally called for community standards to one in which scientific invention, medical technology, specialization, Medicare and Medicaid, and regional heart, cancer, and stroke centers required nationalized standards of care for physicians. This resulted in the routine practice of ordering batteries of diagnostic tests to meet new, stricter standards. Fearing malpractice litigation, physicians began to lose a measure of the autonomy that would allow them to choose only the diagnostic tests they thought were appropriate.

Employment negotiated insurance plans fueled the practice of overspending and added to these pressures. Negotiated as part of employment contracts, many health insurance plans featured first-dollar, one hundred percent coverage of health care costs. As a result, a large percentage of patients did not pay directly for any health care services, thus the cost of the doctor or hospital was rendered irrelevant (Califano, 1986). Everyone expected the most and best. Being indifferent to the costs of the medical services, patients were much more likely to buy more of them, even those that were of marginal utility or duplicative (Gordon, 1992). Hospitals and physicians were more than happy to participate. For hospitals and doctors alike, maximizing services resulted in increased cash flow and consequent smoothing out of financial problems. This trend contributed to the even higher standards of care that required very aggressive diagnosis and treatment, resulted in greater costs, and opened the door for more malpractice litigation.

Health Care Reform

Recognizing these problems in the health care delivery system and sensing a groundswell of public support, the Clinton administration devised a health care reform proposal. Unveiled in the fall of 1993, this proposal called for universal access to health care through managed competition. It also described a system of financing that would be accomplished primarily through mandated coverage at places of employment, with employers required to pay a large percent of the premiums. Subsidies were planned for small businesses, and the federal government assumed the employer responsibility for persons who were not covered by employer-based plans (Drake, 1994).

After months of highly publicized debate, the Clinton health care reform proposal was defeated. Examining the defeat in terms of ethics, Jean deBlois (1995) attributes the failure to four fundamental factors: lack of social consensus on the question of a right to basic health care for all persons, strength and energy of those who argued on behalf of individual rights and liberties over the needs of the community or the nation, unconstrained powerful interest groups, and little or no recognition that substantive reform requires a significant challenge to the values that inform and drive health care.

Having lost features intended to ensure integrity within the new system, managed care was the only piece that emerged unscathed from Clinton's health care reform proposal. Existing as a small part of the United States health care system for several decades, managed care gained prominence as a preferred method of delivery and financing of health care services (deBlois, 1995).

The Move Toward Managed Care

Managed care is an integrated form of health care delivery and financing that represents attempts to control costs by modifying the behavior of providers and patients. Moving away from a system based upon provider and patient autonomy toward one based upon the combination of a focus on payer and provider needs, coupled with overall well-being of particular population groups, managed care requires focused examination of health care ethics. Supporters of managed care assert that the fundamental managed care concept is that lower costs gained through the elimination of waste and excess result in benefits to each patient and the membership as a whole. Aiming toward lower premiums and preventive care benefits, managed care organizations claim that members receive appropriate, quality care. In this regard, managed care is attentive to the needs of the membership as a group as well as the needs of individual patients. As a result of the goal of lower costs, it is said that patients in managed care plans can be saved from unnecessary tests and treatments, which are viewed as a risk inherent in the traditional system (Biblo et al., 1995).

Raising questions about the ethics of managed care, Fiesta (1996) discusses four notable legal cases that have resulted in significant financial losses for managed care organizations. These cases involve patients who have experienced unfavorable outcomes as a result of managed care providers' efforts to follow program policy in cutting costs. One case involves an infant who was febrile, moaning, panting, and flaccid when the parents consulted the managed care emergency line. Even though there were closer hospitals, the parents were instructed to take the child to a hospital that was nearly an hour away because it offered reduced cost to the managed care plan. The infant suffered a cardiac arrest en route. After resuscitation, both of the child's hands were amputated as a result of extraordinary complications. The family was awarded a $45 million verdict in a malpractice suit against the health maintenance organization.

In another case, the court concluded that by limiting enrollees' choice of provider to those on a specified panel, there is an unreasonable risk of harm to members if the selected clinicians are incompetent or unqualified. Another case involved the refusal of a physician assigned to a particular patient to admit the patient to the hospital. Although assigned by the managed care organization as the primary care provider for the patient filing suit, the physician argued that a physician-patient relationship did not exist because he had never seen the patient. Having been refused admission to the hospital as a result of this disagreement, the patient experienced a stroke in the hospital's parking lot. The court held that the plan's designated physician owed the patient a duty of care as a result of an implied physician-patient relationship inherent in the plan's enrollment agreement. In another case, the court rendered a $90 million verdict based upon the managed care organization's refusal to cover a bone marrow transplant. The court held that the managed care organization's internal utilization review decisions were unduly influenced by financial incentives to minimize care. Each of these cases illustrates ethical problems associated with balancing utilitarian views of cost-effective care with a respect for persons and the traditional view of a duty to care.

Ask Yourself

Ethical Problems in Managed Care

- What ethical problems can you foresee with managed care economics?
- How do you think nurses will be affected by managed care?
- How do you think nurses can influence the resolution of ethical problems in managed care?

Ethics in Managed Care.   Particular attention must be paid to the potential for ethical abuses that occur as a result of managed care organizations' unique role of both payer and provider of health care services. Like American society as a whole, the bioethics community was slow in recognizing the profound ethical implications of managed care. Based upon the assumption that the basic ethical criterion for the planned allocation of resources in a managed care setting at the policy level is the well-being of the entire group for whom the decisions are being made, balanced by the requirement of respect for individual health care needs, the Midwest Bioethics

Center developed a list of considerations to be used by managed care organizations for ethically rationing care:

1. Caring is an ethical imperative for health care providers because it is an essential benefit.

2. The first duty or obligation of any health care professional is to provide treatment that is clearly of benefit.

3. It is never ethically defensible to ration palliative care.

4. *Futile* treatment is of no benefit and should not be provided. However, care must be taken when defining a treatment as *futile* that the point of view of the patient is considered.

5. Treatment of marginal benefit needs to be carefully evaluated so that decisions are not inappropriately influenced by concerns such as subjective quality of life judgments of anyone other than the patient, cost constraints, or defensive medicine.

6. Individuals should make for others only those rationing decisions they are willing to impose upon themselves.

7. Populations that are especially needy or vulnerable should be given special consideration in order to be able to compete for the benefits society has to offer.

8. In rationing decisions, people ought not to be discriminated against without cause.

9. Lifestyle choice in and of itself is not a reason for denying care. However, it is ethically justifiable to provide positive incentives to support the development of healthy lifestyles. (Biblo et al., 1995, pp. 19–20)

SUMMARY

Because health care is a scarce resource, citizens rely upon social institutions to make fair and equitable distributive justice decisions. There is little consensus on basic ethical questions such as: Who should receive health care resources? Is there a right to basic health care? How much should be spent on particular health care services? What percentage of the society's overall resources should be invested in health care? Utilitarianism, libertarianism, communitarianism, and egalitarianism are theories that attempt to describe fair means of distributing resources. Recent focus on problems related to the economic aspects of the health care delivery system of the United States has prompted debate on practical issues of distributive justice. Emerging from the struggle to reform the health care system, managed care is becoming a major component of the health care system. Moving from a traditional system that valued patient and provider autonomy to a system that values the economic delivery of health care to a particular population, close attention must be paid to ethical standards in health care.

CHAPTER HIGHLIGHTS

- The history of economic thought is closely associated with the utilitarian movement in the last century.

- The traditional health care system in the United States is fee for service.

- Within a fee-for-service system, there is a strong focus on the principle of autonomy.

- Justice relates to fair, equitable, and appropriate treatment in light of what is due or owed to persons and recognizes that giving to some will deny receipt to others who might otherwise have received these things.

- Distributive justice is the fair, equitable, and appropriate distribution of benefits and burdens. Theories of distributive justice seek to render diverse principles coherent.

- Utilitarian theories are based upon the rule that it is good to maximize the greatest good for the greatest number.

- Libertarian theories propose that the just society protects the rights of property and liberty of each person, allowing citizens to improve their circumstances by their own effort.

- Communitarian theories place the community, rather than the individual, the state, the nation, or any other entity, at the center of the value system.

- Egalitarian theories are related to the concept of equality in which people who are similarly situated should be treated similarly.

- Scarcity of health care resources has led to a rethinking of the structure of health care economics.

- Managed care gives rise to ethical problems associated with balancing utilitarian views of cost-effective care with a respect for persons and the traditional view of a duty to care.

DISCUSSION QUESTIONS AND ACTIVITIES

1. Discuss current problems in health care economics with classmates. Is there a consensus regarding root causes, right to health care, or the role of the government as a payer for health care services?

2. Go to the library and find a basic economics text. How does the health care system differ from other free market systems?

3. Discuss the influence of utilitarian theory on the economics of the current health care system.

4. Why do patient and provider autonomy affect health care delivery and financing?

5. Define distributive justice. In class, discuss the material rules of distributive justice. Which material rule is most popular among classmates?

6. What method of distributing goods and services do you think is fair and equitable? Do your classmates agree with your theories?

7. Discuss health care ethics as related to managed care.

REFERENCES

Bandman, E. L., & Bandman, B. (1978). *Bioethics and human rights: A reader for health professionals*. Boston: Little, Brown.

Beauchamp, T., & Childress, J. (1994). *Principles of biomedical ethics* (4th ed.). New York: Oxford University Press.

Biblo, J. C., Christopher, L. J., & Potter, R. L. (1995). *Ethical issues in managed care: Guidelines for clinicians and recommendations to accrediting organizations.* Kansas City, MO: Bioethics Development Group.

Califano, J. A., Jr. (1986). *America's health care revolution: Who lives? Who dies? Who pays?* New York: Random House.

deBlois, J. (1995, Autumn). Ethical issues and managed care: Asking the right questions. *Health Care Ethics, USA 3*(4), 6–7.

deBlois, J., Norris, P., & O'Rourke, K. (1994, Autumn). *A primer for health care ethics: Essays for a pluralistic society,* pp. 5–6. Washington, DC: Georgetown University Press.

Drake, D. (1994). *Reforming the health care market: An interpretive economic history.* Washington, DC: Georgetown University Press.

Fiesta, J. (1996). Legal update, 1995: Part 2. *Nursing Management, 27*(6), 24–25.

Giesen, D. (1994). A right to health care?: A comparative perspective. *Health Matrix 4*(2), 277–295.

Gordon, J. S. (1992, May/June). How America's health care fell ill. *American Heritage,* 49–65.

Honderich, T. (Ed.). (1995). *The Oxford companion to philosophy.* New York: Oxford University Press.

Morreim, E. H. (1995). *Balancing act: The new medical ethics of medicine's new economics.* Washington, DC: Georgetown University Press.

President's Commission for the Study of Ethical Problems in Medicine and Biomedical and Behavioral Research. (1994). Securing access to health care. In B. L. Beauchamp & L. Walters, *Contemporary issues in bioethics* (4th ed., pp. 683–689). Belmont, CA: Wadsworth.

Rawls, J. (1996). A theory of justice. In J. Feinberg, *Reason and responsibility: Some readings in basic problems of philosophy* (pp. 567–572). Belmont, CA: Wadsworth. (Reprinted from J. Rawls, *A theory of justice,* 1971, Cambridge, MA: Harvard University Press)

Sherrill, R. (1995, January 9–16). Medicine and the madness of the market. *The Nation,* 45–72.

Singer, P. (1972). Famine, affluence, and morality. *Philosophy & Public Affairs 1,* 229–243.

CHAPTER 16

Social Issues

By Mary Jo Butler

In the deserts of the heart let the healing fountain start. . . .

(W. H. Auden, p. 986)

OBJECTIVES

After completing this chapter, the reader should be able to:

1. Explain how the social conditions of poverty, homelessness, domestic violence, an increasing elderly population, and racism affect health.

2. Apply the concept of justice to vulnerable populations, elaborating on the implications for society and the health care system.

3. Discuss the application of beneficence and nonmaleficence to vulnerable groups in light of today's health care system.

4. Identify the pros and cons of promoting autonomy for health care decision making among vulnerable populations.

5. Analyze evidence of victim blaming within the health care system.

6. Illustrate application of the concepts of advocacy and nonviolence to care of vulnerable populations.

7. Examine current research for application to culturally diverse groups.

INTRODUCTION

Health is unquestionably a product of the person and environment interchange. Thus, social conditions that alter the person and environment interchange process are critical concerns for nurses and nursing students. Nurses confront social issues that shape the health and health care management of individuals on a daily basis. These social issues may create conflicts in values and ethical dilemmas that must be addressed in order to determine appropriate health care interventions for involved individuals. The purpose of this chapter is to help elucidate the principles inherent in decision making when social issues create ethical dilemmas for the nurse.

SOCIAL ISSUES

Several pervasive social issues are of special concern to health care providers today. Poverty, homelessness, domestic violence, an increasing elderly population, and racism are particularly important. Each of these issues is reviewed briefly in this chapter along with the dominant guiding principles for related ethical decision making.

Poverty

Poverty and homelessness are on the rise in the United States as a consequence of changes in government assistance programs and taxes (Danziger, 1988). Health care is influenced more and more by poverty as increasing numbers of people lose health insurance due to a voluntary employment based insurance system and a publicly financed health care system for the medically indigent that is becoming available to fewer people and meets only a fraction of the needs of enrolled individuals (Rosenbaum, 1992; United States Department of Commerce, 1990). Without health care coverage, the poor often postpone needed health care or cope with public clinics that are often degrading and impersonal.

Federal programs for the indigent cover only about half of all individuals living on incomes below the poverty level (Johnson, 1990). Individuals without coverage must find health care systems that will provide free care or do without. For this reason, many people below the poverty level do not participate in basic preventive care programs.

Poverty, growing worldwide, is known to have a negative impact on both the health of individuals and the receipt of health care services (Catley, 1992). Poorer people are sicker than people with adequate financial resources. While poverty is detrimental to the health of all individuals living with inadequate resources, it produces a next generation of citizens with more health problems than usual. Children living in poverty have a higher incidence of conditions associated with trauma, drugs, burns, mental illness, and HIV infection (Wessell, 1992). Children living in poverty are more likely to experience poor nutrition, inadequate exercise, and diseases from environmental factors such as vermin or lead. They are more likely to grow up with chronic illnesses that require extensive health care resources. Overall, poverty and health are inextricably enmeshed.

CASE PRESENTATION

Socioeconomic Influences on Health

Martha D is a sixty-nine-year-old African-American woman who lives in a sub-standard third-floor walk up, cold water apartment in a housing project with a high crime rate. She draws a small Social Security check that does not cover living expenses. Her income is supplemented by food stamps, housing assistance, and by working as a nanny for three small children for twenty hours a week. Ms. D earns minimum wage for her job as a nanny and accepts cash for her work to avoid any interference with her Social Security check. She uses public transportation to go to and from her job, spending $2.00 each working day on bus fare.

Ms. D helps her alcoholic single daughter, age forty-seven, with two teenage children, especially when the daughter is experiencing a drinking binge. The children frequently stay with Ms. D and rely on her for food, shelter, and love. Mr. D is an alcoholic and has not been home for two years; however, he does occasionally call from a homeless shelter or treatment facility. Neither the daughter nor Mr. D contribute to household expenses, but Ms. D is very devoted to her family, especially her two grandchildren.

Martha D is 5'8" tall and weighs 285 pounds. She has hypertension, with her blood pressure ranging from 200/90 to 250/110. She is on medication for her blood pressure, and the physician has linked her with a county home health nurse to encourage a diet and simple exercise regime for her obesity and hypertension. Ms. D is beginning to show signs of adult onset diabetes and has been encouraged to lose weight and adhere to a diabetic diet. In addition, Ms. D has some small ulcerations on her left ankle.

The home health nurse visits Ms. D and instructs her in the care of her ulcers, advising her to keep her left foot elevated as much as possible. The nurse spends considerable time explaining a 1200 calorie diabetic diet with moderate sodium restriction to Ms. D and talks with Ms. D about the need to begin walking as soon as the ulcers on her foot heal. Ms. D lets the nurse know she used to attend a weight control group and understands low fat and diabetic diets. However, she says coming home to a nice pot of beans with fried chicken and biscuits is her only daily pleasure. "I've lived sixty-nine years on this diet, don't wish to change, and have nothing to lose if I remain on it the rest of my life." She also points out that it is not safe to walk in her neighborhood so she stays inside. In addition, she indicates that she is too tired to exercise after working all day.

 Think About It

Who Decides What Is Best for a Patient?

- Discuss Ms. D's decision to ignore recommendations regarding diet, exercise, and, perhaps, care of her ankle ulcerations in relation to autonomy, beneficence, and nonmaleficence.

- Since the principle of beneficence requires actively doing good for Ms. D, who decides what is good?

- Discuss implications of justice and health care for Ms. D.

Homelessness

Homeless individuals, although not a homogenous group, are increasing in society. While good census data are hard to obtain, between 250,000 and 3,000,000 people are homeless in the United States (Bowdler, 1989). The homeless are not all mentally ill or substance abusers. The new homeless are often families, single women with children, and the elderly (Bowdler, 1989; Kutza & Keigher, 1991). Like those living in poverty, homeless people suffer from acute and chronic health problems. Burg (1994) categorizes their health problems as those resulting from limited access to care, those coincident with homelessness, and those associated with the psychosocial burden of homelessness. Health problems resulting from limited access to care include exacerbated or advanced conditions that would have responded to early and thorough intervention. Health problems coincident with homelessness include illnesses resulting from living with inadequate nutrition, warmth, hygiene, safety, and other basic needs. Health problems associated with the psychosocial burden of homelessness are primarily mental illnesses, suicide, assault, and substance abuse which can dull the anxiety of homelessness. About sixteen percent of homeless children have a chronic health problem, which is well above the rate for children who are not homeless (National Association, 1989). The homeless, like those living in poverty, have few options for health care, limited access to care, and difficulty with follow-up treatment or compliance. This is due, in part, to the typical model of health care delivery in the United States.

Mondragon (1993) describes the pervasive assumptions that undergird the government's health promotion model. These assumptions view health as the absence of disease and associate common diseases with controllable risk factors. Thus, the key to improved health is deemed to be the provision of knowledge and skills to individuals. It is assumed that people will use self-determination, individualism, and responsibility to secure adequate housing, employment, and proper nutrition. While this model may benefit people with good education, a continuum of options, and resources to elicit change, it is less applicable to those with limited choices who are not in charge of their destinies. It can be hypothesized that poverty and homelessness will contribute to the poor health of American citizens as long as the dominant models for health care delivery inhibit patient participation in care.

 CASE PRESENTATION

No Home to Go To

Ms. Brown comes into the emergency room to secure treatment for a head injury, plus minor bruises and abrasions that she reportedly received during an assault that happened about twenty hours ago. Ms. Brown is thirty-four years old and accompanied by her boyfriend, Roy. She indicates they were sleeping in a protected entrance to an elevator in the city parking garage when two young men began beating and kicking them. The two men took Ms. Brown's purse, a sack of food she and Roy had accumulated, and Roy's wallet which contained $5.00.

Ms. Brown indicates she has been homeless for over a year. She occasionally stays in city shelters but spends most of her time roaming the city and walking to secure meals at the various programs that feed the poor. She is tall and thin, with a variety of skin lesions. She came to the hospital due to dizziness that prevented her from walking to the church where she could eat. She and Roy occasionally work odd jobs but use the bulk of their income to support Roy's drug habit. She is trying to get Roy to quit using.

The physician has the nurse clean Ms. Brown's scalp and tape the traumatic lesion. A contusion is expected, and the physician suggests Ms. Brown rest for a few days and go to the neurological clinic if the dizziness worsens. The nurse points out that Ms. Brown has no place to rest and cannot get to the clinic without access to public transportation. The physician realizes this but indicates it is beyond her control.

Think About It

When Resources Are Lacking

- Apply the concepts of justice, nonmaleficence, and beneficence to Ms. Brown's care.

- Does society have any responsibility for Ms. Brown? If so, what?

- Can thorough treatment be denied if a client has no resources? If not, who pays for the treatment?

Domestic Violence

A third common social condition affecting health and health care delivery is domestic violence, the most common but least reported crime in the United States. Estimated numbers of battered women range from two to twelve million per year (American Medical Association, 1992). Domestic violence flows from a historical position of sexism. Eisler (1987) describes how select tenets of Judaism, Christianity, and Islam support patriarchy, the inferiority of women, and women as the property of men. In the United States it was legal for a husband to beat his wife to maintain his authority until 1899 (Diehm & Ross, 1988). Remnants of these beliefs are still threaded through society, affecting the way families socialize their children and the way communities tolerate gender inequity. Butler and Weatherley (1992) indicate that women have long been defined by the mothering role and dependence on men in American society. While these role definitions are changing, daily events in society continue to perpetuate gender inequity. As long as gender inequity exists, domestic violence will remain a social problem.

The vast majority of abused women eventually leave their abusive partners. However, leaving is a process that takes time, energy, and resources. Many abused women will leave and return to their abusive partners several times before permanently terminating the relationship. Esposito (1993) attributes this to the inability to find housing or suitable jobs; the fear, loneliness, or poverty that results from being out on their own; concern for children who are experiencing relocation and other difficulties; relentless pressure from family and friends to try harder to make the relationship work; or poor support from the criminal justice system. It is sometimes easier to return to a familiar though unpleasant situation than to start over and deal with numerous unknowns.

Since sex is the risk factor, domestic violence affects women of all socioeconomic, racial, and ethnic groups (Esposito, 1993; Ewing, 1987). All women living in violent relationships will experience poorer health. Women living in abusive situations experience acute traumatic injuries and chronic physical and emotional problems (Butler & Weatherley, 1992). They are especially vulnerable to battery during pregnancy and at a higher risk than nonbattered women for poor pregnancy outcomes (Bohn, 1990). The health care system may add insult to abused womens' injuries. The women often feel humiliated by and blamed for the abuse by a health care system that minimizes the abuse, makes insufficient referrals, and fails to acknowledge abuse as the culprit (Campbell, Pliska, Taylor, & Sheridan, 1994). As a result, women leave health care settings without having the domestic violence addressed, remaining isolated and uninformed about their options (Fishwick, 1995).

 ## CASE PRESENTATION

Suspicions of Abuse

Maria P is a twenty-five-year-old Hispanic woman who made an initial visit to the clinic for prenatal care when she was eighteen weeks pregnant. She has returned for a second prenatal visit at twenty-two weeks gestation. Maria has a four-year-old son and a two-year-old daughter. Her record indicates she had several bruises, lacerations, and a black eye during her last pregnancy that she attributed to clumsiness. Her two year old weighed four pounds, eight ounces at birth and was seventeen inches long.

As part of routine prenatal care for the most recent pregnancy, Maria was tested for HIV antibodies. The test was positive, and the physician and nurse conveyed this information to Maria during her second prenatal visit. Maria, of course, was quite upset. She admits that her spouse has been physically abusing her for some time and that both have used intravenous drugs in the past. She has had no sexual partners other than her spouse.

The nurse encourages Maria to tell her spouse that she is HIV positive so that he can be tested for antibodies. She also encourages use of condoms during sexual intercourse to help avoid transmission to her spouse should he not be infected. Maria insists that her husband refuses to use condoms as they interfere with his pleasure. In addition, she says he would kill her if he knew she was HIV positive.

The nurse encourages Maria to go to a shelter for abused women and links her to both a counselor and a social worker who help her devise a safety plan. However, Maria ultimately decides to go home because she cannot abandon her children and she does not want them in a shelter. She knows she cannot make it on her own, as she has neither income nor job skills. She requests that the clinic not interfere and that they allow her to decide if, when, and how she will notify her spouse about her HIV status.

Think About It

When Patient Choices Place Them at Risk for Harm

- Consider the principle of autonomy when determining the appropriate decision in this situation. Remember that confidentiality is an inherent part of autonomy.
- Who is the patient in this situation?
- If Maria's husband is notified by the clinic of her HIV status and he does significant harm to Maria, would liability become an issue?
- If Maria's husband discovers he is HIV positive in the future, blames Maria, and discovers the clinic has known she was HIV positive for some time, is there any liability? Explain.

Increasing Elder Population

In addition to poverty, homelessness, and domestic violence, the elderly are a growing population worldwide (Catley, 1992). By the year 2050, Stark (1991) predicts that sixty nine million Americans will be over age sixty-five. People are living longer due to healthier diets, vaccines, and improvements in the environment (Windom, 1988). Certainly advances in health care knowledge have contributed to greater longevity. However, many elderly, especially from minority populations, live without pensions and on incomes below the poverty level (Hall, 1993). Vast numbers of the elderly are socially isolated, in need of work to survive, and susceptible to economic hardship. Chronic illnesses, pain, especially from arthritic processes, frailties, and disabilities occur with increasing frequency as people age (Tebb, 1995). Health problems contribute significantly to the social isolation, financial burden, and general discomfort that may accompany aging.

The assumption in current prevailing health care models is that the frail elderly will be cared for at home by friends and family to alleviate strain on the health care system. In reality, family members may be unable to provide needed support due to geographical distance from the frail elderly family member or personal responsibilities. Skaff and

Pearlin (1992) describe how caregivers of the elderly experience emotional and financial strain. The caregivers often have to help with finances of the elderly, since their fixed incomes cannot cover the basic cost of living as well as health care expenses. Reliance on friends and family for health care of the frail elderly is especially problematic for the elderly without the necessary social or financial resources. Even though the elderly are known to be vulnerable and at risk, one proposal to control health care costs in the United States is the rationing of care to the aged and a shift to more home care (Arcangelo, 1994).

 CASE PRESENTATION

Aging, Poverty, and Illness

Mr. Chang is a sixty-five-year-old widower with chronic kidney disease. He is supposed to receive dialysis three times a week but frequently misses his appointments due to no transportation or not feeling well. His only hope for a cure is a kidney transplant which Mr. Chang really wants. Mr. Chang is very frail with many health problems. He lives alone in a small garage apartment. The landlord is threatening to evict Mr. Chang because he is behind in his rent payments. Mr. Chang lives on a small pension and Medicare. His prescription costs are excessive.

A home health nurse used to transport Mr. Chang to dialysis occasionally, as Mr. Chang lives outside the township limits and is unable to access public transportation services. The clinic, which does not believe Mr. Chang is a candidate for a transplant, has revised their policies regarding home visits due to changes in reimbursement mechanisms. The home health nurse can no longer visit Mr. Chang unless there is a reimbursable need such as a dressing change; and for liability reasons, she can no longer transport Mr. Chang to dialysis.

 Think About It

What Health Care Should Society Provide for Its Citizens?

- Consider the principle of justice in deciding if health care is a right or a privilege that comes with the ability to pay. If health care must be rationed, who decides what services an individual will receive?
- Is society prepared to pay health care costs for all citizens?
- Is there a level of care that society should provide to all citizens, with private financing providing all care beyond the set level? Explain.
- What is fair for Mr. Chang?

Racism

Racism is another social concern that affects health. The term *race* generally refers to an attribute that allows classifications of human beings on the basis of certain biological characteristics (Melville, 1988). Although no racial group of people ascribes to the same cultural beliefs and practices, it is often race that stereotypes a group of people or engenders ethnocentric beliefs and moral conflicts in values. Brown (1991) believes racism is an ethical problem based on inadequate respect, violation of personal boundaries, and an imbalance of power.

Mondragon (1993) and Fowler and Risner (1994) describe how race affects health. African-Americans, Hispanics, and Native Americans have the worst health status of American groups according to all public health indicators. In addition, they have the highest rates of risk behaviors for disease. Hunger has increased among these three racial groups. They have poorer cancer survival rates and higher incidences of stroke, hypertension, diabetes, and other problems. In addition, African-Americans and Hispanics have the lowest levels of health insurance and the most inappropriate use of expensive emergency rooms. While socioeconomic conditions contribute to these health conditions, it is easy to discern possible racial influences on health.

There is evidence that the health care system itself is racist (Fowler & Risner, 1994; Funkhouser & Moser, 1990; Spigner, 1994). Problems of access and inequity of treatment are frequently cited as evidence of racial bias. In addition, traditional solutions to health problems such as health education and health promotion programs do not seem to be programmed for minority groups (Mondragon, 1993). More importantly, minority groups tend to demonstrate poorer health outcomes in some areas revealing inadequate health care; for example, the infant mortality rate of African-Americans is two times higher than that of the European American population (Hogue & Hargroves, 1993).

There is significant interface of poverty, homelessness, domestic violence, an increasing elderly population, and racism. Poverty underpins homelessness. In addition, the African-American living in poverty is more likely to face homelessness (Davis & Winkleby, 1993). African-Americans, Native Americans, and Hispanics are overrepresented among the homeless. Women experiencing domestic violence move frequently and often deal with homelessness and poverty as they try to improve their situations (Kanna, Singh, Nemil, & Best, 1992). Goodman (1991) provides data that poverty and homelessness are linked to a high abuse rate, and Campbell (1993) indicates that violence and poverty are linked, at least among African-Americans. The elderly are often made homeless as they face mounting health care and living costs on a fixed income. Persons experiencing poverty, homelessness, aging, domestic violence, and racism are vulnerable to poor health and inadequate health care delivery. Often these vulnerable groups are the least powerful and vocal persons in society, yet they are the groups most affected by ethical decisions regarding health (Wessell, 1992).

These social situations represent examples of classism, sexism, and racism. Each indicates prejudice or discrimination against a particular class, gender, or racial group. The implication is that one group of people is held to standards espoused by another group. Statistical data on these social situations and the health of persons experiencing the social situations explain why a feeling of helplessness may emerge when social situations are so intrinsically intertwined with health. Yet treating a person's symptoms without attending to the root causes of the problem may be viewed as inadequate health care.

ETHICAL PRINCIPLES APPLIED TO SOCIAL ISSUES

Ethical dilemmas involving classism, sexism, and racism are difficult to resolve. The common principles most essential in unraveling ethical dilemmas encompassing social issues include justice, nonmaleficence, beneficence, and autonomy. A brief discussion of each principle follows.

Justice

Justice is the duty to treat all people fairly without regard to age, socioeconomic status, race, or gender. This implies a fair distribution of the benefits and burdens among members of a society, with equal treatment to all or to those most in need. This could mean extending necessary treatment to those in need even though they may not have the requisite means to pay for the treatment. A frail elderly gentleman, beloved by his family, might receive an expensive but desired transplant procedure based on justice even though there is only a moderate chance that the extensive surgery will prolong life or improve the quality of life.

Ask Yourself

Who Should Receive Limited Health Care Resources?

- In this day of declining health care resources, should those with the greatest need or those who have contributed to society receive expensive restorative procedures? Or should these procedures be available to all? Support your position.

Nonmaleficence

Nonmaleficence is the duty to prevent or avoid doing harm whether intentional or unintentional. This could mean refusing to discharge an abused woman to her home if there is a possibility of further injury. It might also entail ensuring a safe, hygienic environment before hospital release of a newborn infant and mother suffering from poverty or homelessness.

Beneficence

Beneficence is the duty to actively do good for patients. This principle is described by the Council on Ethical and Judicial Affairs of the American Medical Association (1992) as healing with attention to the psychological, social, and spiritual dimensions of disease or injury as well as the physical problems. Thus, the homeless lady with leg ulcers and diabetes who walks all day and stands in lines in poor shoes and all types of weather to secure free meals and safe sleeping quarters will receive treatment for the leg ulcers that will ensure adequate diet and rest, elevation of the legs, and proper hygiene. Treatment would have to go beyond the usual prescriptions for drugs and address the social conditions contributing to the physical problems.

Autonomy

Autonomy is the patient's right to self-determination without outside control. Related to this principle are the principles of veracity, privacy, confidentiality, and respect for all persons. Autonomy would allow the abused woman, who is made aware of other options and available support, to return home if that is her choice even though her safety is a concern. However, in considering autonomy, Limandri and Tilden (1993) caution that the nurse may need to contemplate whether the abused woman's decision making competency and ability to act autonomously are impaired by the chronic stress of living with abuse.

PERSONAL IMPEDIMENTS TO INTERVENING WITH VULNERABLE GROUPS

Working with people who are poor, homeless, experiencing domestic violence, aged, or of a different race requires exploration of personal values to ensure that negative attitudes do not interfere with health care. Price, Desmond, and Eoff (1989) caution that victim blaming is a real phenomenon that can color attitudes and interactions.

Victim Blaming

Victim blaming tends to hold the people burdened by social conditions accountable for their own situations and responsible for needed solutions. Victim blaming is often evident in language. If there is evidence of personal or systemwide victim blaming, a new world view is needed. A desirable world view would see all persons as autonomous beings who deserve to be treated with dignity and fairness. Of interest, the health care system may not be designed to extend the needed degree of autonomy to all people. Nurses and other health care providers are generally educated to take charge and make decisions. Sines (1994) describes how prominent power relationships interfere with therapeutic practice and desirable client outcomes. To respect others by allowing them to make choices and decisions, when they are capable of doing so, requires an attitude of caring with a focus on advocacy. This implies guarding patient rights, preserving patient values, championing social justice in health care, and serving as the conservator of the patient's best interests (Sines, 1994). Retooling nurses and other providers to enhance the advocate role and foster the needed world view may improve care within a health care agency.

Ask Yourself

How Does Language Reflect One's Values?

How do the values reflected in the language of the following statements imply victim blaming?

- Most young, single, poor women get pregnant to increase their welfare benefits.
- If poor, homeless people would take more responsibility for themselves, they could improve their situation. There are jobs out there for people who want to work.
- The highest calling for a woman is to be the family nurturer.
- If an abused woman wanted help, she would just leave the abusive relationship.
- An important part of assessing for domestic violence is to ask what the woman was doing or if she was drinking right before she was hit.
- Resistance to change is a normal part of aging.
- All five senses tend to decline as a person ages.
- Since most low-income women do not comply with therapies, it is not cost-effective to spend too much time with them on health education.
- What did you expect? Look at how her mother behaved.
- People can get ahead if they take advantage of life's opportunities.

Language of Violence

Another possible impediment to intervening, specifically with the social situation of violence, is the violence mode that colors speech and actions. Ewing (1987) describes how the health care system uses metaphors of violence such as "attacking" germs, "battling" disease, "plotting strategies" against or "defeating" invasive cells and unwanted organisms, and, ultimately, "suffering defeat" or "achieving victory." The prevailing mind set behind this strategy of confrontation is the antithesis of a needed compassionate approach that values nonviolence. This is especially true for women experiencing domestic violence. Language that supports violence can inadvertently lead to victim blaming or covertly encourage futile and dangerous retaliation. Indeed a first step in effective intervention with those experiencing violence is to create a milieu that emphasizes nonviolence. The message has to be clear that violence of any form is wrong and, generally, illegal. This may necessitate a change in how health care providers approach and work therapeutically with people experiencing violence.

SOCIAL ISSUES AND SCHOLARSHIP

Many health care interventions are based, properly, on research; however, nurses need to ask if the underlying research, and therefore the determined therapy, may create problems based on classism, sexism, and racism. For example, growth and development knowledge is based largely on studies of the experiences of white heterosexual men (Gilligan, 1982). Thus, application of growth and development theory to both genders and to other races requires prudence. Campbell (1993) provides excellent data that knowledge of the abuser in domestic violence situations is based on sex role socialization in European American families and therefore does not explain the violence in African-American families. Violence in the African-American family, according to Campbell, may be better explained by role conflict, discrimination, isolation, financial stress, and other variables. Demi and Warren (1995) and Vasquez and Eldridge (1994) explore the issues of valid research for vulnerable populations, pointing out that the way family is defined and the systems for recruiting and retaining families contribute to the inability to generalize research findings. In addition, so many of the research instruments in use are not designed for diverse and vulnerable populations.

Spigner (1994) points out that African-Americans do not participate as readily in research as European Americans due to the way they are represented in the social structure. Their socioeconomic status and the professional hierarchy often impede African-American participation in research studies. Certainly many intelligence tests are under scrutiny for cultural bias. In addition, research that is less than twenty-five years old has viewed women as inferior to men and nonwhite groups as inferior to whites (Vasquez & Eldridge, 1994). These historical roots have contributed to a dearth of scholarly studies on women and minority populations. This means that classroom teachings and clinical knowledge may be based on inadequate research for minority populations.

There is an ethical responsibility to teach how to provide nursing care to diverse cultural groups. Thus, faculty and students must be cognizant of the benefits of selected interventions for all population groups. In addition, they must be vigilant in generalizing research findings to diverse population groups. Research on vulnerable populations needs to be done to ensure an adequate data base for working with those growing populations that are experiencing social issues such as poverty, homelessness, domestic violence, unhealthy aging, and racism.

SUMMARY

This chapter focused on ethical dilemmas that emerge when health care is considered for vulnerable population groups. Ethical decisions related to health care for vulnerable populations confront nurses who work with those experiencing the social conditions of poverty, homelessness, domestic violence, unhealthy aging, and racism on a daily basis. Since values affect professional behavior, nurses must analyze personally held values as well as those of the health care agency where they are employed for appropriate consideration of justice, beneficence, nonmaleficence, and autonomy. Nurses who work with vulnerable groups need to utilize these principles in ethical decision making. Nurses must consider the impact and validity of health care interventions and research on vulnerable populations and ensure that what nurses teach both in the classroom and to patients is based on research applicable to the populations being served and studied.

CHAPTER HIGHLIGHTS

- Poverty, homelessness, domestic violence, aging, and racism affect health in a negative fashion. Limited choices and inappropriate treatment options often interfere with the best health care for these vulnerable populations.

- Applying the concept of justice to vulnerable populations can change the way society and the health care system provide health care. Addressing the social conditions of the individual with an illness or disease is basic to health care.

- Nonmaleficence and beneficence may clash with autonomy when providing care for vulnerable populations.

- Victim blaming, evident in covert or overt beliefs that all people are accountable for their own situations and responsible for solutions, interferes with health care delivery for vulnerable populations and is evidence of sexism, classism, or racism.

- Advocacy and caring, which are ways to avoid delivering health care that is grounded in sexism, classism, and racism, require letting go of the power relationships that often dominate health care delivery.

- Clearing speech patterns and other behaviors of words and actions that are based on violence is a step toward therapeutic interventions with those who experience violence in their lives.

- Findings from research studies may not be applicable to vulnerable populations if the vulnerable are not part of the study population.

DISCUSSION QUESTIONS AND ACTIVITIES

1. Visit a homeless shelter or shelter for abused women. Interview residents about their health and ability to access health care.

2. Spend a few afternoons volunteering in a soup kitchen. Talk with people who come in for free meals about their health problems and ability to secure health care.

3. Spend some time with a home health nurse or Meals-on-Wheels making contact with the elderly who live at home alone. Explore with them their perceptions of quality of life, health dilemmas, and needs.

4. Work with classmates to develop a "health fair" for the homeless, discussing the value of typical activities and materials made available at traditional fairs, while designing a more relevant approach.

5. How many examples of toys, advertisements, acting roles, literature, childrearing practices, and the like can you identify that continue to perpetuate the woman's role as one of caregiver or sexual object? Discuss how the examples contribute to gender inequity for women.

REFERENCES

American Medical Association. (1992). *Diagnostic and treatment guidelines on domestic violence.* Chicago: Author.

Arcangelo, V. (1994). Should age be a criteria for rationing health care? *Nursing Forum, 29,* 25–29.

Auden, W. H. (1986). In memory of W. B. Yeats. In C. Bain, J. Beaty, & J. P. Hunter (Eds.), *The Norton introduction to literature* (4th ed.) New York: Norton.

Bohn, D. K. (1990). Domestic violence and pregnancy: Implications for practice. *Journal of Nurse Midwifery, 35,* 86–98.

Bowdler, J. E. (1989). Health problems of the homeless in America. *Nurse Practitioner, 14*(7), 44–51.

Brown, L. S. (1991). Antiracism as an ethical imperative: An example from feminist therapy. *Ethics and Behavior, 1,* 113–127.

Burg, M. A. (1994). Health problems of sheltered homeless women and their dependent children. *Health and Social Work, 19,* 125–131.

Butler, S. S., & Weatherley, R. A. (1992). Poor women at midlife and categories of neglect. *Social Work, 37,* 510–515.

Campbell, D. W. (1993). Nursing care of African-American battered women: Afrocentric perspectives. *AWHONNS Clinical Issues in Perinatal and Women's Health Nursing, 4,* 407–415.

Campbell, J. C., Pliska, M. J., Taylor, W., & Sheridan, D. (1994). Battered women's experiences in the emergency department. *Journal of Emergency Nursing, 20,* 280–288.

Catley, C. M. (1992). Global considerations affecting the health agenda of the 1990s, *Academic Medicine, 67,* 419–424.

Council on Ethical and Judicial Affairs, American Medical Association. (1992). Physicians and domestic violence. *Journal of the American Medical Association, 267,* 3190–3193.

Danziger, S. (1988). The economy, public policy, and the poor. In H. R. Rodgers (Ed.), *Beyond welfare* (pp. 3–13). Armonk, NY: M.E. Sharpe.

Davis, L. A., & Winkleby, M. A. (1993). Socio-demographic and health related risk factors among African-American, Caucasian, and Hispanic homeless men: A comparative study. *Journal of Social Distress and the Homeless, 2,* 83–101.

Demi, A. S., & Warren, N. A. (1995). Issues in conducting research with vulnerable families. *Western Journal of Nursing Research, 17,* 188–202.

Diehm, C., & Ross, M. (1988). Battered women. In S. Rix (Ed.), *The American woman, 1988–1989* (pp. 292–302). New York: Norton.

Eisler, R. (1987). *The chalice and the blade.* San Francisco: Harper & Row.

Esposito, C. N. (1993). Abuse: Breaking the cycle of violence: The victim's perspective. *Trends in Health Care, Law, and Ethics, 8,* 7–11.

Ewing, W. A. (1987). Domestic violence and community health care ethics: Reflections on systemic intervention. *Family and Community Health, 10,* 54–62.

Fishwick, N. (1995). Getting to the heart of the matter: Nursing assessment and intervention with battered women in psychiatric mental health settings. *Journal of the American Psychiatric Nurses Association, 1,* 48–54.

Fowler, B. A., & Risner, P. B. (1994). A health promotion program evaluation in a minority industry. *ABNF Journal, 5,* 72–76.

Funkhouser, S. W., & Moser, D. K. (1990). Is health care racist? *Advances in Nursing Science, 12,* 47–55.

Gilligan, C. (1982). *In a different voice.* Cambridge, MA: Harvard University Press.

Goodman, L. A. (1991). The prevalence of abuse among homeless and housed poor mothers: A comparison study. *American Journal of Ortho Psychiatry, 61,* 489–500.

Hall, C. (1993). Long term care and the minority elderly. *Pride Institute Journal of Long Term Health Care, 12,* 3–8.

Hogue, C. J. R., & Hargroves, M. A. (1993). Class, race and infant mortality in the United States. *American Journal of Public Health, 83,* 20–33.

Johnson, P. A. (1990). A national health insurance program: A national perspective. *Nursing and Health Care, 11,* 416–418, 427–429.

Kanna, M., Singh, N., Nemil, M., & Best, A. (1992). Homeless women and their families: Characteristics, life circumstances, and needs. *Journal of Child and Family Studies, 1,* 155–165.

Kutza, E. A., & Keigher, S. M. (1991). The elderly "new homeless": An emerging population at risk. *Social Work, 36,* 288–293.

Limandri, B. J., & Tilden, V. P. (1993). Domestic violence: Ethical issues in the health care system. *AWHONNS Clinical Issues in Perinatal and Women's Health Nursing, 4,* 493–502.

Melville, M. B. (1988). Hispanics: Race, class, or ethnicity? *The Journal of Ethnic Studies, 16*(1), 67–83.

Mondragon, D. (1993). No more "Let them eat admonitions": The Clinton administration's emerging approach to minority health. *Journal of Health Care for the Poor and Underserved, 4,* 77–82.

National Association of Children's Hospitals and Related Institutions. (1989). *Assuring children's access to health care: Fixing the Medicaid safety net.* Alexandria, VA: Author.

Price, J. H., Desmond, S. M., & Eoff, T. A. (1989). Nurses' perceptions regarding health care and the poor. *Psychological Reports, 65,* 1043–1052.

Rosenbaum, S. (1992). Child health and poor children: Special issue. The impact of poverty on children. *American Behavioral Scientist, 35,* 275–289.

Sines, D. (1994). The arrogance of power. A reflection on contemporary mental health nursing practice. *Journal of Advanced Nursing, 20,* 894–903.

Skaff, M. M., & Pearlin, L. J. (1992). Caregiving: Role engulfment and the loss of self. *Gerontologist, 32,* 656–664.

Spigner, C. (1994). Black participation in health research: A functionalist overview. *Journal of Health Education, 25,* 210–214.

Stark, P. L. (1991). Health care under seige: Challenge for change. *Nursing and Health Care, 12,* 26–30.

Tebb, S. (1995). An aid to empowerment: A caregiver well being scale. *Health and Social Work, 20,* 87–92.

United States Department of Commerce. (1990). *Statistical abstract of the United States, 1989* (109th ed). Washington, DC: U.S. Government Printing Office.

Vasquez, M. J. T., & Eldridge, N. S. (1994). Bringing ethics alive: Training practitioners about gender, ethnicity, and sexual orientation issues. *Women & Therapy, 15,* 1–6.

Wessell, M. L. (1992). Said another way: An ethical issue for a profession for all seasons. *Nursing Forum, 27,* 29–33.

Windom, E. (1988). An aging nation presents new challenges to the health care system. *Public Health Reports, 103,* 1–2.

CHAPTER 17

Gender Issues

By Sandra L. Cotton

The women must learn to dare to speak,
The men must learn to bother to listen.
The women must learn to say I think this is so.
The men must learn to stop dancing solos on the
  ceiling.

(Marge Piercy, 1982)

OBJECTIVES

After completing this chapter, the reader should be able to:

1. Describe historical bases of gender issues in nursing.
2. Discuss the relationship between issues of gender and race.
3. Describe factors associated with and the impact of sex discrimination in nursing.
4. Discuss sexual harassment within a nursing context.
5. Discuss communication issues related to gender.
6. Describe nursing issues related to modern sexism.

INTRODUCTION

In a perfect world people would consistently relate to each other with mutual respect and empathy. Unfortunately, the reality of our lives is that our interactions are sometimes clouded by prejudice or lack of understanding. The workplace is a common arena for many societal issues to manifest. Issues such as pay equity, employment opportunities, sexual harassment, role strain, and race relations are but a few examples of gender influenced conflicts that may be encountered in professional relationships. There are two basic approaches to dealing with these social justice issues. One can simply pretend that these issues do not exist. This approach may result in increased frustration as unresolved feelings and issues play out on the job. Alternatively, one can become aware of the issues and define ways to deal with the realities of our society head-on. This chapter focuses on the latter approach and explores issues concerning gender in the nursing workplace.

HISTORICAL PERSPECTIVES AND OVERVIEW OF GENDER BASED ISSUES

The American Nurses Association (ANA) expanded its definition of nursing from "the diagnosis and treatment of human responses to actual or potential health problems" to include the "application of scientific knowledge, integration of objective data, inclusion of the full range of human experiences, and provision of a caring relationship that facilitates health and healing" (ANA, 1995, p. 6). While some authors contend that most have come to accept the term *nurse* as "a person who cares for or tends to the needs of the sick" (Ellis and Hartley, 1995, p. 6), controversy remains concerning exactly what a person who provides nursing care should be called and how this relates to the gender of the person providing the care (Bernardi, 1996).

In her comprehensive work, *Woman as Healer*, Achterberg (1990) chronicles the journey of women in healing professions. Citing the masculinization of American medicine as one of many issues that challenge nurses, Achterberg states that although nursing has gained professional status, it suffers because of issues of "nurses' functioning subordinate to multiple layers of authority" (p. 177).

Lewenson (1996) notes that nurses have constantly had to struggle with paternalistic ideology that continues to permeate the profession. **Paternalism** has been defined as "the system, principle, or practice of managing or governing individuals, businesses, or nations, etc. . . . in the manner of a father dealing benevolently and often intrusively with his children" (*Webster's*, 1995). Lewenson (1996) contends that paternalism coupled with **nursism,** "a form of sexism that specifically maligns the caring role in society [has led to] discrimination in nursing by virtue of the role undertaken, regardless of gender" (pp. 226, 228).

Societal Expectations

As nursing continues to be a predominantly female profession, societal issues that have affected women have also been reflected in nursing. In a turn of the century commentary entitled *The Hospital Hotel*, nurses were noted for being "well-bred, well-educated specimens of womanhood" (JAMA, 1996, p. 324). Women have been socialized to achieve or be less than they are capable of becoming. This reluctance to achieve is evident in the lack of women in positions of power, especially in the political arena (Hamilton, 1996). Although more recent societal influences have had a positive impact in this regard, nursing is still a female dominated profession, which unfortunately has a history of oppression that many believe it has yet to overcome.

Ask Yourself

Is There Gender Stereotyping in Nursing?

Based upon recent survey data, a growing number of Americans would approve of nursing as a career choice for their sons (Begany, 1994). Of those opposed to having their sons in nursing, "a nurse should be a woman" was cited as the most frequent response for opposition to the profession.

- In what ways do you think nurses can help dispel this declining but continuing stereotype?

- How would you respond if your son or daughter chose nursing as a profession? Would you encourage him or her? Why or why not?

Authors such as Achterberg (1990), Baldwin (1995), Kavanagh (1996), Lewenson (1996), and Stromberg (1988) believe that nurses have been forced to work within a framework that focuses on societal expectations of women and what is considered women's work. In what has been termed the *medicalization* of American society, nursing has been forced to overcome the prejudices of a society that has historically embraced the biomedical curative model of health care. As diversified consumers of health care are demanding more sophisticated and culturally congruent care, nurses are in a prime position to provide cost-effective, high quality care. If nursing is to be successful in this and other arenas, it must concomitantly address issues of territoriality, power, and authority within its own ranks as well as with other health care professionals. A model of interdependence that seeks to create a positive situation for all providers and consumers of care may be most desirable (Baldwin, 1995).

GENDER AND RACE

Issues concerning race are closely linked to gender as they relate to access to educational preparation, employment opportunities, and wage inequities (Amott & Matthaei, 1991; Kavanagh, 1996; Lewenson, 1996). Amott and Matthaei additionally discuss class as it relates to gender and race in their extensive review of *A Multicultural Economic History of Women in the United States*. Based on their conceptual framework that race, gender, and class are intrinsically interconnected, Amott and Matthaei believe that the explanatory power of each concept, in itself, is limited, but together may broaden our understanding of the lives of women who enter nursing. As noted by Achterberg

(1990), Amott and Matthaei concur that the "development of the nursing profession coincided with the takeover of medicine by white men, who forced midwives and other women healers out of health care" (p. 121).

An increasing number of persons from diverse racial and ethnic backgrounds are joining the nursing profession (National League of Nursing [NLN], 1995). A rich history of the African-American nurse experience in the United States is depicted by Lewenson (1996) as she describes the establishment of educational programs for African-American nurses in the late 1800s and the forty-three-year history of the National Association of Colored Graduate Nurses (NACGN) (1908–1951). The NACGN eventually integrated with the American Nurses Association (ANA) because the ANA did not discriminate as many state organizations did when African-American nurses tried to join.

Racism, the assumption that members of one race are superior to those of another (Kavanagh, 1996) was an everyday experience for African-American nurses at the turn of the century. Despite Title VII of the Civil Rights Act of 1964, some African-Americans continue to experience racism today (Malveaux, 1987; 1988). African-American nurses are disproportionately employed in institutions that serve African-Americans and in public as opposed to private organizations (Stromberg, 1988). Discussion related to transcultural nursing is raising the awareness of nurses working with culturally diverse populations and will potentially improve patient outcomes. Foolchand (1995) notes that research efforts need to "move beyond the view that it is sufficient to understand Black people's cultural practices in order to improve service delivery" (p. 104). Foolchand expresses the caution of another educator that too much emphasis placed upon culture may divert "attention away from the central issue of racism in professional institutions and training" (p. 102). Strategies Foolchand identifies for improving racial equality in the nursing profession include incorporating race equality issues in school of nursing curriculums, educating staff in equal opportunities and antiracist strategies, and the recruitment, selection, and career progression of African-American faculty. If nursing is a reflection of society at large, issues related to racial inequalities within the broader context of society must also be examined.

SEX DISCRIMINATION IN NURSING

Historically, women have worked for lower pay than their male counterparts (Reskin & Padavic, 1994). Although pay equity is generally protected by state laws, issues of comparable worth, which have long been associated with traditionally female dominated professions such as nursing, a profession that requires a high level of "education, skill, and responsibility and yet has low salaries" (Ellis & Hartley, 1995, p. 403), have not had the same protection. It has been suspected that men in nursing are raising salaries; however, other economic considerations, such as nursing shortages, fair labor related legislation, and collective bargaining, may be responsible (Ellis & Hartley, 1995). Although a disparity in earnings known as a *pay gap* exists between men and women of many occupations, the gap is considerably narrower for nurses (Reskin & Padavic, 1994). When compared to other occupations, the fact that nurses have historically earned less may account for this lack of difference (Stromberg, 1988). However, the fact that a gap exists at all is striking in that men make up only six percent of the nursing profession (Benokraitis & Feagin, 1995). As Gilloran (1995) notes, the development of a patriarchal structure within nursing, with fewer women in senior management positions, may account for this.

According to sociologist Christine Williams (1995), issues of comparable worth are a real concern for nurses. Williams identifies several hidden advantages to being a man in nursing, particularly related to hiring and promotion. Williams's work supports Gilloran's (1995) assertions of gender disequity as men are typically *tracked* into higher paying and more prestigious positions. Even in a predominantly female profession, women may be experiencing a form of economic gender discrimination.

Gender Issues in Women's Health

Although men may have hidden advantages in nursing, some areas, primarily in women's health, have remained closed (Ketter, 1994). California bans prices based upon gender, for example, for services such as haircuts, dry cleaning, or tailoring ("California Bans Prices," 1995), but exempts labor and delivery rooms from state job discrimination laws by upholding a hospital's ban on employing nurses who are men in these areas (Letizia, 1994). California's Fair Employment and Housing Commission cited "invasion of a woman's privacy" as justification for the exemption, but one nurse called it "the most outlandish ruling" she had ever encountered (Thompson, 1995, p. 9).

In court proceedings that addressed this issue, the fact that most obstetricians are male was not deemed analogous to the situation of the nurse who is male (Ketter, 1994). Most courts cited that the doctor was chosen by the patient, while the nurse was not. Several state courts addressed this aspect of gender discrimination; however, none sided with the nurse. Section 703(e)(1) of the Civil Rights Act allows for gender based discrimination if gender "is a bona fide occupational qualification reasonably necessary to the normal operation of that particular business or enterprise" (Ketter, p. 24). Many men in nursing believe this form of discrimination is reinforced in educational settings when faculty members seek the permission for male student nurses to observe or participate in procedures with female patients but do not seek the permission of male patients when female students are involved. It is postulated that women are more universally accepted by patients because they are viewed as nurturers (Ellis & Hartley, 1995). Although no data support these assumptions, institutions continue to promote this form of gender discrimination when they proactively provide for the modesty and privacy of their female patients. Some nurses agree with this position. Others do not (Spancraft, 1995; Thompson, 1995).

Expanding Numbers of Men in the Profession

Although the number of men in nursing has steadily increased, men still comprise a relatively small number of all practicing RNs (NLN, 1995). Citing societal stereotyping as one of the major limiting factors for men in nursing, Squires (1995) may be categorizing men further when he asserts that health care reform that increases responsibility and autonomy will attract more men to the nursing profession. Perhaps what Williams (1995) perceives as hidden advantages for men in nursing adds some credence to

Squires's assertions. Despite these and other stereotypes, Squires considers the lure of nursing to be universal regardless of gender. Noting the challenge, variety, and excitement of nursing, Squires is quick to acknowledge that the road men in nursing have traveled thus far has not been without controversy. One professional organization formed in 1974, the American Assembly for Men in Nursing (AAMN), addresses these issues with a goal to "encourage men to become nurses, support those men already in nursing, and educate society as to the benefits of male nurses" (AAMN, 1996).

Gender and Caring

Men now comprise over twelve percent of students entering schools of nursing (NLN, 1995). Nursing graduate degree programs also report a steady increase in the number of male students entering their programs (NLN). As the number of men in nursing increases, research directed toward gender related issues in the profession has begun to emerge (Gilloran, 1995; Paterson, Crawford, Saydak, Venkatesh, Tschikota, & Aronowitz, 1995). For example, many authors have focused nursing research on caring as it relates to gender. Although much of this work is in its infancy, research questions related to possible differences in the learning or expression of caring as it relates to the gender of the student, educator, or recipient of care demonstrate the attention these and other issues in nursing has commanded. Recognition of the need to explore gender became evident for Peter and Gallop (1994) in their comparative study designed to examine whether caring uniquely reflected the moral orientation of nursing students. They discovered that differences in caring noted between medical and nursing students appeared to be related to gender differences. Further research including nursing students who are male is needed to support their findings, as their sample did not include this group.

Ironically, a gender bias may already exist in the literature that focuses on caring. Reverby (1987) offers an historical perspective of caring as it relates to women but does not address any possible implications in relation to the addition of men to the profession. Chinn (1991) devoted an entire anthology to caring but did not explore gender in relation to caring, except as it related to economic gains (or lack thereof) for male faculty members in male dominated academic centers. The exclusion of men by Grigsby and Megel (1995) as they explored the caring experiences of nursing faculty is another example of current nursing research that does not include men.

Despite an increased interest in the caring aspect of nursing, Begany (1994) perpetuates a nursing stereotype by equating the positive attribute of caring to images of nurturer or handmaiden. Some men in nursing may already experience a form of gender discrimination with regard to the stereotypical belief that all men in nursing are homosexuals. This stereotype is rooted in gender based role assumptions, such as Begany's, related to the caring attributes that many perceive as feminine. Because nursing has historically been viewed as "woman's work," men in nursing have been categorized as feminine and have subsequently been labeled as homosexuals. Even though Williams (1995) found there were hidden advantages in nursing for men, she also discovered that, ironically, these "opportunities . . . may extend only to those who exhibit conventional masculine characteristics, including a heterosexual orientation" (p. 65).

Do Men and Women Express Caring in Different Ways?

- What do you think of Begany's (1994) images of caring? What does caring mean to you?

- Williams (1995) believes that organizations are gender biased in how they regard *masculine* behaviors versus *feminine* ones. She suggests the development of gender sensitive evaluation tools that would acknowledge women's contributions to the profession. If you were appointed to develop such an evaluation tool, what attributes would your tool reward and recognize as unique to women? What justice issues may be involved in using gender-sensitive evaluation processes?

- Goals of the American Assembly for Men in Nursing include supporting men already in nursing and educating society about the benefits of male nurses. What do you think are the benefits of nurses who are men? How do these differ from the benefits of nurses who are women?

As more men enter the profession, additional gender issues may be identified. For example, once in the workforce, men in nursing may experience difficulty when cross-gender mentoring relationships exist (Feist-Price, 1994). Feist-Price notes several potential adversities in cross-gender mentoring relationships, mainly related to communication differences among men and women (Tannen, 1990). Feist-Price further notes that cross-gender mentoring relationships have successful outcomes, especially when formal mechanisms are in place to deal with issues as they arise. One implication for nursing may be in the area of caring. If differences in the development or expression of caring in male nurses indeed exist, these and other differences need to be recognized and utilized to improve the practice of nursing.

SEXUAL HARASSMENT IN NURSING

Bullough (1990) describes Florence Nightingale's encounters with harassment and the prevailing strategy of the day "to gain respect" through being a lady (Nightingale, 1859). Bullough contends that sexual harassment has been a dominant theme in American nursing. The Equal Employment Opportunity Commission (EEOC) has defined **sexual harassment** as "all unwelcome sexual advances, request for sexual favors, and other conduct of a sexual nature when (1) submission to such conduct is made a condition of a woman's employment or academic advancement; (2) submission to or rejection of such conduct by a woman is used as a basis for employment decisions or academic decisions affecting the individual; or (3) such conduct has the purpose or effect of unreasonably interfering with a woman's work or academic performance or creating an intimidating work environment" (Benokraitis & Feagin, 1995, p. 73). Bullough suggests that nurses need to employ specific strategies to combat sexual harassment. The National Organization for Women (NOW) recommends being assertive, seeking support from other workers, keeping a diary to document each incident, filing a complaint or grievance, keeping performance documents, seeking counseling, initiating legal action, and seeking a new job as strategies to deal with sexual harassment on the job (NOW, 1993).

Ask Yourself

Women's Rights

The National Organization for Women (NOW) is the largest women's rights organization in the country, actively working to achieve full and meaningful equality for all women.

- How do issues of women's rights relate to nursing?
- What issues remain for women in the nursing profession?
- How do these issues differ from issues that may impact men in the nursing profession?

One does not need to venture far to find images that reinforce the view that nurses are sexual objects. A quick tour of the *get well* section at your local greeting card shop graphically illustrates this point. Although sexual harassment does not recognize gender boundaries, clearly sexual harassment has historically been the bane of women. As more men enter the nursing profession, issues concerning sexual harassment directed toward them or from them may emerge. Research is needed that is directed toward understanding issues concerning sexual harassment in nursing, how best to address the needs of men in nursing, and implications for the women with whom they work.

COMMUNICATION ISSUES RELATED TO GENDER

How nurses communicate with each other, their patients, and their colleagues has long been discussed in the nursing literature (Campbell-Heider & Hart, 1993; Sweet & Norman, 1995). With changing societal roles and expectations, it is important for nurses to address how these changes relate to the practice of nursing and what areas of research are needed to effect positive changes.

The Doctor-Nurse Game

A gender division of labor has been a significant factor in how nurses, who are primarily women, and physicians, who are primarily men, relate to each other in health care settings. Initially described as the *doctor-nurse game* (Stein, 1967), issues regarding communication with physicians remain an area of primary concern for many nurses (Anderson, Maloney, Oliver, Brown, & Hardy, 1996). Favorable patient outcomes have been positively associated with successful nurse-physician communication (Shortell, Zimmerman, Rousseau, Gillies, Wagner, Draper, Knaus, & Duffy, 1994; Zimmerman, Shortell, Rousseau, Duffy, Gillies, Knaus, Devers, Wagner, & Draper, 1993).

Many nurses still use less than straightforward methods to manage conflict among themselves or between nurses and physician colleagues (Valentine, 1995). Valentine indicates that staff nurses are most comfortable using avoidance, while nurse managers tend to use compromise as their primary method of conflict management. These methods may be reinforced by nursing educators who Valentine found also employed avoidance as their primary conflict management tool. According to Tannen (1990), the primary reason for these and other communication conflicts relates to identifying and understanding gender differences in communication. Previously linked to societal roles and expectations of women, the "doctor-nurse game" was re-examined by Stein, Watts, and Howell (1990). The authors found that a more humanistic public image of physicians and the increasing numbers of female physicians and male nurses have generally improved physician-nurse relations.

 Think About It

Do Men and Women Communicate Differently?

Tannen (1990) asserts that men and women communicate from such differing frames of reference that their communication could be considered a cultural clash of sorts.

- What has your experience been in this area?
- What communication concerns with fellow students, faculty, patients, or physicians have you experienced in your program of study?
- How would you rate the nurse-physician communication in your clinical agencies? Describe why.
- Describe potential gender based differences in communication.

With females comprising nearly fifty percent of students entering medicine and males comprising twelve percent of students entering nursing school, perhaps the patriarchal system of health care will shift. The implications this may have for nursing remain unknown. Several studies focus on the traditional nurse-doctor relationship. None to date have examined the interactions of nurses, male or female, with physicians who are female.

Communicating with Patients

Through informal dress and communications, nurses may in fact be sending powerful negative messages to their patients and medical colleagues (Campbell-Heider & Hart, 1993). The bedside manner of nurses is discussed by these authors who note that the tone of familiarity expressed by nurses who use their first names with patients may translate sociologically into persistent stereotypic themes and become a mechanism of social control. While superior nursing care may reduce these stereotypes, Campbell-Heider and Hart discuss the role of deliberative communications strategies, both verbal and nonverbal, in accelerating professional recognition.

Successful interpersonal communications with patients is recognized as a feature central to the practice of nursing. Registered nurses' communication practices are found to be lacking, though, in relation to sensitive issues and sexuality (Propst, 1996). Propst found that only half of the respondents in her sample of women's health nurses discussed issues concerning sexuality with their patients. It is important to note that even in a specialty practice area, such as women's health, nurses are not immune to communication issues when sensitive topics are involved.

Gossip

Another area of communication related to gender involves the use of gossip. Laing (1993) proposes that gossip, as viewed from a feminist perspective, plays an important role in the socialization process of nurses. Discussed as a legitimate form of communication, gossip has many purposes and serves many functions. In the context of nurses, Laing believes that gossip may be a critical variable when defined as a "healing form of communication derived from trust which only develops over time" (p. 40). Laing does not explore implications for men in nursing; she is quick to note that although gossip is primarily associated with women, both sexes engage in gossip, often about similar topics.

MODERN SEXISM

Even though women have made tremendous inroads in the workplace, Benokraitis and Feagin (1995) report that sex inequality is still a major problem. In fact it may be on the rise in some areas. **Sexism** is "the assumption that members of one sex are superior to those of the other" (Kavanagh, 1996, p. 296). In our predominantly male oriented health care system, issues concerning sexism may evidence themselves in power struggles for reimbursement as nurses take on advanced practice roles (Baldwin, 1995). Unfortunately, even within the nursing profession, issues of sexism related to men in nursing are present. An example of this is the male colleague who feels he has a hiring edge over women in nursing because he never needs to be off for maternity leave or stay home from work to care for sick children.

Ask Yourself

Are Male Nurses Perceived as More Competent?

Benokraitis and Feagin (1995) interviewed male nurses. The authors report that physicians view male nurses as more competent than their female counterparts. They also found that female nurses were often ignored whereas male nurses' opinions were valued.

- Have you observed this behavior in your clinical or classroom settings?
- How could you best deal with this form of modern sexism?

Heterosexism, "the assumption that everyone is or should be heterosexual, and that heterosexuality is superior and expectable" (Kavanagh, 1996, p. 296), as experienced by some men in nursing (Williams, 1995) and our clients (Stevens, 1995) is an additional area of concern. Van Ooijen and Charnock (1995) note that very little attention is given to addressing this and other gender issues within the nursing curriculum, despite the belief that developing an understanding of these issues may have a tremendous impact upon nursing care.

SEXUAL ORIENTATION

Lesbians and gay men may be the largest minority group in nursing. Though no one knows exactly how many of the nearly two million nurses in America are lesbian or gay, there are probably between one hundred thousand and two hundred thousand (Zurlinden, 1997). These nurses are likely to be practicing in every state and working in every hospital. Fearing sexual harassment and discrimination from coworkers, superiors, and bureaucratic systems, many remain reluctant to have their sexual orientation known.

Sexual harassment and bigotry is a fact of life for many lesbians and gay men. Twenty-five years after the birth of the modern gay rights movement, a poll in *Time* reveals that fifty-two percent of respondents consider same-gender relationships between consenting adults to be morally wrong (Henry, 1994). This culturally prevalent attitude can range from prejudice to homophobia. Prejudice that is operationalized on the institutional level leads to discrimination. More extreme forms of bigotry include harassment and physical violence. Zurlinden (1997) writes, "Unmasked, homophobia is really hatred, willful ignorance, mean-spiritedness, and narrow-mindedness. People suffering from homophobia do not run screaming in terror when they encounter a lesbian or gay man. Instead, they assume they are justified to be cruel; to discriminate in housing, employment, and education; and to pass laws to prevent gay men and lesbians from enjoying the civil liberties that other Americans take for granted" (p. 11).

Within institutions, bigotry can be insidious, damaging, and difficult to change. Some employers systematically discriminate against lesbians and gay men through hiring, promotion, and disciplinary practices. This may be the result of institutional policy (as in the military), discriminatory administrative practice, punitive supervisors, or discrimination by coworkers (Zurlinden, 1997). Discrimination may also take the form of absence of employment benefits available to heterosexuals. Though a few university hospitals have agreed to extend spousal benefits such as health insurance, life insurance, and maternity leave to same-gender couples, these are not available in most institutions.

There are also legal implications for nurses who are gay or lesbian. Nearly half of all states still have laws that forbid particular types of sexual relationships, including same-gender sex and sodomy. In some states lesbian and gay men may risk losing their nursing licenses. Being accused of a felony is enough to lead to suspension of a nurse's license in some states; conviction can lead to permanent loss of license (Zurlinden, 1997). Additionally, a number of state boards of nursing have provisions that require "good moral character" to retain a nursing license (National Council of State Boards of Nursing, 1992). This policy is potentially troublesome in that many consider same-gender relationships to be morally wrong.

Though discriminatory practices remain, most health care professions have publicly endorsed a nonjudgmental attitude toward sexual orientation. The American Nurses Association (ANA), American Psychiatric Association, American Psychological Association, National Association of Social Workers, and the American Medical Association all include statements related to nonjudgmental recognition of sexual orientation (Zurlinden, 1997). Additionally, the ANA *Code for Nurses with Interpretive Statements* (1985) promotes the nondiscriminatory practice of nursing.

SUMMARY

Nursing has been faced with gender issues since the early days of the profession. Nursing role and status has been colored by societal expectations of women and paternalistic ideology permeating the health care arena. Considerations of gender can be related to lower salaries for nurses compared to primarily male professions, communication patterns with physicians and patients, perceptions of abilities to carry out nursing's caring imperative, and stereotypical expectations of how nurses should look and act. While men in the profession face the challenge of dealing with societal stereotypes, they are also often tracked into higher paying and more prestigious positions. Issues concerning discrimination based on sexual orientation occur on many fronts and may be underrecognized. Awareness of these issues enables nurses of both genders to be alert for inequities and to develop strategies for change.

CHAPTER HIGHLIGHTS

- Controversy exists regarding how the title of the person caring for the sick relates to the gender of the person providing care. Both women and men in nursing must deal with social stereotyping regarding expected roles and behaviors.

- Societal expectations of women and paternalistic ideology throughout history have led to discrimination in nursing, though gender discrimination may exist for both women and men in different nursing settings.

- Issues concerning race and gender are closely related and must be addressed in nursing.

- Issues of comparable worth relative to gender are of concern in nursing, particularly in areas of salary and positions of prestige and responsibility.

- Nurses need to be alert to and employ strategies to combat sexual harassment.

- Gender based differences in styles and patterns of communication can affect all areas of nursing practice, requiring attentiveness to effective communication with patients and colleagues in order to foster better patient outcomes.

- Sexism, occurring in both subtle and overt ways, continues to be an issue in nursing; and harassment and discrimination based on sexual orientation may be under-recognized.

DISCUSSION QUESTIONS AND ACTIVITIES

1. One frequently cited political action strategy is to build coalitions with "powerful persons of like mind" (Hamilton, 1996). If nurses in your community are to become empowered, with whom would they build coalitions?

2. Considering Foolchand's (1995) strategies, in what ways does your school or curriculum address issues of improving racial equality in the nursing profession?

3. Patterson et al. (1995) discuss ways in which nursing students who are males learn to care. Read an article on how nursing students learn to care. Do men learn about or express caring differently than women? How does this relate to your experiences as a student nurse? How does this relate to Begany's (1994) images of nurturer or handmaiden?

4. What stereotypes of nurses are present in your community or national media? What types of *get well* cards are in your local card shop? What do you think it will take to change these and other stereotypes about nurses?

5. What is the gender makeup of your local nursing administration? How many women are in positions of authority or power within your health care setting? What are their salary ranges? How do their salaries compare with men in positions of similar responsibility?

6. Observe gender based communication patterns between nurses and physicians. Consider your own style of communication with same gender and other gender friends and colleagues. What patterns do you identify? How might these patterns affect your professional interactions? Are there areas that need to be modified in order to promote more effective communication?

REFERENCES

Achterberg, J. (1990). *Woman as healer.* Boston, MA: Shambhala.

American Assembly for Men in Nursing. (1996). *Membership* [Brochure]. Pensacola, FL: Author.

American Nurses Association. (1985). *Code for nurses with interpretive statements.* Washington, DC: Author.

American Nurses Association (1995). *Nursing's social policy statement* [Brochure]. Washington, DC: Author.

Amott, T., & Matthaei, J. (1991). *Race, gender, and work; A multicultural economic history of women in the United States.* Boston: South End Press.

Anderson, F., Maloney, J., Oliver, D., Brown, D., & Hardy, M. (1996). Nurse-physician communi-cation: Perceptions of nurses at an army medical center. *Military Medicine, 161,* 411–415.

Baldwin, D. (1995). Territoriality and power in the health professions. In Final report of the Council on Graduate Medical Education, National Advisory Council on Nurse Education and Practice, *Report on primary care workforce projections* (pp. 1–36). Washington, DC: U.S. Department of Health and Human Services.

Begany, T. (1994). Your image is brighter than ever. *RN, 57,* 28–35.

Benokraitis, N. V., & Feagin, J. R. (1995). *Modern sexism: Blatant, subtle, and covert discrimina-tion* (2nd ed.). Englewood Cliffs, NJ: Prentice-Hall.

Bernardi, A. (1996, Winter). Untitled. [Letter to the editor]. *Interaction, Newsletter of the American Assembly for Men in Nursing,* p. 3.

Bullough, V. (1990). Nightingale, nursing, and harassment. *Image, 22,* 4–7.

California bans prices based on gender. (1995, October 14). *The Dominion Post,* p. A2.

Campbell-Heider, N., & Hart, C. (1993). Updating the nurse's bedside manner. *Image, 25,* 133–139.

Chinn, P. L. (1991). *Anthology on caring.* New York: National League of Nursing Press.

Ellis, J., & Hartley, C. (1995). *Nursing in today's world* (5th ed.). Philadelphia, PA: Lippincott.

Feist-Price, S. (1994). Cross-gender mentoring relationships: Critical issues. *Journal of Rehabilitation, 60,* 13–17.

Foolchand, M. (1995). Promoting racial equality in the nursing curriculum. *Nurse Education Today, 15,* 101–105.

Gilloran, A. (1995). Gender differences in care delivery and supervisory relationship: The case of psychogeriatric nursing. *Journal of Advanced Nursing, 21,* 652–658.

Grigsby, K., & Megel, M. (1995). Caring experiences of nurse educators. *Journal of Nursing Education, 34,* 411–418.

Hamilton, P. (1996). *Realities of contemporary nursing.* Menlo Park, CA: Addison-Wesley.

Henry, W. (1994, June 17). Pride and prejudice. *Time, 143*(26), 57–59.

JAMA (1996). The hospital hotel. *Journal of the American Medical Association, 275,* 324.

Kavanagh, K. (1996). Social and cultural dimensions of health and health care. In J. Creasia & B. Parker (Eds.), *Conceptual foundations of nursing practice* (pp. 285–308). St. Louis, MO: Mosby.

Ketter, J. (1994, April). Sex discrimination targets men in some hospitals. *The American Nurse, 26,* 1, 24.

Laing, M. (1993). Gossip: Does it play a role in the socialization of nurses? *Image, 25,* 37–43.

Letizia, B. (1994, December). Ban on male nurses in labor and delivery is upheld. *RN, 57,* 16.

Lewenson. (1996). *Taking charge: Nursing suffrage & feminism in America, 1873–1920.* New York: National League of Nursing Press.

Malveaux, J. (1987). Are black women taking jobs from others? *Essence, 18*(11), 116.

Malveaux, J. (1988). When poverty hits home. *Essence, 19*(11), 118.

National Council of State Boards of Nursing. (1992). *Profiles of member board: 1992.* Chicago: Author.

National League of Nursing (1995). *1995 Nursing data review; NLN division of research*. New York: Author.

National Organization for Women. (1993). *Sexual harassment survival skills* [Brochure]. Morgantown, WV: Author.

Nightingale, F. (1859). *Notes on nursing: What it is, and what it is not*. London: Harrison & Sons.

Paterson, B., Crawford, M., Saydak, M., Venkatesh, P., Tschikota, S., & Aronowitz, T. (1995). How male nursing students learn to care. *Journal of Advanced Nursing, 22,* 600–609.

Peter, E., & Gallop, R. (1994). The ethic of care: A comparison of nursing and medical students. *Image, 26,* 47–51.

Piercy, M. (1982). Councils. *Circles on the water.* New York: Knopf.

Propst, M. (1996). Registered nurses' practice and perspective toward sexuality in women's health. *Southern Nursing Research Society Abstracts,* 83.

Reskin, B., & Padavic, I. (1994). *Women and men at work.* Thousand Oaks, CA: Pine Forge Press.

Reverby, S. (1987). A caring dilemma: Womanhood and nursing in historical perspective. *Nursing Research, 36,* 5–10.

Shortell, S., Zimmerman, J., Rousseau, D., Gillies, R., Wagner, D., Draper, E., Knaus, W., & Duffy, J. (1994). The performance of intensive care units: Does good management make a difference? *Medical Care, 32,* 508–525.

Spancraft, E. (1995, February). Banning male RNs from L & D is blatantly unfair [Letter to the editor]. *RN, 58,* 9.

Squires, T. (1995). Men in nursing. *RN, 58,* 26–28.

Stein, L. (1967). The nurse-doctor game. *Archives of General Psychiatry, 16,* 699–703.

Stein, L., Watts, D., & Howell, T. (1990). The doctor-nurse game revisited. *New England Journal of Medicine, 322,* 546–549.

Stevens, P. (1995). Structural and interpersonal impact of heterosexual assumptions on lesbian health care clients. *Nursing Research, 44,* 25–30.

Stromberg, A. (1988). Women in female-dominated professions. In A. Stromberg & S. Harkess (Eds.), *Women working: Theories, and facts in perspective* (pp. 206–224). Mountain View, CA: Mayfield.

Sweet, S., & Norman, I. (1995). The nurse-doctor relationship: A selective literature review. *Journal of Advanced Nursing, 22,* 165–170.

Tannen, D. (1990). *You just don't understand: Women and men in conversation.* New York: Ballantine.

Thompson, J. (1995, February). Banning male RNs from L & D is blatantly unfair [Letter to the editor]. *RN, 58,* 9.

Valentine, P. (1995). Management of conflict: Do nurses/women handle it differently? *Journal of Advanced Nursing, 22,* 142–149.

van Ooijen, E., & Charnock, A. (1995). How men and women view the world: A sexual perspective. *Nursing Times, 91,* 38–39.

Webster's college dictionary (1995). New York: Random House.

Williams, C. (1995). Hidden advantages for men in nursing. *Nursing Administration Quarterly, 19,* 63–70.

Zimmerman, J., Shortell, S., Rousseau, D., Duffy, J., Gillies, R., Knaus, W., Devers, K., Wagner, D., & Draper, E. (1993). Improving intensive care: Observations based on organizational case studies in nine intensive care units. *Critical Care Medicine, 21,* 1443–1451.

Zurlinden, J. (1997). *Lesbian and gay nurses.* Albany, NY: Delmar.

CHAPTER 18

Transcultural and Spiritual Issues

Written in collaboration with Mary Gail Nagai-Jacobson

> *God is a spirit, a mystery beyond human understanding, and therefore we can only approach that mystery through metaphor. Our metaphors come, of course, from human and cultural understandings of the good, the loving, the just. . . . More surely than anything else, we are defined by our stories—the cultural myths we hear from our earliest days.*
>
> **(Sewell, 1991, pp. 237, 261)**

OBJECTIVES

At the end of this chapter, the reader should be able to:

1. Describe factors associated with cultural sensitivity within nursing.
2. Discuss the influence of culture on health and health care decisions.
3. Identify approaches for dealing with transcultural issues in nursing.
4. Discuss issues related to the use of complementary therapies by patients.
5. Identify legal considerations related to transcultural issues.
6. Discuss the relationship between spirituality and health.
7. Describe issues associated with spirituality and religion.
8. Identify the nursing role in addressing patients' spiritual concerns.
9. Discuss considerations regarding nurturing one's spirit.

INTRODUCTION

The influence of culture, religion, and spirituality are major factors in the development of values. Because nurses deal with people from varied cultural and spiritual backgrounds, it is important that they be alert for issues relating to these areas. This chapter presents general considerations regarding culture and spirituality and discusses related issues that may arise when caring for patients.

TRANSCULTURAL ISSUES

We live in a multicultural society, alive with diversity. Such diversity of people and backgrounds provides a richness to our lives, yet challenges our abilities to appreciate, rather than judge or fear, differences. **Diversity** is encountered wherever there are differences, whether these be gender, age, socioeconomic position, sexual orientation, health status, ethnicity, race, or culture (Kavanagh, 1993). Dealing with diversity is an essential component of nursing care. Nurses need competence in providing culturally appropriate care. **Cultural competence** (Waters, 1996) includes **cultural awareness**—knowledge about values, beliefs, behaviors, and the like of cultures other than one's own—and **cultural sensitivity**—the ability to incorporate the patient's cultural perspective into nursing assessments and to modify nursing care in order to be as congruent as possible with the patient's cultural perspective.

The same phenomenon may be viewed differently by people from different cultures because culture teaches us to understand a perception of reality. For example, the *man in the moon* that most people in this country have been taught to "see" is identified in other cultures as a *frog in the moon*, a *woman in the moon*, or a *rabbit in the moon* (Tafoya, 1996). Another way of appreciating different perspectives is to consider what one sees when one is in the valley compared to what is seen from halfway up the mountain or the view from the top of the mountain. Different perceptions of the same reality derive from the perspectives from which it is viewed. One view of reality is not more correct than the other; the different views merely come from different perspectives.

Ask Yourself

How Do You Deal with Diversity?

Consider a situation in which you were afraid of or judged someone you did not know because she or he was different from you.

- What about the person or situation triggered your judgment or fear?

- Why do you think you reacted to the person or situation the way you did?

- How and from whom did you learn to react in this way?

- What has helped you to understand diversity and overcome fear?

- How can nurses learn to appreciate rather than fear diversity among colleagues and patients?

Understanding Culture

Self-awareness is a key factor in dealing with transcultural issues. The best starting point for becoming sensitive to the culture of another is to understand one's own culture and its influence on one's perceptions and behaviors. **Culture** refers to the total lifeways of a group of interacting individuals, consisting of *learned* patterns of values, beliefs, behaviors, and customs shared by that group (Tripp-Reimer, 1987). These *learned patterns* are transmitted from one generation to the next in formal ways, such as through educational settings, and in informal ways, such as through role modeling. Unique cultural expressions can be observed within many groups of interacting individuals, for example, the culture of the deaf community, prison culture, or the culture of health care. It is important to recognize that we are each part of a culture and to identify values, beliefs, and behaviors that we hold dear, as these reflect our own cultural perspective. In this process we each must be alert to our own **ethnocentrism,** reflected in the tendency to judge behaviors of someone from another culture by the standards of one's own culture.

In its *Position Statement on Cultural Diversity in Nursing Practice*, the American Nurses Association (ANA) (1991) states that ethnocentric approaches to nursing practice are ineffective in meeting health and nursing needs of diverse cultural groups, and encourages nurses in all settings to be knowledgeable about cultures and their impact on interactions with health care. Nurses must develop cultural sensitivity, which implies understanding behaviors and values of another culture within the context of that culture, without imposing one's own cultural values on others. In this process it is important to avoid **stereotyping,** which is expecting all persons from a particular group to behave, think, or respond in a certain way based on preconceived ideas. Every culture contains variation, and some people within the group may not ascribe to all beliefs and values attributed to that culture.

Ask Yourself

How Might Ethnocentrism Affect Nursing Care?

Consider the varied meanings the following behaviors may have depending upon the cultural context in which they occur: direct eye contact may connote honesty or intrusion; a firm handshake may be viewed as confidence or hostility; and frequent bathing may be considered to be necessary or unhealthy.

- How might behaviors such as these be judged by people within the dominant culture in this country?

- How do practices and expectations within health care settings reflect ethnocentrism regarding behaviors such as these?

- How might ethnocentrism or stereotyping affect interaction with others, especially within a nursing setting?

Cultural Values and Beliefs

Because culture is one of the key organizing concepts of nursing, nurses need to be knowledgeable about:

> how cultural groups understand life processes; how cultural groups define health and illness; what cultural groups do to maintain wellness; what cultural groups believe to be the causes of illness; how healers cure and care for members of cultural groups; and how the cultural background of the nurse influences the way in which care is delivered. (ANA, 1991)

Cultural values and beliefs guide one's thinking, being, and doing in patterned ways. Beliefs about health and practices related to health and healing are some of the patterns influenced by culture that are significant in the provision of health care. Such beliefs and practices are evidenced in both direct and subtle ways, and sensitivity to them can affect patient outcomes and satisfaction with care. It is helpful to recognize a distinction between **disease,** which is the biomedical explanation of sickness, and **illness,** which is a personal response to the disease flowing from how one's culture teaches one to be sick (Burkhardt, 1985; Tafoya, 1996). Transcultural issues are often present in nursing situations but may not be identified as such. Instead, patients may be labeled as stoic, uncooperative, noncompliant, strange, or "crazy" because of choices they make; and their health and care may be compromised. Leininger (1991) has delineated principles of transcultural care, human rights, and ethical considerations that offer guidance for nurses in dealing with transcultural issues. Although she offers these principles as a guide particularly to transcultural nurses, they apply as well to other nurses. They are listed in Figure 18–1, Transcultural Care Principles, Human Rights, and Ethical Considerations. In light of these principles, many nursing practices derived from the Western biomedical model may benefit from reevaluation.

Figure 18–1 **Transcultural Care Principles, Human Rights, and Ethical Considerations**

1. Human beings of any culture in the world have a right to have their cultural care values known, respected and appropriately used in nursing and other health care services.
2. Human cultures have diverse and universal modes of caring and healing practices that need to be recognized and used by professional nurses to function effectively and therapeutically with people of different cultures.
3. Care is the essence of nursing and a basic human need for growth, healing, well-being, recovery, and survival.
4. Cultural care is a critical component influencing human health, well-being, and recovery from illnesses or disabilities.
5. Every culture has at least two major types of health care systems namely, the *folk (generic, lay or indigenous) care system* and the *professional care*

system which influences their health outcomes, and the transcultural nurse is challenged to use this knowledge to guide nursing care decisions and actions.

6. All professional nurses are challenged to respect common human needs and humanistic aspects of people care worldwide, and also the divergent care expressions, meaning, and practices.

7. Transcultural nurses are expected to respect Western and non-Western cultures who often have different values, beliefs, and norms to assess and understand human beings.

8. Transcultural nursing principles and practices are the arching framework for all nursing care practices which differ from nursing practices that rely on traditional medical symptoms, diseases and treatment regimes.

9. Since transcultural nursing focuses upon *comparative cultural care* values, beliefs and practices of cultures, the nurse is expected to work with individuals, families, groups, cultures, subcultures and institutions that reflect cultural care variabilities.

10. Nurses with transcultural knowledge are expected to respond appropriately to *culture care differences* and *similarities* in order to ease or ameliorate a human condition or lifeway, and to help clients face death.

11. Ethical and moral differences and similarities exist among human cultures which necessitates that nurses recognize, respect and respond appropriately to such variabilities.

12. It is essential that transcultural nurses be open-minded and willing to learn from cultural informants about their human values, beliefs, needs and practices in order to make appropriate nursing care plans, judgments and actions.

13. The ability of the nurse to listen, use silence and envision the client's or family's human condition or cultural circumstance with its positive or less positive features is important in transcultural nursing.

14. Transcultural nursing often requires that nurses communicate with clients in their native language to know, learn and understand individuals, families and groups of different cultures.

15. Transcultural nurses are challenged to identify what constitutes ethical or moral principles and norms of cultures and not assume that all cultures are alike.

16. Transcultural nurses are expected to guide other nurses who have not been prepared in transcultural nursing in order to prevent marked ethnocentrism, cultural imposition practices, and inappropriate ethical and moral judgments about clients.

17. Transcultural nursing reflects that an individual or group of a designated culture are active participants and decision-makers in culture care practices in order to develop and maintain creative and effective professional care practices.

18. Clients of diverse or similar cultures have a right to have their caring life styles and expressions known and used in transcultural nursing in order to promote client health or well-being.

19. Transcultural nursing takes into account the world view, environmental context, ethnohistory, social structure features (including the religious, kinship, philosophic, economic, political, technological and cultural values), language, expressions, gender and age difference of people.

20. Transcultural nursing is concerned with the assessment of caregiver and carereceiver expressions, beliefs and lifeways that often go beyond nurse-client dyadic relationship to that of care relationships with families, groups, institutions and communities in order to facilitate congruent care practices and to avoid unfavorable culture care conflicts, stress and negligent care practices.

21. Since ethical, moral and legal systems of human values, and rights exist in all cultures, it is the task and responsibility of transcultural nurses to discover these dimensions with key and general informants and in diverse cultural contexts.

22. Human care rights tend to be covert and embedded in social structure, cultural values and world view of clients, and so the transcultural nurse is challenged to discover these dimensions mainly through qualitative research methods.

23. Transcultural nurses recognize that cultures are complex, dynamic and change over time and in varying ways.

24. Transcultural nurses recognize that many cultures and subcultures in the world have not been studied and yet nurses are expected to care for all peoples including minorities.

25. Transcultural nursing is a major breakthrough for new nursing knowledge and practices that do not follow the traditional nursing or medical disease, symptom and illness models.

Leininger, M. (1991). *Journal of Transcultural Nursing, 3*, 21–23. Reprinted with permission of the *Journal of Transcultural Nursing*.

Incorporating cultural assessment into care with patients is an important part of a comprehensive nursing assessment and can facilitate better understanding of sometimes overlooked factors that influence health behaviors and decisions. Cultural assessment helps nurses to appropriately identify and understand the meaning of behaviors that might otherwise be judged negatively or be confusing to the nurse (Giger and Davidhizar, 1995). It is important to recognize that each person is culturally unique and that not all persons in a particular cultural group believe or respond the same way. The model for cultural assessment presented by Giger and Davidhizar includes exploration of six cultural phenomena that are evident in all cultural groups: communication, space, social organization, time, environmental control, and biological variation. Such exploration enables nurses to identify areas where modifications in care can be incorporated so that care is more culturally congruent. Although the process may also reveal divergent beliefs that are difficult to accommodate within the current health care system, acknowledging differences may help the patient and family to feel more comfortable within the system. For example, when assessing eating patterns and food preferences, the nurse might discover that the patient commonly eats only two meals a day consisting of burritos in the morning and rice and beans in the evening. Typical hospital food and a three-meals-a-day pattern might not be appetizing for this patient. The patient's nutrition may suffer, and she may perceive that she is not being fed. By arranging for the patient to have culturally similar foods at similar times, the nurse provides more culturally congruent care.

 CASE PRESENTATION

Cultural Differences

Brenda White is a home health nurse caring for seventy-two-year old Mrs. Cortez who is living with her daughter and family while recovering from a stroke. Part of the care involves working with the patient on coordination and strengthening exercises. Brenda has found Mrs. Cortez to be very cooperative and uncomplaining in doing the exercises under her direction, indicating that she would do what was needed to get well. One day Brenda's supervisor, Maria Lopez, tells her that the agency has received a complaint from Mrs. Cortez's family that Brenda is being too rough on the patient. Brenda responds that she does not understand this because Mrs. Cortez has never complained. Brenda further explains that she was trying to have the patient work to her maximum capability and to give her instructions in a clear and direct manner. Ms. Lopez says that in her culture elders are considered very precious and are treated with gentleness and respect. Perhaps the family perceived that Brenda's direct ways indicated disrespect for their mother, even though the patient did not indicate this.

 Think About It

How Can Nurses Develop Cultural Competence?

- How is cultural diversity evident in this situation?
- Where is there evidence of a lack of cultural competence?
- What might Brenda do to make her care more culturally sensitive?
- How do you think you would respond in a similar situation?
- How can nurses develop cultural competence?

Culture and the Health Care System

Transcultural issues arise when nurses, patients, and families hold differing views of what is important or necessary regarding health, recovery, illness, or the dying process. The contemporary health care system is not user-friendly when it comes to incorporating diversity. By virtue of its history, the system reflects predominantly middle-class, European American, Judeo-Christian, paternalistic values and perspectives (Kavanagh, 1993). This system includes the attitude that the health care provider knows what is "best for the patient," as viewed from the health provider's perspective.

The health provider's perspective generally derives from a combination of two cultural orientations. The primary cultural orientation is the biomedical model, and the secondary cultural orientation is the provider's personal cultural background. If the patient's perspective is different from this model and is not considered, dilemmas may emerge. Consider, for example, a situation in which the physician, who is schooled in the Western biomedical model, views death as "the enemy" to be overcome at all costs, while the patient, who comes from a Native American culture, views death as a part of life that one prepares for by being in harmony with one's surroundings. Medical or surgical interventions that may prolong the patient's life a few weeks, which would be very important in the physician's world view, may be very low on the list of considerations for the patient.

One must be aware that the health care system is a different culture from that of most of the patients served by the system. The language, values, norms, behaviors, rituals, and environment is generally unfamiliar to those who seek its services. Even people who belong to the same dominant culture in society as their health care providers are often strangers when they enter the institutions of the system. For those who do not belong to the dominant culture, negotiating the system can be a formidable task. Lack of understanding of language, procedures, expectations, and other elements of the culture can lead to miscommunication, unclear decisions, and a sense of powerlessness or lack of control. Ethical or legal dilemmas may arise due to misunderstandings. Consider again the case of Mrs. Cortez. Misunderstanding of the nurse's intent might lead the family to decide to terminate nursing care or bring legal action against the nurse because of their perception that their mother is being mistreated.

When one speaks of values such as autonomy, beneficence, justice, or the right to self-determination, it is important to ask from whose perspective these values are understood—that of the nurse or that of the patient. This same question is appropriate regarding definitions of health. Cultural assessment provides insight into the congruence, or lack thereof, between patients' and nurses' understandings of health. Consider, for example, a situation in which the nurse believes that health includes being able to be a productive member of society and that health problems provide opportunities for one to grow and become more self-actualized, while the patient believes that his work related injury is an act of *fate* and focuses on being free of pain and able to "get around." If the differing perceptions of health are not recognized and addressed, efforts to have the patient participate in rehabilitation and job retraining or to utilize nonpharmacological measures for pain control may meet with much resistance and patient dissatisfaction.

Complementary Therapies

Culture guides one's choice of when to go for health care, what kind of care to seek, to whom to go, and how long to participate in care. Many people who utilize conventional health care settings also utilize alternative or complementary therapies (Eisenberg, Kessler, Foster, Norlock, Calkins, & Delbanco, 1993). Such therapies may derive from traditions in the patient's own culture or may be borrowed from traditions of another culture. Complementary therapies include a wide variety of modalities, such as: relaxation techniques, healing touch and other energy based healing techniques, spiritual healing, biofeedback, nutritional practices, herbal treatments, massage and other body work, meditation, prayer, homeopathy, acupuncture, and biofeedback.

These therapies are often used concurrently with conventional therapies, but they may be chosen in lieu of conventional therapies. In order to have a broad picture of the many factors affecting a patient's health and healing, nurses need to be aware of various therapies being utilized by the patient. It is wise for nurses to incorporate discussion of complementary therapies into nursing assessment in an open way, since patients may be hesitant to bring up the subject. Nurses do not need to ascribe to such therapies in order to become knowledgeable about them. Complementary therapies often derive from paradigms that differ from, and may not make sense in, the conventional medical model, yet may be very useful in the healing process. Hufford (1996) suggests that the patient has the major responsibility for seeking information regarding alternative therapies and making health choices in this regard, but that health care providers need to have some knowledge about risks and benefits involved. When patients are interested in complementary therapies, it is important to determine whether there are risks associated with their use. If there are significant risks involved and the patient is committed to utilizing the therapy, nurses need to work with other health team members to minimize risks and maximize benefits. When there is not a strong commitment to the nonconventional modality, it is wise to encourage ongoing discussion of known risks and benefits related to various options (Hufford, 1996). When conventional health care providers can work with traditional systems and their healers, the overall care becomes more culturally congruent.

Think About It

How Should Nurses Deal with Complementary Therapies?

Conventional medicine and medical practitioners tend to be skeptical of healing modalities that have not been subjected to empirical scientific study; thus, discussion of nonconventional modalities is not included in lists of alternatives for patients, nor are these modalities available in most conventional health care settings.

- What do you think about this attitude toward complementary therapies?
- What experiences have you had with complementary therapies?

- How might attitudes toward complementary therapies affect the ability of nurses to provide culturally congruent care for their patients?
- What are the ethical implications related to limiting a patient's access to complementary therapies and practitioners when they are in conventional health care institutions?
- What is your view of complementary therapies within nursing practice?

Factors important for the healing process are often culturally prescribed. For example, the involvement of family in the care of a sick member may be very important in some cultures. It can be quite distressing for nursing staff on a hospital unit when multiple family members "camp out" in a patient's room or the nearby hallway, or bring food from home that is not on a patient's diet. Providing culturally congruent care in such situations may include relaxing visiting regulations and collaborating with the family regarding appropriate foods from home. If the needs of one patient are different from those of the roommate, dilemmas may arise that require diplomatic interventions by the nurse.

Legal Considerations Related to Transcultural Issues

Cultural misunderstandings can provide fertile ground for litigation. Communication—verbal, nonverbal, and written—is always of utmost importance. When a patient's first language is different from that of the nurse, it is essential to determine the extent of the patient's understanding of the nurse's language. When the patient uses another language (including sign language), having an interpreter fluent in the patient's language is essential. If the interpreter is a member of the patient's family, the translation may be filtered through the perspective of the family member. Consider, for example, an elderly Cambodian man who is in the hospital and not doing well. His grandson serves as interpreter. The grandson was born in this country and is embarrassed by his grandfather's "old" ways. When the man says that he needs a particular traditional herbal tea each afternoon in order to get well (which is available in a local ethnic store), the grandson translates this generically as "tea." Even though the nurse responds by making sure that the patient has tea each afternoon, the patient's needs are not met.

The language of explanation of procedures and consent forms presents other issues. Be sure that the patient or family member is able to read the language in which the form is written and that all terms used are understood. If the form needs to be interpreted for the patient, it is essential that the interpreter understands the procedure and that an appropriate person is available to clarify any areas of uncertainty. People may indicate that they understand when they do not in order to avoid offending the nurse or being considered ignorant. One way of dealing with this is having patients describe in their own words what they have been told.

ISSUES RELATED TO SPIRITUALITY AND RELIGION

Spirituality is a universal human experience that transcends culture, although it may be colored and shaped by cultural experiences. It is vital that nurses at all levels of practice are attentive to spirituality and recognize the individual as a body-mind-spirit being who experiences health concerns in all these dimensions. In the midst of advances in technology and scientific discoveries, which have increased our understanding of the nature of illness and disease, attunement to the role of spirituality in health and healing has diminished. Perhaps the limited scientific knowledge of former times made the role of the spirit and the intangible forces deriving from that spirit more apparent. Many persons were cared for in their homes, even in the case of serious illness. Touching, praying, and presence were a natural part of such environments. Historically, institutions such as hospitals were often staffed by religious orders concerned for both spiritual and physical needs.

Healing and health care has long been connected with the spirituality of a people. With indigenous peoples, healing rituals frequently are spiritual in nature. Although medicine's embrace of the Cartesian duality separating body and spirit allows little place for the spirit in health care, people seeking medical care continue to incorporate spiritual and religious rituals and practices into their care for self and others. It is noteworthy that the words health, holy, and whole all derive from the same old Saxon, *Hal*, and Greek, *Holos*, which mean whole. By their nature, then, health and healing are associated with that which is holy and whole. A question to ponder is whether contemporary health care culture, now vested in technology, managed care, mergers, and the like, can once again incorporate spirituality within its vision of healing.

Approaching Spirituality

By nature, humans are body-mind-spirit beings. The uniqueness of each person a nurse encounters encompasses the spiritual as well as physical, mental, and emotional manifestations of that person. **Spirituality** is the animating force, life principle, or essence of being that permeates life and is expressed and experienced in multifaceted connections with self, others, nature, and God or Life Force (Burkhardt, 1994; Burkhardt & Nagai-Jacobson, 1994). Meaning and purpose in life and life events flows from the spirit and is manifested in open or private ways. All persons are spiritual, whether they ascribe to a religious orientation or deny the existence of the Divine. Beliefs and values are molded and shaped by one's spirituality as well as by societal and cultural conditioning.

Nursing espouses a holistic, body-mind-spirit view of persons. With this understanding, that persons are indeed body-mind-spirit beings, intertwined and whole, nurses know that, as they respond from their own wholeness, they are always dealing with the spiritual manifestation of others. An ethical response to this awareness requires that an appreciation of spiritual aspects of care be part of all nursing interactions. Nurses must include behaviors that care for spiritual as well as physical and mental concerns.

Because spirituality is at once universal and often very personal and private, nurses may find this area difficult to approach. It is important, however, that nurses develop competence in addressing spiritual needs. Recognizing that spirituality is basic to health enables nurses to listen for language, observe behavior, and gather information related to spiritual concerns.

Spirituality assessment can provide nurses with information about how patients view life, death, health, and health concerns. Such assessment provides insight into important connections, beliefs, practices, or rituals that may influence a person's choices or affect healing. Processes that incorporate open-ended questions and allow patients to tell their stories are more effective than check-lists for spirituality assessment (Burkhardt & Nagai-Jacobson, 1994; 1997; Dossey, Keegan, Guzzetta, & Kolkmeier, 1995; Nagai-Jacobson & Burkhardt, 1996). Although expression of spiritual concerns may include talk of God or faith, patients communicate their spiritual needs and concerns in many other ways as well. They may express questions related to the meaning of present or past experiences, fears or worries about what is happening, or how they will find the strength they need. They may talk about important relationships, the need for reconciliation, experiences of peace or anxiety, or the desire to put their lives in order. Religious articles may be evident, or the nurse may observe the patient engaging in practices such as prayer or meditation. Effective spirituality assessment requires nurses to attend with their whole beings to indicators of spirituality occurring within routine interactions with patients. Opportunities to explore spirituality with patients present in many situations.

 Think About It

Recognizing Spiritual Concerns

Spiritual issues reflect core experiences that often defy explanation. Such experiences may relate to suffering, forgiveness, hope, love, or mystery. In the midst of care with patients, nurses often hear comments or questions or observe behaviors reflective of spiritual concerns. Consider the following examples:

A patient or family member says:

"I don't know why God is doing this to me (or her)."
"I should have locked the gate."
"Will you pray for me?"
"I don't know why, but having surgery worries me."
"I wish I had been willing to go to the beach when he wanted to."
"I think I need to trust God and not take chemotherapy. God wants me to trust Him completely."
"Without my income I don't know how my family will make it."
"We told him not to buy that motorcycle."
"Do you believe in miracles?"

Patients or family members may be observed:

Reading a sacred text.
Wearing religious jewelry or articles of clothing.
Praying or meditating.
Staring out a window with a worried or pensive expression.

• How are spiritual concerns reflected in these comments or behaviors?

- What personal beliefs or experiences might affect your feelings and responses to comments or behaviors such as these?

- Describe aspects of each comment or behavior that might raise questions or concerns for you.

- How would you respond to each of these comments or behaviors? In which circumstances would you feel more comfortable or less comfortable?

Spirituality and Religion

Although spirituality may be expressed through religious beliefs and practices, it is not synonymous with these terms. **Religion** is the codification of beliefs and practices concerning the Divine and one's relationship with the Divine that are shared by a group of people. Religion may be quite intertwined within a dominant culture, as with Judaism in Israel or Hinduism in India, or it may be counterculture, as with the Amish in the United States. Some religions, such as many Christian sects, include people from different cultures. Religious teachings generally include rules regarding right and wrong and guidelines for dealing with issues related to these areas. Because religious beliefs and teachings flow from a particular world view, rules and values can be quite variable among different religions. A minor consideration within one religion or sect may constitute a serious dilemma in another. Norms for proper dress for women is one example. For instance, although most Christian denominations have few, if any, restrictions regarding womens' dress, some Christian sects teach that women should wear only skirts or dresses and not use makeup nor cut their hair. Orthodox Muslims have very strict rules regarding how women are to dress in public.

What is considered right or wrong within a particular religion is not always congruent with ethical perspectives of the greater society. Consider, for example, an infant girl brought to a hospital in the United States with severely infected wounds from trauma to her labial area following a clitorectomy procedure performed by her father. From the perspective of the nurse and the institution, this might be viewed as severe mutilation, constituting abuse, whereas the family would consider this an important religious practice. Another example is the Jehovah Witness belief that blood transfusions are wrong, and the ensuing dilemma when a transfusion is medically indicated as a life saving measure.

Ask Yourself

How Does Spirituality Affect Your Nursing Practice?

- What religious or spiritual beliefs or practices are important to you?

- How has your spirituality or religious perspective been influential in your choice of nursing as a profession?

- How do you think your spirituality or religious perspective might affect or be incorporated into your nursing practice?

Religiosity refers to beliefs and practices that are the expressive aspects of religion. These include, among others, prayer, ritual, dietary practices, modes of dress, and study of sacred texts. Awareness of religious practices and beliefs that are important to patients and families enables nurses to incorporate religious needs into care planning. Familiarity with beliefs and practices of different religions that may affect health care is important in order to be better able to incorporate particular needs into patient care (Andrews & Hanson, 1989). This information provides a basis from which nurses can explore with patients what is necessary to support or meet their spiritual needs, taking care not to presume a need until it is verified with the patient. For example, a Catholic patient may not wish to have a priest called, a Jewish patient may have no problem with eating ham, or a patient who lists no religious affiliation may practice daily meditation.

Although many people express their spirituality through religion, spiritual expression is not limited to this context. Many people will note that they believe in God but do not go to church. Instead they pray on their own, or experience the Divine through nature, or relate to a Higher Power or Universal Being that is found in all of life. It is important to plan nursing care according to how each patient expresses and experiences spirituality.

Creating Sacred Space. Addressing religious concerns within a health care setting does not require nurses to share the same religious perspective as their patients. What is necessary is that nurses create an environment that is open to a variety of religious and spiritual expression. Creating sacred space in the midst of science and technology can challenge a nurse's creativity. Nursing care may include providing the quiet a patient needs for meditation, arranging a private space for a particular ritual, contacting an appropriate spiritual support person, or ensuring that specific dietary requirements are met. Praying with or reading scripture to patients may be included in nursing care, providing it is done with the patient's permission and within the context of the patient's tradition. Prayer can be an important intervention, and research suggests that prayer reflecting an attitude of "Thy will be done" is particularly effective (Dossey, 1993; 1996). It is good for nurses who are so inclined to include prayer for patients in their personal prayer, with an openness to what is for the patient's highest good. Nurses need to be aware of acting out of their own spiritual or religious perspectives while taking care not to impose these views on another.

Dilemmas Related to Religious Beliefs. When patients refuse conventional medical treatments based on religious beliefs or spiritual perspective, dilemmas can arise. Patients who decide to rely on prayer for healing rather than chemotherapy for treatment of cancer, for example, may be considered irrational, and their competence to make decisions may be questioned. If an adult refuses a blood transfusion due to religious beliefs, after all risks have been explained, it is considered an informed decision. If a parent refuses a transfusion for a child based on the same belief, it may be taken to court as neglect or abuse. A woman who refuses to leave a dangerously abusive marriage because of religious convictions may find that frustrated health care providers are less responsive to her cries for help.

Ask Yourself

What Happens When Religious Beliefs and Medical Care Conflict?

- How do you think you would react to patient decisions in the examples noted above?

- What principles would guide you in dealing with dilemmas arising from religious convictions?

- What personal religious or spiritual practices are important to your health?

- What personal convictions might affect your health care decisions?

Nurturing Spirit

Caregiving is influenced by a nurse's spiritual, as well as physical and emotional, well-being. The ability to attend to spirituality with another requires that nurses first attend to their own spirits (Burkhardt & Nagai-Jacobson, 1997). Self-awareness, which includes appreciation of oneself as a unique body-mind-spirit being, underlies the nurse's recognition of this same wholeness in others.

Just as sustenance and care are necessary for the health of body and mind, so too does the spirit require nurture. Caring for one's spirit includes mindfulness and taking time to attend to one's inner being. The spirit can be nurtured in many ways, and we must each discover what our own spirit needs in order to thrive. Prayer, meditation, music, religious worship, or shared ritual may be important. The spirit may be nurtured through special time with friends or family or by giving oneself alone time at home, in nature, or in some other sacred space. Attending to one's need for rest, play, or creative activity are other ways to care for spirit. The spirit can be nurtured in a very profound way through sharing one's story. As nurses become more adept at nurturing their spirits, they are better able to recognize and support the process with patients and families.

SUMMARY

Attentiveness to spiritual and cultural aspects of care with patients is an important part of holistic nursing care. The diversity of cultures and spiritual expressions within our society requires that nurses be able to identify concerns and issues in these areas and address them competently and confidently. Familiarity with values, beliefs, and practices of various cultures and religions is a useful adjunct to careful cultural and spiritual assessments with patients. Self-awareness regarding one's own cultural and spiritual values, beliefs, and expressions is necessary in order to address these areas with patients. Such awareness allows nurses to act from their own spiritual or cultural perspectives, while taking care not to impose these views on others. In this way care planning can more readily flow from assessments that identify issues and needs regarding the patient's cultural and spiritual expressions and experiences.

CHAPTER HIGHLIGHTS

- Since culture influences beliefs and behaviors regarding health and healing, cultural assessment is integral to a comprehensive nursing assessment.

- Providing effective nursing care within the diversity of our multicultural society requires cultural competence on the part of nurses. Cultural competence can help prevent dilemmas from arising when there are differences in cultural perspective between patient and nurse.

- The culture of health care institutions may vary greatly from the people served by these systems. Values such as autonomy, beneficence, or the right to self-determination need to be considered from the cultural perspectives of patient, family, and health care providers.

- Complementary therapies are utilized by many people encountered in conventional health care settings. Nursing care is enhanced when nurses are aware of various therapies being utilized by patients. Knowledge of and working with traditional healing systems and healers can help nurses promote more culturally congruent care.

- Communication is a key factor in providing culturally congruent and spiritually sensitive care and in averting associated legal and other dilemmas.

- Health and healing are associated with that which is holy and whole. Spirituality has long been a component of healing and health care, since by nature, humans are body-mind-spirit beings.

- Grounded in a holistic view of persons, nursing care must include spirituality assessment and interventions addressing spiritual needs, recognizing that religious or spiritual perspective may influence health care choices.

- Expressions of spirituality are many and varied and may include, but are not limited to, the context of religion. Religious values are not always congruent with ethical perspectives of the greater society.

- Providing spiritual care requires that nurses be attentive to their own spirits and the spiritual concerns of patients and create an environment that is open to a variety of religious and spiritual expressions. Nurses need awareness of acting from their own cultural, spiritual, or religious perspectives while not imposing these views on others.

DISCUSSION QUESTIONS AND ACTIVITIES

1. Consider how your cultural, spiritual, or religious values affect personal choices regarding health and healing. Discuss this with other students, noting similarities and differences.

2. What aspects of the culture of the health care system are difficult for you as a nurse? Identify conflicts and the beliefs and values underlying them.

3. Recall a time when you or someone you know experienced a conflict with persons within the health care system. What values, beliefs, or understandings contributed to this conflict?

4. Discuss with other students nonconventional therapies, or folk remedies, that you or someone you know have used. Why was the therapy used? How did you know about the therapy? Was it used in place of or along with conventional therapies? What was the outcome?

5. List ten things that nurture you spiritually. Consider how often you have done these in the past day, week, month. Make a plan to include at least one each day for the next week.

6. Choose a religious tradition or a nonconventional therapy with which you are unfamiliar. Explore this tradition or therapy through readings and discussions with members, practitioners, or persons who have practiced the religion or utilized the therapy. Share your findings with classmates.

7. Discuss how nurses can create sacred space within health care settings.

8. Discuss patient health care choices or behaviors which are based on religious beliefs that might present a dilemma for you. Consider how you would approach the situation in a professional manner and describe the ethical stance that would guide your decisions.

REFERENCES

American Nurses Association. (1991). *Position paper on cultural diversity in nursing practice.* Kansas City, MO: Author.

Andrews, M. M., & Hanson, P. A. (1989). Religious beliefs: Implications for nursing practice. In J. S. Broyle & M. M. Andrews (Eds.), *Transcultural concepts in nursing care* (pp. 357–418). Glenview, IL: Scott, Foresman/Little, Brown College Division.

Burkhardt, M. A. (1985). Nursing, health, and wholeness. *Journal of Holistic Nursing, 3,* 35–36.

Burkhardt, M. A. (1994). Becoming and connecting: Elements of spirituality for women. *Holistic Nursing Practice, 8,* 12–21.

Burkhardt, M. A., & Nagai-Jacobson, M. G. (1994). Reawakening spirit in clinical practice. *Journal of Holistic Nursing, 12,* 9–12.

Burkhardt, M. A., & Nagai-Jacobson, M. G. (1997). Spirituality and healing. In B. M. Dossey (Ed.), *AHNA core curriculum for holistic nursing* (pp. 42–51). Gaithersburg, MD: Aspen.

Dossey, B. M., Keegan, L., Guzzetta, C. E., & Kolkmeier, L. G. (1995). *Holistic nursing: A handbook for practice.* Gaithersburg, MD: Aspen.

Dossey, L. (1993). *Healing words: The power of prayer and the practice of medicine.* San Francisco: HarperCollins.

Dossey, L. (1996). *Prayer is good medicine.* San Francisco: HarperCollins.

Eisenberg, D. M., Kessler, R. C., Foster, C., Norlock, F. E., Calkins, D. R., & Delbanco, T. L. (1993). Unconventional medicine in the United States. *New England Journal of Medicine, 328,* 246–252.

Giger, J. N., & Davidhizar, R. E. (1995). *Transcultural nursing: Assessment and intervention* (2nd ed.). St. Louis, MO: Mosby.

Hufford, D. J. (1996, January 18–21). *Ethical dimensions of alternative medicine.* Presentation at the First Annual Alternative Therapies Symposium: Creating Integrated Healthcare, San Diego, CA.

Kavanagh, K. H. (1993). Transcultural nursing: Facing the challenges of advocacy and diversity/universality. *Journal of Transcultural Nursing, 5,* 4–13.

Leininger, M. (1991). Transcultural care principles, human rights, and ethical considerations. *Journal of Transcultural Nursing, 3,* 21–22.

Nagai-Jacobson, M. G., & Burkhardt, M. A. (1996). Viewing persons as stories: A perspective for holistic care. *Alternative Therapies in Health and Medicine, 2,* 54–58.

Sewell, M. (Ed.). (1991). *Cries of the spirit: A celebration of women's spirituality.* Boston: Beacon Press.

Tafoya, T. (1996, May). *Embracing the shadow: Mending the sacred hoop.* Paper presented at the South Texas AIDS Training (STAT) for Mental Health Providers: The Human, Transcultural, and Spiritual Dimensions of HIV/AIDS, San Antonio, TX.

Tripp-Reimer, T. (1987). Cultural assessment. In J. P. Bellak & P. A. Bamford (Eds.), *Nursing assessment: A multidimensional approach.* Boston: Jones & Bartlett.

Waters, C. (1996). Professional development in nursing—A culturally diverse postdoctoral experience. *Image, 28,* 47–50.

PART **V**

THE POWER TO MAKE A DIFFERENCE

Part V discusses the importance of empowerment of nurses and patients. To deal with the complex issues facing nursing today, the nurse is required to exercise integrity, accountability, and courage. Nurses have the responsibility, authority, and power to make principled choices. Additionally, empowerment of patients is an important element of nursing care that derives from an appreciation that patients have the ability to discern their needs and make decisions about their lives and health. Being an enabler of empowerment requires the nurse to relinquish power and embrace the patient as an equal partner. Nurses can facilitate empowerment by working directly with patients and through addressing social, political, and environmental factors affecting empowerment of individuals and communities. In the midst of an ever changing and challenging health care environment in which issues of power and control continue to affect patient care, it is imperative that nurses be both empowered and competent enablers of patient empowerment.

CHAPTER 19

Empowerment for Nurses

Written in collaboration with Barbara C. Banonis

Copper Woman warned Hai Nai Yu that the world would change and times might come when Knowing would not be the same as Doing. And she told her that Trying would always be very important.
(Cameron, 1981, p. 53)

OBJECTIVES

After completing this chapter, the reader should be able to:

1. Discuss the effect of mind sets on expectations regarding nursing practice and ethical stances.
2. Describe metaphors for nursing and discuss their impact on nursing ethics.
3. Explain the impact on nursing practice of perceptions of nursing both within and outside the profession.
4. Describe the concepts of power and empowerment.
5. Discuss personal empowerment and its importance within nursing.
6. Discuss the relationship among professional empowerment, principled behavior, and nursing practice.
7. Describe the role of diversity in empowerment.
8. Discuss the importance of nursing's vision of nursing to professional practice.

INTRODUCTION

Dealing in a principled way with issues facing nursing today requires integrity, accountability, and courage. Presumptions underlying discussion of issues in this book are: (1) nurses have the power to make choices and to act in responsible and principled ways, and (2) nurses have authority to make decisions and recommendations regarding activities that are within the scope of their practice. However, the parameters of nursing's power and authority are not always clear, and many nurses feel constrained by the systems within which they work and by persisting paternalistic attitudes that promote disempowerment. This chapter discusses the concept of empowerment as a process through which nurses are enabled to clarify and claim their ability to make decisions regarding issues related to nursing practice. Elements of personal empowerment are addressed, and factors associated with professional empowerment are considered. Principles regarding empowerment for nurses that are discussed in this chapter are also foundational for empowering patients, which is the focus of Chapter 20.

INFLUENCES ON NURSING'S PERCEPTIONS OF PRINCIPLED PRACTICE

Nurses, patients, and other health care providers may vary greatly in their perceptions of ideals for nursing and nursing practice. These perceptions influence expectations and decisions regarding care, authority, and accountability. Expectations regarding good nursing care or taking an ethical stance flow from such perceptions. Aroskar (1982) notes that decision making is affected by factors in a nurse's external and internal environments. A nurse's external environment includes norms, ideals, and expectations of patients, families, other health care providers, and the professional and social systems with which a nurse interacts. The internal environment includes a nurse's *mind set* or inner world of personal beliefs and perceptions.

Influence of Mind Sets

Aroskar (1982) suggests that nurses' mind sets or characterizations of and beliefs about the health care system influence how nurses identify and respond to ethical issues and dilemmas in practice. She discusses issues related to different mind sets regarding health care that are common within nursing. For example, when nurses view health care in terms of medical cases focused on the cure of disease, the physician is seen as the dominant authority. Following the physician's orders (whether or not the nurse agrees with them) and loyalty to the physician and institution are considered the legitimate and ethical focus of nursing activities. Aroskar states that "this mind set may well impede efforts to achieve more ethical practice which requires critical, reflective thinking and challenges the decision-making structure of the present system" (p. 26). If nurses view health care as a commodity in which nursing and medical care are sold to patients by institutions, the nurse's primary responsibility is to the employing institution. Within this view, needs of individual patients may be subordinated to the utilitarian goal focused on the good of the greatest number of people or the institutional goal of making a profit. Nurses who hold this view may not challenge the rightness or wrongness of nursing actions provided they are congruent with goals and policies of the institution. This mind set finds fertile ground in managed care arenas.

Metaphors of Nursing

People often use *metaphors* to focus attention on particular aspects of reality in order to enhance understandings of roles, events, and experiences. Metaphors may also influence one's perceptions of these events and experiences. For example, likening nurses to *angels in white* calls attention to nursing roles of caring, protecting, and serving; yet viewing nurses as angels may set up the expectation that they be somewhat distant and above human frailties. Numerous metaphors have been associated with nursing that reflect different mind sets regarding roles and responsibilities in health care and various approaches to determining appropriate ethical stances for nursing care delivery.

Winslow (1984) discusses the impact on nursing ethics of a shift from a military metaphor for nursing, which stresses loyalty, to a legal metaphor for nursing as advocate for patient rights. The military metaphor is associated with obedience to higher authority, a view of disease as the enemy, discipline, respect for those of higher rank, uniform dress, and, above all, loyalty. Winslow notes that "loyalty meant refusal to criticize the nurse's hospital or training school, fellow nurses, and most importantly, the physician under whom the nurse worked . . . being loyal to the physician by preserving the patient's confidence was the same as being loyal to the patient" (p. 33). Ethical imperatives that flow from this metaphor include following physician orders, even if the nurse questions their appropriateness, upholding the patient's faith in the physician, even if the nurse questions the doctor's competence, and being loyal to health care colleagues, even at the expense of the patient.

In the early history of nursing, following the physician's order without question would have absolved the nurse from guilt, even in the event of a deleterious outcome. Today, however, this is not the case. Nursing's move from vocation to profession requires that nurses be more personally accountable for their actions. Court rulings have held nurses legally responsible for their decisions and actions. Legal decisions, changes in the health care delivery system, and feminist awarenesses within the nursing profession have encouraged the transition from the metaphor of loyal soldier to that of patient advocate. Winslow (1984) notes that a significant revision in nursing's self-image began in the 1960s and 1970s. Greater emphasis on consumerism and patient rights, coupled with growing dissatisfaction with increased costs and depersonalization of health care, helped to open the door for nurses to expand their roles as patient advocates. As advocates for patient rights, nurses are responsible to those who require nursing care. This obliges nurses to be alert to situations in which patients may be endangered by incompetent, unethical, or illegal practice by any member of the health care team or the health care system and to take appropriate actions to safeguard the patient (American Nurses Association, 1985). Current nursing codes and standards that stress responsibility to patients through collegial membership in the health team reflect ethical imperatives flowing from the metaphor of advocacy.

Loyalty remains a valued virtue for nurses within the advocacy metaphor. Although ideally the nurse's first loyalty is to the patient, circumstances of conflicting loyalty are apt to occur. Loyalty to colleagues and to employers is also important, and nurses may at times be faced with making difficult decisions between advocacy for patients or loyalty to colleagues. Personal integrity, knowledge, and courage are all required in such situations.

How Do Mind Sets Affect Perceptions?

You are the vice president for nursing at a large medical center. Recently one of the physicians, who holds a lot of power in the system and is generally very open and easy to work with, expressed considerable displeasure about a particular nurse refusing to carry out a medical order and referring concerns about certain physician practice decisions to the ethics committee. The physician says that you should fire the nurse for insubordination. You are aware that the nurse's decisions were reasonable, in the patient's interest, and based on sound principles and standards of nursing practice.

- How would you respond to the physician?
- Where do you see potential for conflicting loyalties in this situation?
- Discuss how differing perceptions of nursing might affect this situation.
- Describe what you see as the most realistic outcome in this situation. What about the ideal outcome?

How Nursing Is Perceived by Others

Factors such as mind sets and metaphors influence a nurse's perceptions of and choices regarding principled behavior. Perceptions of others also affect considerations regarding appropriate or ethical nursing actions. Although nursing as a profession has claimed the metaphor of advocate in lieu of that of loyal soldier, many nurses within the profession have not fully embraced the change. Operationalizing the advocacy role may put nurses at risk in some institutions and situations, as evidenced in cases such as that of Jolene Tuma discussed in Chapter 11. Although nursing has made a paradigm shift regarding its role and responsibilities, awareness of nursing's current professional imperatives is often lacking among patients, families, physicians, and health care administrators. The role of nursing as perceived by many outside of the profession remains embedded in the loyal soldier metaphor and health care as medical cases or commodity mind sets. As a result, many physicians still expect nurses to follow their bidding and take offense when their decisions or actions are challenged. The hierarchical, patriarchal system remains the norm in many health care institutions, and since physicians are perceived to be of higher rank, their influence often holds more sway than that of nurses who may challenge them. Although patients and families often have more continual and direct contact with nurses, they may have limited understanding that the nurse is their advocate and function instead from the mind set that the physician is the captain of a ship in which the nurse is a member of the crew. Images in the media depicting nurses in ancillary, subordinate roles also affect perceptions of patients and others regarding expectations of nurses.

UNDERSTANDING POWER AND EMPOWERMENT

Nurses have the power to make a difference by acting in principled ways in all areas of their lives and practice. However, as has been evident throughout the discussions in this book, many factors mitigate against nurses claiming this power. Nurses need to develop skills in dealing with these factors in order to function fully in their legitimate roles within health care. It is essential that nurses be aware of values, beliefs, and other factors affecting personal decision making and expand their knowledge of ethical principles, legal considerations, and issues facing nursing. Understanding **power** and **empowerment** can help in developing strategies for action in this regard.

Although the word *power* is often understood in terms of strength, force, or control, a primary dictionary definition of the term, derived from its Latin root *potere*, is "the ability to do or act, capability of doing or accomplishing something" (*The Random House Dictionary of the English Language*, 1987). To have power, then, implies having the ability to do or act; and to *empower* would be to facilitate the ability of another person to do or to act.

Rodwell (1996) suggests that empowerment is a "helping process whereby groups of individuals are enabled to change a situation, given skills, resources, opportunities and authority to do so. It is a partnership which respects and values self and others— aiming to develop positive beliefs in self and the future" (p. 309). Gurka (1995) reflects that empowerment is a philosophy or world view flowing from belief in each person's inherent worth and process of self-discovery which involves creating a vision, taking risks, making choices, and behaving in authentic ways. Empowerment requires respect for an individual's personal beliefs and goals and trust in the person's ability to make decisions, take action, and be accountable for the actions. Although sharing of knowledge through education is important for empowerment, emotional and social support is essential (Gibson, 1991; Rodwell, 1996).

Through their in-depth analyses of the concept, Gibson (1991) and Rodwell (1996) suggest that empowerment is both process and outcome, taking different forms within different people and contexts. Because of this, empowerment needs to be defined by the people concerned. Empowerment is a transactional process involving relationship with others. This relationship includes mutually beneficial interactions aimed at strengthening rather than weakening; power sharing through mutual sharing of knowledge, resources, and opportunities; and respect for self and others. Empowerment is nurtured by collaborative efforts that focus on solutions rather than problems and on strengths, rights, and abilities rather than deficits. Empowerment derives from a feminine perspective of *power with* or *power to*, which implies sharing responsibility, knowledge, and resources; collaboration for goal achievement; incorporating diversity; valuing the contributions of each person; and valuing the process. In contrast is the masculine view of *power over* that incorporates a sense of paternalistic control, struggle for and protection of limited resources, separation of leaders and followers, expediency, and results even at the expense of persons (Chinn, 1995).

Empowerment implies choice on the part of those being empowered. One cannot empower another because to presume to do so removes the element of choice. Individuals and groups must ultimately motivate and empower themselves. This process requires self-awareness, positive self-esteem, commitment to self and others, and both the desire and ability to make decisions. Responsibility and accountability for one's actions and having the authority to act are implicit in the ability to choose.

Through the empowerment process, one can enable others to develop awareness of areas that need change, foster a desire to take action, and share resources, skills, and opportunities that support the change. Rodwell (1996) notes that it is self-awareness and resources rather than the services provided to persons that self-empower. Enhanced self-esteem, personal satisfaction, sense of connectedness, the ability to set and reach goals, a sense of control over life and change processes, and a sense of hope and direction are outcomes of empowerment (Gibson, 1991; Rodwell, 1996).

Ask Yourself

What Makes You Feel Empowered?

- Consider a situation in which you felt empowered. Describe factors contributing to your sense of empowerment.

- Recall a time when you felt disempowered. What contributed to this sense? How might you have felt more empowered in the situation?

PERSONAL EMPOWERMENT

Nursing's power to make a difference in care with patients derives from many factors. In order to serve as credible models of empowerment for others, nurses must demonstrate congruence between values and behaviors in their own lives. Personal integrity implies an ability to be honest with and care for oneself, as well as respond to the needs of others. Often nurses, and especially women, have learned to value care for others before or instead of care for self. A true value for human life must include value for one's own life as well. The biblical adage is: "Love thy neighbor *as* thyself," not instead of thyself or before thyself (Leviticus 19:18). One must attend to oneself and treat oneself with the same respect and dignity as one treats others. Personal empowerment begins with actions that support the meeting of one's own needs and self-actualization. It is from one's personal stores of creativity, empowerment, and health that one is able to inspire, teach, and assist others in achieving their potential.

In principle many nurses would agree with the concept of care for self; however, actions often conflict with this acknowledged belief. Nurses often agree to work additional hours even when they are exhausted; consume large amounts of caffeine and sugar to boost waning energy; go home to care for children, spouse, and friends; and collapse into bed only to get up and do it all again the next day because they feel limited power to do otherwise. What causes a person to behave in this kind of conflict with their stated values? Often the person has learned conflicting messages. A belief in caring for oneself may conflict with a learned belief that caring for others is more admirable or important than caring for oneself.

Some people feel very little control over any area of their lives. Others may feel empowered to make decisions in some situations but not in others, for example, a person may actively make decisions in the home environment while feeling like a pawn of the system at work. The sense of power that nurses have in their personal lives may affect their perception of empowerment in the professional arena. Burnout, job dissatisfaction, and limited professional commitment affect the quality of patient care and are often associated with feelings of powerlessness (Moss, 1995). Attributes of empowerment noted in the previous section reflect important considerations for self-empowerment of nurses on both personal and professional levels.

Attending to personal empowerment underlies the ability to enable empowerment in others. This requires valuing oneself and "listening inwardly to your own senses as well as listening intently and actively to others, consciously taking in and forming strength" (Chinn, 1995, p. 3). Self-awareness is necessary, since self-perception has a direct link to quality of patient care (Moss, 1995). Such awareness requires attentiveness to factors that influence one's thoughts, feelings, actions, and reactions in the present circumstance and reflective considerations of such influences on past experiences. Empowerment involves taking ownership of one's inner life and recognizing that one has full control over one's thoughts, feelings, and actions.

Owning one's thoughts involves recognizing old or repetitive thought patterns and changing those that are no longer supporting a creative, actualizing life. Self-critical, judgmental, and negative thinking are particularly confining. Old thinking can be updated with new knowledge. Questioning the origin of particular thoughts can reveal ideas that were true at one time but are no longer true. For example, a child who was always told that she did not know enough to make a decision, and that mother knew best, may become an adult who still consults her mother before making decisions. Seeking alternative views of situations and learning logical or critical thinking skills are other ways to restructure thought patterns.

Feelings are transient signals that alert us to what is supportive or offensive in a situation. Owning feelings means acknowledging and investigating the internal source of the message rather than blaming other persons or situations for one's feelings. People may experience different feelings in similar situations. For example, a death can elicit feelings of sadness, despair, hope, relief, joy, and others, depending upon the unique inner response of each person. Feelings and the reactions they elicit are in the person, not in the event.

It is important to name and take ownership of personal values and to claim one's ability to make choices. When experiencing a lack of control in life, a person should determine internal and external barriers to having control, consider whether one wants control, and explore what one needs to do and is willing to risk in order to take control. Consciously acting based upon clear evaluation of the current situation rather than acting automatically is one way to own one's behavior. Taking ownership of behavior requires being able to see options. Believing there are no options can result in feeling powerless, trapped, or victimized. Even when one does not believe one can change a current unacceptable situation immediately, chances are one can make a plan for change and set that plan into motion one step at a time. A *victim* waits and hopes something or someone else will change; makes excuses for not taking action (time, cost, fatigue, and the like); blames people, places, or things for their situation; is trapped and unaware of options. An *empowered person* decides to be accountable for personal responses, makes plans, considers options, develops strategies for change, and acts on plans by doing what is necessary to succeed.

Personal empowerment "is growth of personal strength, power, and ability to enact one's own will and love for self in the context of love and respect for others . . . [and] is only possible when individuals express respect and reverence for all other forms of life and ground the energy of the Self as one with the earth" (Chinn, 1995, p. 3). A commitment to personal growth and self-care, developing a positive sense of self, awareness of strengths and abilities as well as limitations, and drawing on one's supports and sources of connectedness foster this process. It is essential that one trust oneself and one's knowledge and abilities and is courageous in taking risks. Empathy with others, appreciation of diversity, tolerance, flexibility, and willingness to compromise empower a person. Empowerment requires being true to oneself and one's values in the midst of a loving response to the choices of others. Congruence among one's being, knowing, and doing reflects personal integrity. This means that one's actions flow from one's essence, and one's choices derive from what one knows to be good and true.

PROFESSIONAL EMPOWERMENT

In order to deal in a principled way with issues and dilemmas arising within health care settings, nurses must feel personally and professionally empowered to act on sometimes difficult choices. Many factors affect nursing actions in the professional arena, including personal attitudes and self-concept; the structural and functional interrelatedness of health care systems; political, economic, and social forces; and interactions with patients and colleagues. Barriers to empowerment exist within the community of nursing and are also imposed from external sources. Curtin (1982) reminds us that "many nurses are unwilling to assume responsibility for decision making and that nursing has failed to develop an adequate support system for nurses" (p. 10). Professional empowerment is built upon the foundational elements of personal accountability and support of nursing colleagues.

Nurses need to recognize that empowerment requires becoming knowledgeable about and addressing system issues as well as interpersonal issues. Such issues include recognizing the need for changing the power base within the current health care system, moving from a paternalistic, hierarchical model of control toward one that values collaboration, and the power of the collective. Nurses must become involved in shared decision making and in forming institutional policies as part of this process (Chandler, 1991; Gaul, 1995; Moss, 1995).

When nurses feel disempowered in their work settings, they can choose the *victim* stance, which relinquishes power to the system, or they can challenge the system.

Challenging social and economic constraints on nursing and health care through political activity or involvement in professional organizations fosters professional empowerment. Developing conflict management, negotiating, and effective communication skills enables a nurse to more effectively deal with both system and interpersonal issues.

Unity in Diversity

Empowerment incorporates divergent and conflicting solutions to problems based on value in support of others rather than in divisiveness (Chinn, 1995; Gibson, 1991). It implies embracing diversity and moving from fear of that which is different to appreciation of the strength derived from and unity contained in diversity. Nurses need to recognize that systems exert control, in part, by fostering divisiveness among workers so as to deter unity of opposition to system policies. When nurses unite with and support colleagues who challenge harmful or potentially harmful practices, they are personally and professionally empowered.

Challenging unjust, unprofessional, or unethical practices may entail risk for nurses. Feeling empowered to take a stand requires personal integrity and support from others. Nurses need to be willing to struggle with difficult questions and arrive at decisions that flow from their internal values and perspective rather than looking for the *right* answer from an external source. Empowerment implies accountability for one's own choices and actions. Jameton (1984) reflects that people pretend they are forced to do things when they are not. He gives the example of a nurse who instructs a patient to take a medication because the physician ordered it, noting that both patient and nurse pretend that they must act because of the physician's order, although each could make another choice. Reflecting that nurses who choose to work in systems such as hospitals are accountable for their actions despite the existence of systemic problems affecting health care, Jameton (1984) writes,

> If one fails to resist exploitation, incompetence, and corrupt practices, one becomes responsible for them. If one resists them, one enters into conflict with conventional conceptions of behavior for employees and thereby risks reprisals. One has to choose between complicity and self-sacrifice, or enter the uncomfortable middle ground of irony. Ethics does not give a clear answer as to which one must choose. Instead, one is free to move in the direction of the kind of world one personally desires to create. (p. 289)

It is imperative that nurses decide whether they prefer a world in which they are empowered in the professional arena or one in which they are controlled by others. The choices nurses make affect the outcome.

RE-VISIONING NURSING

Empowerment within the profession requires a renewed vision of nursing. As nurses we need to redefine nursing according to our own vision, rather than accepting the definition imposed by the dominant groups in health care, that is, physicians and institutions. When nurses draw pictures of their vision of nursing, what emerges are images of caring, light, comfort, and love. These images reflect the heart of the vision of nursing within nurses. Making choices based on the vision and values of the profession fosters congruence between nursing's knowing and doing, which strengthens personal and professional effectiveness. In contrast, nurses who work in situations in which they feel a lack of synchronicity with their values often experience burnout, become nasty, take on attributes and values of the dominant group, and look for someone to blame (behaviors reflective of oppressed groups). Remaining in a victim role involves a choice to give away one's power and allow someone else to define one's reality. Re-defining nursing according to nursing's own vision is an act of empowerment.

Empowerment involves risk and commitment and requires both courage and compassion. Curtin (1996) illustrates this through a parable about a baby eagle who broke his wing after falling from his nest and was found by a mountain climber who took him home, nursed the broken wing, and put him in with the chickens. Not knowing what or how to eat, the eagle learned from the chickens how to peck at the feed on the ground. Even as he grew larger and stronger he continued to peck away like the chickens and forgot that he was an eagle. When a friend of the climber noted that the eagle should be flying up in the mountains with other eagles, the climber responded that the eagle knew he had good situation with free food and a warm coop, and would not fly away even if he could. The friend offered to teach the eagle to fly and took him to the top of the barn, telling him that he was an eagle and could fly and be free. The eagle heard this but remembered what happened the last time he tried to fly, and, seeing the chickens below, remembered the food and shelter, and would not fly. The friend tried another approach of taking the eagle to the mountains, teaching him how to spread and flap his wings, and encouraging his efforts, telling him repeatedly that he was an eagle and could fly. Finally the eagle took the risk and flew, delighting in the experience; but as he flew over the chicken yard, he remembered that he was hungry and returned to peck for food with the chickens. This distressed the friend who disparaged the eagle for continuing to act like a chicken when he could be free. Eventually a new plan was devised in which the friend carefully crept up to the eagle and, putting a hood over his head, carried him to an area where there were other eagles. The eagle saw their nests and watched them hunt, eat, feed their young, and fly. The friend showed him the beauty of his homeland, encouraged him to hunt and fly, and reminded him that he was an EAGLE. After several days the eagle got the idea, and when the friend took him to the top of the highest mountain, he took off and soared high, never looking back, and never eating chicken feed again, because he was an EAGLE, and he knew it. (Summarized from Curtin, 1996.)

Curtin (1996) reflects that this parable offers many insights regarding empowerment for nurses. The story demonstrates that empowerment is not easy for either the one trying to empower or the one being empowered, but that it is important not to give up. One must also realize that empowerment costs money, time, and effort.

> It (empowerment) isn't easy. Telling the eagle to fly wasn't enough. It isn't easy. Changing the eagle's environment and even teaching him to fly wasn't enough. It isn't easy. You have to start at the beginning and recreate an attitude in a new environment. It's tough on the eagle

too. The eagle was frightened: he had been hurt. The eagle knew the old, safe ways of pecking and free grain and warm nest. And he could have that with no effort! It was hard for the eagle to believe that the easy way sooner or later would destroy him. And it was really tough on the eagle when [the friend] blamed him for being what he'd been taught to be all his life. (Curtin, 1996, p. 210)

Curtin notes that neither freedom nor risk are easy, and that they are not for everyone. It is important, however, not to "blame the chickens for what they are. It's unfair—and it's a waste of time. But never give up on the eagles. They can fly—and they will" (p. 210). Empowerment for nurses means recognizing *who* we are, knowing that, like the eagle, we have both the ability and the freedom to fly!

SUMMARY

Empowerment is a multifaceted concept. Awareness of attitudes about nursing's role in health care and factors that shape these attitudes enables nurses to be better able to identify that which supports or diminishes both personal and professional empowerment. Attentiveness to personal empowerment, which includes integrity, accountability, and courage, is foundational for addressing empowerment issues within the profession. No one can empower another, but the inner process can be facilitated when knowledge and resources are offered within an environment of mutual respect and support. Empowerment for nurses requires remembering *who* we are, recognizing that *knowing* must be the same as *doing*, and following our own vision of nursing.

CHAPTER HIGHLIGHTS

- Mind sets regarding health care influence how nurses identify and respond to ethical issues and dilemmas in practice settings.
- Nursing's contemporary self-perception reflects the legal metaphor of patient advocate rather than the military metaphor of loyal soldier. Each of these metaphors implies different ethical imperatives for nursing.
- Ethical imperatives flowing from the advocacy metaphor are reflected in current nursing codes and standards of practice.
- Empowerment, which is both process and outcome, derives from a feminine perspective of *power to* or *power with*, reflecting a supportive partnership based on mutual love and respect that enables persons to change situations given necessary resources, knowledge, skills, and opportunities. Empowerment comes from within a person and involves choice; one cannot empower another.
- The ability to deal with health care issues and dilemmas in a principled way derives from personal and professional empowerment and requires attentiveness to intrapersonal, interpersonal, and systems issues.
- Personal empowerment requires self-awareness and is characterized by maintaining personal integrity in the midst of a loving response to the choices of others.

Self-concept and sense of power in a nurse's personal life affects nursing care and a nurse's ability to enable empowerment in others.

- Recognizing unity in diversity and incorporating divergent views and solutions empowers nurses and others.

- Defining nursing according to nursing's own vision is an act of empowerment that implies accountability for one's own choices and actions, with awareness that each choice helps create the kind of world and environment within which nurses must practice.

DISCUSSION QUESTIONS AND ACTIVITIES

1. Talk with both retired and practicing nurses about ethical imperatives that guide (or guided) their nursing practice. Identify mind sets and metaphors reflective of these imperatives.

2. Where in your life do you feel most personally empowered? Discuss the circumstances surrounding your feelings of empowerment with other students.

3. Review Chapters 5 and 6 and reflect on how your values and current phase of development affect your sense of personal empowerment.

4. Describe a situation in which you took ownership for your own thoughts, feelings, or actions. Describe a time when you found yourself blaming others or assuming a victim stance. Discuss with classmates factors prompting each stance and how you felt in each situation.

5. Discuss differences in others that might engender fear or caution in you and limit your ability to embrace the diversity.

6. What aspects of empowerment do you think are most important in nursing practice settings? Support your perspective.

7. Interview practicing nurses regarding personal and professional power, including situations where they feel empowered to make decisions, where they derive authority to make decisions, and situations in which they have experienced dilemmas around the issue of power. Ask them to describe their ideal image of nursing and compare that to their current reality.

8. Illustrate your vision of nursing and develop strategies for making nursing's self-vision better known to others. Implement one strategy.

REFERENCES

American Nurses Association. (1985). *Code for nurses with interpretive statements.* Washington, DC: Author.

Aroskar, M. A. (1982). Are nurses' mind sets compatible with ethical practice? *Topics in Clinical Nursing, 4,* 22–32.

Cameron, A. (1981). *Daughters of copper woman.* Vancouver, BC: Press Gang.

Chandler, G. E. (1991). Creating an environment to empower nurses. *Nursing Management, 22,* 20–23.

Chinn, P. (1995). *Peace and power: Building communities for the future*. New York: National League of Nursing Press.

Curtin, L. (1982). Autonomy, accountability and nursing practice. *Topics in Clinical Nursing, 4,* 7–14.

Curtin, L. (1996). *Nursing into the 21st century*. Springhouse, PA: Springhouse.

Gaul, A. L. (1995). Casuistry, care, compassion, and ethics data analysis. *Advances in Nursing Science, 17,* 47–57.

Gibson, C. H. (1991). A concept analysis of empowerment. *Journal of Advanced Nursing, 16,* 354–361.

Gurka, A. M. (1995). Transformational leadership: Qualities and strategies for the CNS. *Clinical Nurse Specialist, 9,* 169–174.

Jameton, A. (1984). *Nursing practice: The ethical issues*. Englewood Cliffs, NJ: Prentice-Hall.

Moss, M. T. (1995). Foundations of nursing empowerment. *Nursing Economics, 13,* 112–114.

Rodwell, C. M. (1996). An analysis of the concept of empowerment. *Journal of Advanced Nursing, 23,* 305–313.

The Random House dictionary of the English language, second edition unabridged. (1987). New York: Random House.

Winslow, G. R. (1984). From loyalty to advocacy: A new metaphor for nursing. *The Hastings Center Report, 14,* 32–40.

CHAPTER 20

Enabling Patient Empowerment

Power is the energy *from which action arises.*
(Chinn, 1995, p. 8)

OBJECTIVES

After completing this chapter, the reader should be able to:

1. Discuss the meaning of patient empowerment.
2. Discuss the nursing role in empowerment of patients.
3. Describe attitudes of nurses that enable empowerment.
4. Identify nursing knowledge and skills basic to empowerment.
5. Describe factors that enhance or block patient empowerment.
6. Discuss approaches to fostering empowerment with patients.

INTRODUCTION

The concept of empowerment relates to the principle of autonomy and to the nursing role of patient advocate. Fostering empowerment in others requires nurses to be attentive to both personal and professional empowerment. This chapter focuses on nursing's role in facilitating empowerment of patients. Understandings of power and empowerment, which are discussed in Chapter 19 relative to nursing empowerment, apply as well to patients. The discussion of empowerment in this chapter flows from these same understandings.

PATIENTS AND EMPOWERMENT

The concept of empowering patients has emerged as nursing has directed its ethical focus to advocacy for patients. Adherence to principles discussed throughout this book, particularly respect for persons, autonomy, justice, and beneficence, makes it incumbent upon nurses to involve patients in making decisions about their health and care. Some patients have both desire and skills to take charge of their lives, some have desire but need to improve their skills, while others have limitations in ability and desire. Negotiating within a system that has traditionally placed decision making authority and power primarily within the hands of physicians requires skill, support, and a strong sense of personal empowerment. Factors discussed in Chapter 19 regarding personal empowerment for nurses apply as well to patients. Patient empowerment is both a process and outcome in which nurses have an active role.

NURSES AND PATIENT EMPOWERMENT

One cannot empower another, as that would strip them of their ability to choose. Although empowerment is something that comes from within a person, nurses can serve as enablers of the process. Enabling the empowerment process requires a paradigm shift away from the paternalistic attitude of knowing what is best for the patient and toward the recognition and acceptance that patients are essentially responsible for their own health and have the ability to discern what they need, make decisions, and direct their own destinies. In order to make appropriate decisions, however, people may need information and support.

Gibson (1991) describes empowerment in the health care arena as "a social process of recognizing, promoting and enhancing people's abilities to meet their own needs, solve their own problems and mobilize the necessary resources in order to feel in control of their own lives . . . a process of helping people to assert control over the factors which affect their health" (p. 339). In light of this description and nursing's focus on patient advocacy, nurses are called to be enablers of the empowerment process with patients, families, and communities. Certain attitudes, knowledge, and skills are basic to fulfilling this role.

Attitudes of Nurses That Enable Empowerment

A view of the nurse as a facilitator and resource rather than merely that of provider of services for patients is basic to enabling empowerment with patients (Gibson,

1991). Nurses must learn to surrender their need for control, developing instead attitudes of collaboration and mutual participation in decision making. This requires self-reflection on the part of the nurse, through which the nurse confronts personal values and subtle, and not so subtle, benefits gained from being in a position of power. It is essential that nurses make a commitment to being with patients as they struggle with their questions and issues and seek meaning in the process. Relinquishing control also means that nurses need to accept decisions made by patients and families, even when they are different from what the nurse might do or suggest. Respect for persons, which includes valuing others and mutual trust, is key (Gibson, 1991; Rodwell, 1996).

Nursing Knowledge and Skills Necessary for Enabling Empowerment

Information presented throughout this book provides a foundation for facilitating the empowerment process. Attention to ethical principles and processes of decision making fosters empowerment. Awareness of the development of values and their impact on choices allows nurses to be more clear about their own perspectives, so as to foster integrity and avoid imposing personal values on others. Knowledge of social, cultural, political, economic, and other forces affecting a person's options and health choices is essential.

Empowerment is an interactive process. As in many other areas of nursing, effective communication is necessary for facilitating empowerment. The ability to listen with one's whole being and to trust intuitive as well as intellectual understanding is important. Reflective listening allows the nurse to help people to recognize their own strengths, abilities, and personal power, as well as to develop awareness of root causes of problems and to determine their readiness to take action for change. If it is determined that the patient does not want to be empowered, nursing interventions need to be provided in a style of empowerment rather than control (Gibson, 1991). This means approaching patients with an attitude of trust in their abilities to know, at some place within themselves, what they need, and to incorporate behaviors such as offering choices about aspects of care over which they can have control.

Having opportunities and resources necessary for understanding and changing one's world is part of the empowerment process. Nurses must have knowledge of factors affecting a patient's health and health care decisions in order to help provide or share the necessary resources. Recognizing that individual responsibility for health is necessarily tempered by social and environmental factors, such knowledge includes awareness of patient and family values and decision making style; cultural context; social, political, and economic influences on one's options; and health care system constraints. Gibson (1991) suggests that nurses need to focus health promotion efforts on the macro social level, attending to conditions that control, influence, and produce health or illness in people. Efforts as individuals, within professional organizations, and within communities, aimed at providing access to health care for all, provide a broad base of support for empowerment.

It is important that nurses approach patients as equal partners. Skillful collaboration and negotiation, which incorporate power sharing and mutually beneficial interactions, enable empowerment. Relinquishing professional power returns power to the patient.

ENHANCING PATIENT CAPACITY FOR DECISION MAKING

The ability to make decisions regarding one's life and destiny requires a basic level of cognitive functioning and sense of control over life and change processes. Empowerment originates in self-esteem; is developed through love, a sense of connectedness, responsibility, and opportunities for choice; and is supported through perceived meaning and hope in life (Rodwell, 1996).

Helping patients to know who they are is an enabler to empowerment. The process of self-discovery enables patients to decide what they want to do based on appreciation of who they are. Thus "the patient's empowerment to make decisions comes from the deepest understanding of the self" (Purtilo & Meier, 1993). This may require facilitating a patient's self-awareness on many levels, such as identifying personal values, sources of these values, where and with whom they feel connected, and where and how they experience control in life. Utilizing the decision making process discussed in Chapter 4 can facilitate empowerment with patients.

Determining whether a person functions primarily from a sense of internal or external locus of control can be useful. **Locus of control** refers to beliefs about the ability to control events in one's life. People who believe that they are able to influence or control things that happen to them are considered to have an **internal locus of control.** On the other hand, people who feel that forces outside of themselves direct or rule their lives, whether these be generalized forces such as fate or other persons who are perceived as more powerful, are considered to have an **external locus of control.** Persons who are internally motivated are more likely to perceive themselves as having power to make choices and control their lives, and to be motivated to make necessary changes. Those who are externally motivated tend to be more fatalistic, expecting their lives to be controlled by powerful others, and less likely to enact personal power (Dawson, 1994; Miller, 1993).

Ask Yourself

How Does Locus of Control Affect Empowerment?

- Reflect on how you have deliberated significant decisions in your life. Do you consider that you are more internally or externally motivated? Give specific examples to support your self-assessment.
- In working with patients what would you consider indications of internal and external locus of control?

- How would your approach to facilitating empowerment be different with persons who exhibit internal locus of control compared to those with external locus of control?

Barriers to Empowerment

Empowerment involves a willingness to take risks, to move beyond that which is known and perhaps comfortable, to the unknown. It often requires a change in self-perception, developing a different vision of who one is. This can stimulate anxiety and fear. Nurses need to recognize such barriers and appreciate that not everyone wants to take the risks and assume the responsibility that empowerment demands. Paternalistic attitudes within the health care system have fostered reliance on health care providers to determine what patients need for health. Other barriers include patient lack of knowledge of resources or strategies that promote empowerment, dependency, apathy, mistrust, and being labeled by staff (Connelly, Keele, Kleinbeck, Schneider, & Cobb, 1993). Social, cultural, economic, or political factors can present barriers such as limitation of resources, control of knowledge about options, locking people into traditional roles and expectations, social labeling that stereotypes and devalues certain people or behaviors, and restriction of access to resources. Lack of empowerment of professionals and their inability to relinquish power to patients affect patient empowerment as well. Honoring patient decisions may be very threatening to nurses who do not appreciate that patients know what they need.

FOSTERING PATIENT EMPOWERMENT

Role modeling self-empowerment is a good starting point for facilitating the process in others. As noted previously, belief that patients have the right and ability to make choices regarding their health, as well as regarding other areas of their lives, is basic to empowerment. Patients need to be given opportunities for choice regarding small as well as major decisions. This means that there needs to be participatory decision making, involving collaboration and negotiation, in all areas of health care. For example, involving patients in making decisions about when they will bathe, what foods to include in their diet, or when to take their medications is as important to empowerment as their participation in decision making regarding life support measures. Because of social, environmental, and other factors, some people have had limited opportunities for making choices and may need education, practice, and nurture in this area. Offering options and developing strategies to enhance the patient's ability to set and reach goals are important parts of the nursing role. Connelly et al. (1993) suggest that choosing implies having both the freedom and the courage to choose from different options. Support is an important part of the encouraging process.

Support can take many forms. It may mean determining what patients identify as being empowering to them and encouraging such choices, behaviors, or attitudes. Caring relationships, in which experiences are shared and patients are accepted for who they are, offer support. Having at least one other person who supports a choice made or a stance that a person takes enhances the likelihood that the person will follow through on the decision.

Considering options and making choices implies having both knowledge and availability of needed resources. Enabling empowerment may require nurses to provide or help patients discover how to access resources. In some instances this may mean becoming politically and socially active regarding health care issues affecting vulnerable populations. Strategies that enhance a patient's ability to acquire necessary knowledge are empowering forces. This may mean working with patients or communities to identify both health concerns and socioculturally relevant approaches to dealing with these concerns. Processes that encourage mutually respectful exchange of ideas and analysis of concerns and potential solutions are needed. Success in achieving goals must be defined from the perspective of the patient or community.

Think About It

Outcomes of Patient Empowerment

Upholding the view that patients know what they need opens nurses to the probability that some patients will make decisions that are not consistent with what the nurse or other health team members think is best. Such decisions may have a relatively minor impact on a patient's or family's health and well-being or may be judged to have potentially serious outcomes for the patient or family.

- What factors need to be considered when dealing with decisions involving differing values between patients and nurses?

- Give examples of situations in which patient empowerment might potentiate an ethical dilemma for you.

- If you feel a patient is making an unwise decision, how would you respond?

- Discuss your view regarding any limits or constraints on patient empowerment.

SUMMARY

Patient empowerment is an important element of nursing care that derives from an appreciation that patients have the ability to discern their needs and make decisions about their lives and health. Being an enabler of empowerment requires that nurses learn to relinquish power and embrace the patient as an equal partner. Self-awareness, respect for others, and effective communication skills serve as foundations for the process. Knowledge about and availability of resources, support, and opportunities for choice are necessary for empowerment. Nurses can facilitate empowerment by working directly with patients and through addressing social, political, and environmental factors affecting empowerment of individuals and communities. In the midst of an ever changing and challenging health care environment in which issues of power and control continue to affect patient care, it is imperative that nurses be competent enablers of patient empowerment.

CHAPTER HIGHLIGHTS

- Patient empowerment, which is both a process and an outcome, relates to ethical principles and flows from nursing's focus on patient advocacy.
- Although nurses cannot empower patients, they can be enablers of empowerment, a process that requires recognition and acceptance that patients have the ability to discern what they need, to make decisions, and to direct their own destinies.
- Empowerment is interactive and requires knowledge of personal values and needs for control, mutual trust and respect, effective communication and reflective listening skills, and a willingness to accept patient decisions regardless of whether the nurse thinks they are best.
- Fostering patient empowerment requires knowledge of social, political, cultural, economic, and environmental factors affecting a person's options and health choices and may involve addressing health promotion efforts on the macro social level.
- Empowerment is fostered through self-discovery, enhanced self-esteem, a sense of connectedness, support, opportunities for choice, and having needed resources, knowledge, and skills.
- Empowerment strategies that mesh with a person's or community's sociocultural context are more effective.

DISCUSSION QUESTIONS AND ACTIVITIES

1. Describe a personal experience as a patient within the health care system in which you felt that you were empowered. What contributed to the empowerment process for you?
2. Describe a patient or family with whom you have worked who exhibited empowerment. Give specific examples of evidences of empowerment from your perspective.
3. Observe practicing nurses in a clinical setting and describe attitudes and behaviors that foster or block empowerment with patients.
4. Discuss factors within the health care system that inhibit patient empowerment.
5. Describe the relationship between patient empowerment and principled behavior in nursing.
6. Describe a situation in which you believe you fostered empowerment with a patient or family. How did you enable the process? Describe the outcome.
7. What would indicate to you that a patient might not want to be empowered? How would you approach and work with this patient?

REFERENCES

Chinn, P. L. (1995). *Peace & power: Building communities for the future* (4th ed.). New York: National League of Nursing Press.

Connelly, L. M., Keele, B. S., Kleinbeck, S. V. M., Schneider, J. K., & Cobb, A. K. (1993). A place to be yourself: Empowerment from the client's perspective. *Image, 25,* 297–303.

Dawson, M. S. (1994). Using locus of control to empower student nurses to be professional. *Nursing Forum, 29,* 10–15.

Gibson, C. H. (1991). A concept analysis of empowerment. *Journal of Advanced Nursing, 16,* 354–361.

Miller, C. M. (1993). Trajectory and empowerment theory applied to care of patients with multiple sclerosis. *Journal of Neuroscience Nursing, 25,* 343–348.

Purtilo, R. B., & Meier, R. H. (1993). Team challenges: Regulatory constraints and patient empowerment. *American Journal of Physical Medicine & Rehabilitation, 72,* 327–330.

Rodwell, C. M. (1996). An analysis of the concept of empowerment. *Journal of Advanced Nursing, 23,* 305–313.

Code for Nurses with Interpretive Statements
American Nurses Association

Copies are available for purchase through American Nurses Publishing (800) 637-0323

Reprinted with permission of the American Nurses Association, copyright 1985

PREAMBLE

A code of ethics makes explicit the primary goals and values of the profession. When individuals become nurses, they make a moral commitment to uphold the values and special moral obligations expressed in their code. The Code for Nurses is based on a belief about the nature of individuals, nursing, health, and society. Nursing encompasses the protection, promotion, and restoration of health; the prevention of illness; and the alleviation of suffering in the care of clients, including individuals, families, groups, and communities. In the context of these functions, nursing is defined as the diagnosis and treatment of human responses to actual or potential health problems.

Since clients themselves are the primary decision makers in matters concerning their own health, treatment, and well-being, the goal of nursing actions is to support and enhance the client's responsibility and self-determination to the greatest extent possible. In this context, health is not necessarily an end in itself, but rather a means to a life that is meaningful from the client's perspective.

When making clinical judgments, nurses base their decisions on consideration of consequences and of universal moral principles, both of which prescribe and justify nursing actions. The most fundamental of these principles is respect for persons. Other principles stemming from this basic principle are autonomy (self-determination), beneficence (doing good), nonmaleficence (avoiding harm), veracity (truth-telling), confidentiality (respecting privileged information), fidelity (keeping promises), and justice (treating people fairly).

In brief, then, the statements of the code and their interpretation provide guidance for conduct and relationships in carrying out nursing responsibilities consistent with the ethical obligations of the profession and with high quality in nursing care.

INTRODUCTION

A code of ethics indicates a profession's acceptance of the responsibility and trust with which it has been invested by society. Under the terms of the implicit contract between society and the nursing profession, society grants the profession considerable autonomy and authority to function in the conduct of its affairs. The development of a code of ethics is an essential activity of a profession and provides one means for the exercise of professional self-regulation.

Upon entering the profession, each nurse inherits a measure of both the responsibility and the trust that have accrued to nursing over the years, as well as the corresponding obligation to adhere to the profession's code of conduct and relationships for ethical practice. The *Code for Nurses with Interpretive Statements* is thus more a collective expression of nursing conscience and philosophy than a set of external rules imposed upon an individual practitioner of nursing. Personal and professional integrity can be assured only if an individual is committed to the profession's code of conduct.

A code of ethical conduct offers general principles to guide and evaluate nursing actions. It does not assure the virtues required for professional practice within the character of each nurse. In particular situations, the justification of behavior as ethical must satisfy not only the individual nurse acting as a moral agent but also the standards for professional peer review.

The Code for Nurses was adopted by the American Nurses Association in 1950 and has been revised periodically. It serves to inform both the nurse and society of the profession's expectations and requirement in ethical matters. The code and the interpretive statements together provide a framework within which nurses can make ethical decisions and discharge their responsibilities to the public, to other members of the health team, and to the profession.

Although a particular situation by its nature may determine the use of specific moral principles, the basic philosophical values, directives, and suggestions provided here are widely applicable to situations encountered in clinical practice. The Code for Nurses is not open to negotiation in employment settings, nor is it permissible for individuals or groups of nurses to adapt or change the language of this code.

The requirements of the code may often exceed those of the law. Violations of the law may subject the nurse to civil or criminal liability. The state nurses' associations, in fulfilling the profession's duty to society, may discipline their members for violations of the code. Loss of the respect and confidence of society and of one's colleagues is a serious sanction resulting from violation of the code. In addition, every nurse has a personal obligation to uphold and adhere to the code and to ensure that nursing colleagues do likewise.

Guidance and assistance in applying the code to local situations may be obtained from the American Nurses Association and the constituent state nurses' associations.

CODE FOR NURSES WITH INTERPRETIVE STATEMENTS

1 The nurse provides services with respect for human dignity and the uniqueness of the client, unrestricted by consideration of social or economic status, personal attributes, or the nature of health problems.

1.1 Respect for Human Dignity

The fundamental principle of nursing practice is respect for the inherent dignity and worth of every client. Nurses are morally obligated to respect human existence and the individuality of all persons who are the recipients of nursing actions. Nurses therefore must take all reasonable means to protect and preserve human life when there is hope of recovery or reasonable hope of benefit from life-prolonging treatment.

Truth telling and the process of reaching informed choice underlie the exercise of self-determination, which is basic to respect for persons. Clients should be as fully involved as possible in the planning and implementation of their own health care. Clients have the moral right to determine what will be done with their own person; to be given accurate information, and all the information necessary for making informed judgments; to be assisted with weighing the benefits and burdens of options in their treatment; to accept, refuse, or terminate treatment without coercion; and to be given necessary emotional support. Each nurse has an obligation to be knowledgeable about the moral and legal rights of all clients and to protect and support those rights. In situations in which the client lacks the capacity to make a decision, a surrogate decision maker should be designated.

Individuals are interdependent members of the community. Taking into account both individual rights and the interdependence of persons in decision making, the nurse recognizes those situations in which individual rights to autonomy in health care may temporarily be overridden to preserve the life of the human community; for example, when a disaster demands triage or when an individual presents a direct danger to others. The many variables involved make it imperative that each case be considered with full awareness of the need to preserve the rights and responsibilities of clients and the demands of justice. The suspension of individual rights must always be considered a deviation to be tolerated as briefly as possible.

1.2 Status and Attributes of Clients

The need for health care is universal, transcending all national, ethnic, racial, religious, cultural, political, educational, economic, developmental, personality, role, and sexual differences. Nursing care is delivered without prejudicial behavior. Individual value systems and life-styles should be considered in the planning of health care with and for each client. Attributes of clients influence nursing practice to the extent that they represent factors the nurse must understand, consider, and respect in tailoring care to personal needs and in maintaining the individual's self-respect and dignity.

1.3 The Nature of Health Problems

The nurse's respect for the worth and dignity of the individual human being applies, irrespective of the nature of the health problem. It is reflected in care given the person who is disabled as well as one without disability, the person with long-term illness as well as one with acute illness, the recovering patient as well as one in the last phase of life. This respect extends to all who require the services of the nurse for the promotion of health, the prevention of illness, the restoration of health, the alleviation of suffering, and the provision of supportive care of the dying. The nurse does not act deliberately to terminate the life of any person.

The nurse's concern for human dignity and for the provision of high quality nursing care is not limited by personal attitudes or beliefs. If ethically opposed to interventions in a particular case because of the procedures to be used, the nurse is justified in refusing to participate. Such refusal should be made known in advance and in time for other appropriate arrangements to be made for the client's nursing care. If the nurse becomes involved in such a case and the client's life is in jeopardy, the nurse is obliged to provide for the client's safety, to avoid abandonment, and to withdraw only when assured that alternative sources of nursing care are available to the client.

The measures nurses take to care for the dying client and the client's family emphasize human contact. They enable the client to live with as much physical, emotional, and spiritual comfort as possible, and they maximize the values the client has treasured in life. Nursing care is directed toward the prevention and relief of the suffering commonly associated with the dying process. The nurse may provide interventions to relieve symptoms in the dying client even when the interventions entail substantial risks of hastening death.

1.4 The Setting for Health Care

The nurse adheres to the principle of nondiscriminatory, nonprejudicial care in every situation and endeavors to promote its acceptance by others. The setting shall not determine the nurse's readiness to respect clients and to render or obtain needed services.

 The nurse safeguards the client's right to privacy by judiciously protecting information of a confidential nature.

2.1 The Client's Right to Privacy

The right to privacy is an inalienable human right. The client trusts the nurse to hold all information in confidence. This trust could be destroyed and the client's welfare jeopardized by injudicious disclosure of information provided in confidence. The duty of confidentiality, however, is not absolute when innocent parties are in direct jeopardy.

2.2 Protection of Information

The rights, well-being, and safety of the individual client should be the determining factors in arriving at any professional judgment concerning the disposition of confidential information received from the client relevant to his or her treatment. The standards of nursing practice and the nursing responsibility to provide high quality health services require that relevant data be shared with members of the health team. Only information pertinent to a client's treatment and welfare is disclosed, and it is disclosed only to those directly concerned with the client's care.

Information documenting the appropriateness, necessity, and quality of care required for the purposes of peer review, third-party payment, and other quality assurance mechanisms must be disclosed only under defined policies, mandates, or protocols. These written guidelines must assure that the rights, well-being, and safety of the client are maintained.

2.3 Access to Records

If in the course of providing care there is a need for the nurse to have access to the records of persons not under the nurse's care, the persons affected should be notified and, whenever possible, permission should be obtained first. Although records belong to the agency where the data are collected, the individual maintains the right of control over the information in the record. Similarly, professionals may exercise the right of control over information they have generated in the course of health care.

If the nurse wishes to use a client's treatment record for research or nonclinical purposes in which anonymity cannot be guaranteed, the client's consent must be obtained first. Ethically, this ensures the client's right to privacy; legally, it protects the client against unlawful invasion of privacy.

3 The nurse acts to safeguard the client and the public when health care and safety are affected by incompetent, unethical, or illegal practice by any person.

3.1 Safeguarding the Health and Safety of the Client

The nurse's primary commitment is to the health, welfare, and safety of the client. As an advocate for the client, the nurse must be alert to and take appropriate action regarding any instances of incompetent, unethical, or illegal practice by any member of the health care team or the health care system, or any action on the part of others that places the rights or best interests of the client in jeopardy. To function effectively in this role, nurses must be aware of the employing institution's policies and procedures, nursing standards of practice, the Code for Nurses, and laws governing nursing and health care practice with regard to incompetent, unethical, or illegal practice.

3.2 Acting on Questionable Practice

When the nurse is aware of inappropriate or questionable practice in the provision of health care, concern should be expressed to the person carrying out the questionable practice and attention called to the possible detrimental effect upon the client's welfare. When factors in the health care delivery system threaten the welfare of the client, similar action should be directed to the responsible administrative person. If indicated, the practice should then be reported to the appropriate authority within the institution, agency, or larger system.

There should be an established process for the reporting and handling of incompetent, unethical, or illegal practice within the employment setting so that such reporting can go through official channels without causing fear of reprisal. The nurse should be knowledgeable about the process and be prepared to use it if necessary. When questions are raised about the practices of individual practitioners or of health care systems, written documentation of the observed practices or behaviors must be available to the appropriate authorities. State nurses' associations should be prepared to provide assistance and support in the development and evaluation of such processes and in reporting procedures.

When incompetent, unethical, or illegal practice on the part of anyone concerned with the client's care is not corrected within the employment setting and continues to jeopardize the client's welfare and safety, the problem should be reported to other appropriate authorities such as practice committees of the pertinent professional organizations or the legally constituted bodies concerned with licensing of specific categories of health workers or professional practitioners. Some situations may warrant the concern and involvement of all such groups. Accurate reporting and documentation undergird all actions.

3.3 Review Mechanisms

The nurse should participate in the planning, establishment, implementation, and evaluation of review mechanisms that serve to safeguard clients, such as duly constituted peer review processes or committees and ethics committees. Such ongoing review mechanisms are based on established criteria, have stated purposes, include a process for making recommendations, and facilitate improved delivery of nursing and other health services to clients wherever nursing services are provided.

 The nurse assumes responsibility and accountability for individual nursing judgments and actions.

4.1 Acceptance of Responsibility and Accountability

The recipients of professional nursing services are entitled to high quality nursing care. Individual professional licensure is the protective mechanism legislated by the public to ensure the basic and minimum competencies of the professional nurse. Beyond that, society has accorded to the nursing profession the right to regulate its own practice.

The regulation and control of nursing practice by nurses demand that individual practitioners of professional nursing must bear primary responsibility for the nursing care clients receive and must be individually accountable for their own practice.

4.2 Responsibility for Nursing Judgment and Action

Responsibility refers to the carrying out of duties associated with a particular role assumed by the nurse. Nursing obligations are reflected in the ANA publications *Nursing: A Social Policy Statement* and *Standards of Nursing Practice.* In recognizing the rights of clients, the standards describe a collaborative relationship between the nurse and the client through use of the nursing process. Nursing responsibilities include data collection and assessment of the health status of the client; formation of nursing diagnoses derived from client assessment; development of a nursing care plan that is directed toward designated goals, assists the client in maximizing his or her health capabilities, and provides for the client's participation in promoting, maintaining, and restoring his or her health; evaluation of the effectiveness of nursing care in achieving goals as determined by the client and the nurse; and subsequent reassessment and revision of the nursing care plan as warranted. In the process of assuming these responsibilities, the nurse is held accountable for them.

4.3 Accountability for Nursing Judgment and Action

Accountability refers to being answerable to someone for something one has done. It means providing an explanation or rationale to oneself, to clients, to peers, to the nursing profession, and to society. In order to be accountable, nurses act under a code of ethical conduct that is grounded in the moral principles of fidelity and respect for the dignity, worth, and self-determination of clients.

The nursing profession continues to develop ways to clarify nursing's accountability to society. The contract between the profession and society is made explicit through such mechanisms as (a) the Code for Nurses, (b) the standards of nursing practice, (c) the development of nursing theory derived from nursing research in order to guide nursing actions, (d) educational requirements for practice, (e) certification, and (f) mechanisms for evaluating the effectiveness of the nurse's performance of nursing responsibilities.

Nurses are accountable for judgments made and actions taken in the course of nursing practice. Neither physicians' orders nor the employing agency's policies relieve the nurse of accountability for actions taken and judgments made.

5 **The nurse maintains competence in nursing.**

5.1 Personal Responsibility for Competence

The profession of nursing is obligated to provide adequate and competent nursing care. Therefore it is the personal responsibility of each nurse to maintain competency in practice. For the client's optimum well-being and for the nurse's own professional development, the care of the client reflects and incorporates new techniques and knowledge in health care as these develop, especially as they relate to the nurse's particular field of practice. The nurse must be aware of the need for continued professional learning and must assume personal responsibility for currency of knowledge and skills.

5.2 Measurement of Competence in Nursing Practice

Evaluation of one's performance by peers is a hallmark of professionalism and a method by which the profession is held accountable to society. Nurses must be willing to have their practice reviewed and evaluated by their peers. Guidelines for evaluating the scope of practice and the appropriateness, effectiveness, and efficiency of nursing practice are found in nursing practice acts, ANA standards of practice, and other quality assurance mechanisms. Each nurse is responsible for participating in the development of objective criteria for evaluation. In addition, the nurse engages in ongoing self-evaluation of clinical competency, decision-making abilities, and professional judgments.

5.3 Intraprofessional Responsibility for Competence in Nursing Care

Nurses share responsibility for high quality nursing care. Nurses are required to have knowledge relevant to the current scope of nursing practice, changing issues and concerns, and ethical concepts and principles. Since individual competencies vary, nurses refer clients to and consult with other nurses with expertise and recognized competencies in various fields of practice.

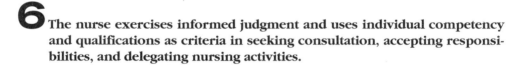

6 The nurse exercises informed judgment and uses individual competency and qualifications as criteria in seeking consultation, accepting responsibilities, and delegating nursing activities.

6.1 Changing Functions

Nurses are faced with decisions in the context of the increased complexity of health care, changing patterns in the delivery of health services, and the development of evolving nursing practice in response to the health needs of clients. As the scope of nursing practice changes, the nurse must exercise judgment in accepting responsibilities, seeking consultation, and assigning responsibilities to others who carry out nursing care.

6.2 Accepting Responsibilities

The nurse must not engage in practices prohibited by law or delegate to others activities prohibited by practice acts of other health care personnel or by other laws. Nurses determine the scope of their practice in light of their education, knowledge, competency, and extent of experience. If the nurse concludes that he or she lacks competence or is inadequately prepared to carry out a specific function, the nurse has the responsibility to refuse that work and to seek alternative sources of care based on concern for the client's welfare. In that refusal, both the client and the nurse are protected. Inasmuch as the nurse is responsible for the continuous care of patients in health care settings, the nurse is frequently called upon to carry out components of care delegated by other health professionals as part of the client's treatment regimen. The nurse should not accept these interdependent functions if they are so extensive as to prevent the nurse from fulfilling the responsibility to provide appropriate nursing care to clients.

6.3 Consultation and Collaboration

The provision of health and illness care to clients is a complex process that requires a wide range of knowledge, skills, and collaborative efforts. Nurses must be aware of their own individual competencies. When the needs of the client are beyond the qualifications and competencies of the nurse, consultation and collaboration must be sought from qualified nurses, other health professionals, or the appropriate sources. Participation on intradisciplinary or interdisciplinary teams is often an effective approach to the provision of high quality total health services.

6.4 Delegation of Nursing Activities

Inasmuch as the nurse is accountable for the quality of nursing care rendered to clients, nurses are accountable for the delegation of nursing care activities to other health workers. Therefore, the nurse must assess individual competency in assigning selected components of nursing care to other nursing service personnel. The nurse should not delegate to any member of the nursing team a function for which that person is not prepared or qualified. Employer policies or directives do not relieve the nurse of accountability for making judgments about the delegation of nursing care activities.

7 The nurse participates in activities that contribute to the ongoing development of the profession's body of knowledge.

7.1 The Nurse and Development of Knowledge

Every profession must engage in scholarly inquiry to identify, verify, and continually enlarge the body of knowledge that forms the foundation for its practice. A unique body of verified knowledge provides both framework and direction for the profession in all of its activities and for the practitioner in the provision of nursing care. The accrual of scientific and humanistic knowledge promotes the advancement of practice and the well-being of the profession's clients. Ongoing scholarly activity such as research and the development of theory is indispensable to the full discharge of a profession's obligations to society. Each nurse has a role in this area of professional activity, whether as an investigator in furthering knowledge, as a participant in research, or as a user of theoretical and empirical knowledge.

7.2 Protection of Rights of Human Participants in Research

Individual rights valued by society and by the nursing profession that have particular application in research include the right of adequately informed consent, the right to freedom from risk of injury, and the right of privacy and preservation of dignity. Inherent in these rights is respect for each individual's rights to exercise self-determination, to choose to participate or not, to have full information, and to terminate participation in research without penalty.

It is the duty of the nurse functioning in any research role to maintain vigilance in protecting the life, health, and privacy of human subjects from both anticipated and unanticipated risks and in assuring informed consent. Subjects' integrity, privacy, and rights must be especially safeguarded if the subjects are unable to protect themselves because of incapacity or because they are in a dependent relationship to the investigator. The investigation should be discontinued if its continuance might be harmful to the subject.

7.3 General Guidelines for Participation in Research

Before participation in research conducted by others, the nurse has an obligation to (a) obtain information about the intent and the nature of the research and (b) ascertain that the study proposal is approved by the appropriate bodies, such as institutional review boards.

Research should be conducted and directed by qualified persons. The nurse who participates in research in any capacity should be fully informed about both the nurse's and the client's rights and obligations.

8 The nurse participates in the profession's efforts to implement and improve standards of nursing.

8.1 Responsibility to the Public for Standards

Nursing is responsible and accountable for admitting to the profession only those individuals who have demonstrated the knowledge, skills, and commitment considered essential to professional practice. Nurse educators have a major responsibility for ensuring that these competencies and a demonstrated commitment to professional practice have been achieved before the entry of an individual into the practice of professional nursing.

Established standards and guidelines for nursing practice provide guidance for the delivery of professional nursing care and are a means for evaluating care received by the public. The nurse has a personal responsibility and commitment to clients for implementation and maintenance of optimal standards of nursing practice.

8.2 Responsibility to the Profession for Standards

Established standards reflect the practice of nursing grounded in ethical commitments and a body of knowledge. Professional standards or guidelines exist in nursing practice, nursing service, nursing education, and nursing research. The nurse has the responsibility to monitor these standards in daily practice and to participate actively in the profession's ongoing efforts to foster optimal standards of practice at the local, regional, state, and national levels of the health care system.

Nurse educators have the additional responsibility to maintain optimal standards of nursing practice and education in nursing education programs and in any other settings where planned learning activities for nursing students take place.

9 The nurse participates in the profession's efforts to establish and maintain conditions of employment conducive to high quality nursing care.

9.1 Responsibility for Conditions of Employment

The nurse must be concerned with conditions of employment that (a) enable the nurse to practice in accordance with the standards of nursing practice and (b) provide a care environment that meets the standards of nursing service. The provision of high quality nursing care is the responsibility of both the individual nurse and the nursing profession. Professional autonomy and self-regulation in the control of conditions of practice are necessary for implementing nursing standards.

9.2 Maintaining Conditions for High Quality Nursing Care

Articulation and control of nursing practice can be accomplished through individual agreement and collective action. A nurse may enter into an agreement with individuals or organizations to provide health care. Nurses may participate in collective action such as collective bargaining through their state nurses' association to determine the terms and conditions of employment conducive to high quality nursing care. Such agreements should be consistent with the profession's standards of practice, the state law regulating nursing practice, and the Code for Nurses.

10 The nurse participates in the profession's effort to protect the public from misinformation and misrepresentation and to maintain the integrity of nursing.

10.1 Protection from Misinformation and Misrepresentation

Nurses are responsible for advising clients against the use of products that endanger the clients' safety and welfare. The nurse shall not use any form of public or professional communication to make claims that are false, fraudulent, misleading, deceptive, or unfair.

The nurse does not give or imply endorsement to advertising, promotion, or sale of commercial products or services in a manner that may be interpreted as reflecting the opinion or judgment of the profession as a whole. The nurse may use knowledge of specific services or products in advising an individual client, since this may contribute to the client's health and well-being. In the course of providing information or education to clients or other practitioners about commercial products or services, however, a variety of similar products or services should be offered or described so the client or practitioner can make an informed choice.

10.2 Maintaining the Integrity of Nursing

The use of the title *registered nurse* is granted by state governments for the protection of the public. Use of that title carries with it the responsibility to act in the public interest. The nurse may use the title *R.N.* and symbols of academic degrees or other earned or honorary professional symbols of recognition in all ways that are legal and appropriate. The title and other symbols of the profession should not be used, however, for benefits unrelated to nursing practice or the profession, or used by those who may seek to exploit them for other purposes.

Nurses should refrain from casting a vote in any deliberations involving health care services or facilities where the nurse has business or other interests that could be construed as a conflict of interest.

11 The nurse collaborates with members of the health professions and other citizens in promoting community and national efforts to meet the health needs of the public.

11.1 Collaboration with Others to Meet Health Needs

The availability and accessibility of high quality health services to all people require collaborative planning at the local, state, national, and international levels that respects the interdependence of health professionals and clients in health care systems. Nursing care is an integral part of high quality health care, and nurses have an obligation to promote equitable access to nursing and health care for all people.

11.2 Responsibility to the Public

The nursing profession is committed to promotion of the welfare and safety of all people. The goals and values of nursing are essential to effective delivery of health services. For the benefit of the individual client and the public at large, nursing's goals and commitments need adequate representation. Nurses should ensure this representation by active participation in decision making in institutional and political arenas to assure a just distribution of health care and nursing resources.

11.3 Relationships with Other Disciplines

The complexity of health care delivery systems requires a multidisciplinary approach to delivery of services that has the strong support and active participation of all the health professions. Nurses should actively promote the collaborative planning required to ensure the availability and accessibility of high quality health services to all persons whose health needs are unmet.

APPENDIX B

A Patient's Bill of Rights
American Hospital Association

Reprinted with permission of the American Hospital Association, copyright 1992

INTRODUCTION

Effective health care requires collaboration between patients and physicians and other health care professionals. Open and honest communication, respect for personal and professional values, and sensitivity to differences are integral to optimal patient care. As the setting for the provision of health services, hospitals must provide a foundation for understanding and respecting the rights and responsibilities of patients, their families, physicians, and other caregivers. Hospitals must ensure a health care ethic that respects the role of patients in decision making about treatment choices and other aspects of their care. Hospitals must be sensitive to cultural, racial, linguistic, religious, age, gender, and other differences as well as the needs of persons with disabilities.

The American Hospital Association presents *A Patient's Bill of Rights* with the expectation that it will contribute to more effective patient care and be supported by the hospital on behalf of the institution, its medical staff, employees, and patients. The American Hospital Association encourages health care institutions to tailor this bill of rights to their patient community by translating and/or simplifying the language of this bill of rights as may be necessary to ensure that patients and their families understand their rights and responsibilities.

BILL OF RIGHTS*

1. The patient has the right to considerate and respectful care.

2. The patient has the right to and is encouraged to obtain from physicians and other direct caregivers relevant, current, and understandable information concerning diagnosis, treatment, and prognosis.

   Except in emergencies when the patient lacks decision-making capacity and the need for treatment is urgent, the patient is entitled to the opportunity to discuss and request information related to the specific procedures and/or treatments, the risks involved, the possible length of recuperation, and the medically reasonable alternatives and their accompanying risks and benefits.

   Patients have the right to know the identity of physicians, nurses, and others involved in their care, as well as when those involved are students, residents, or other trainees. The patient also has the right to know the immediate and long-term financial implications of treatment choices, insofar as they are known.

3. The patient has the right to make decisions about the plan of care prior to and during the course of treatment and to refuse a recommended treatment or plan of care to the extent permitted by law and hospital policy and to be informed of the medical consequences of this action. In case of such refusal, the patient is entitled to other appropriate care and services that the hospital provides or transfer to another hospital. The hospital should notify patients of any policy that might affect patient choices within the institution.

4. The patient has the right to have an advance directive (such as a living will, health care proxy, or durable power of attorney for health care) concerning treatment or designating a surrogate decision maker with the expectation that the hospital will honor the intent of that directive to the extent permitted by law and hospital policy.

   Health care institutions must advise patients of their rights under state law and hospital policy to make informed medical choices, ask if the patient has an advance directive, and include that information in patient records. The patient has the right to timely information about hospital policy that may limit its ability to implement fully a legally valid advance directive.

5. The patient has the right to every consideration of privacy. Case discussion, consultation, examination, and treatment should be conducted so as to protect each patient's privacy.

6. The patient has the right to expect that all communications and records pertaining to his/her care will be treated as confidential by the hospital, except in cases such as suspected abuse and public health hazards when reporting is permitted or required by law. The patient has the right to expect that the hospital will emphasize the confidentiality of this information when it releases it to any other parties entitled to review information in these records.

---

*These rights can be exercised on the patient's behalf by a designated surrogate or proxy decision maker if the patient lacks decision-making capacity, is legally incompetent or is a minor.

7. The patient has the right to review the records pertaining to his/her medical care and to have the information explained or interpreted as necessary, except when restricted by law.

8. The patient has the right to expect that, within its capacity and policies, a hospital will make reasonable response to the request of a patient for appropriate and medically indicated care and services. The hospital must provide evaluation, service, and/or referral as indicated by the urgency of the case. When medically appropriate and legally permissible, or when a patient has so requested, a patient may be transferred to another facility. The institution to which the patient is to be transferred must first have accepted the patient for transfer. The patient must also have the benefit of complete information and explanation concerning the need for, risks, benefits, and alternatives to such a transfer.

9. The patient has the right to ask and be informed of the existence of business relationships among the hospital, educational institutions, other health care providers, or payers that may influence the patient's treatment and care.

10. The patient has the right to consent to or decline to participate in proposed research studies or human experimentation affecting care and treatment or requiring direct patient involvement, and to have those studies fully explained prior to consent. A patient who declines to participate in research or experimentation is entitled to the most effective care that the hospital can otherwise provide.

11. The patient has the right to expect reasonable continuity of care when appropriate and to be informed by physicians and other caregivers of available and realistic patient care options when hospital care is no longer appropriate.

12. The patient has the right to be informed of hospital policies and practices that relate to patient care, treatment, and responsibilities. The patient has the right to be informed of available resources for resolving disputes, grievances, and conflicts, such as ethics committees, patient representatives, or other mechanisms available in the institution. The patient has the right to be informed of the hospital's charges for services and available payment methods.

The collaborative nature of health care requires that patients, or their families/surrogates, participate in their care. The effectiveness of care and patient satisfaction with the course of treatment depend, in part, on the patient fulfilling certain responsibilities. Patients are responsible for providing information about past illnesses, hospitalizations, medications, and other matters related to health status. To participate effectively in decision making, patients must be encouraged to take responsibility for requesting additional information or clarification about their health status or treatment when they do not fully understand information and instructions. Patients are also responsible for ensuring that the health care institution has a copy of their written advance directive if they have one. Patients are responsible for informing their physicians and other caregivers if they anticipate problems in following prescribed treatment.

Patients should also be aware of the hospital's obligation to be reasonably efficient and equitable in providing care to other patients and the community. The hospital's rules and regulations are designed to help the hospital meet this obligation. Patients and their families are responsible for making reasonable accommodations to the needs of the hospital, other patients, medical staff, and hospital employees. Patients are responsible for providing necessary information for insurance claims and for working with the hospital to make payment arrangements, when necessary.

A person's health depends on much more than health care services. Patients are responsible for recognizing the impact of their life-style on their personal health.

CONCLUSION

Hospitals have many functions to perform, including the enhancement of health status, health promotion, and the prevention and treatment of injury and disease; the immediate and ongoing care and rehabilitation of patients; the education of health professionals, patients, and the community; and research. All these activities must be conducted with an overriding concern for the values and dignity of patients.

APPENDIX C

Code of Ethics for Registered Nurses
Canadian Nurses Association

Reprinted with permission of the Canadian Nurses Association, copyright 1997

PREAMBLE

The *Code of Ethics for Registered Nurses* gives guidance for decision-making concerning ethical matters, serves as a means for self-evaluation and reflection regarding ethical nursing practice, and provides a basis for peer review initiatives. The code not only educates nurses about their ethical responsibilities, but also informs other health care professionals and members of the public about the moral commitments expected of nurses.

The Canadian Nurses Association (CNA) periodically revises its code to address changing societal needs, values, and conditions that challenge the ability of nurses to practice ethically. Examples of such factors are: the consequences of economic constraints; increasing use of technology in health care; and, changing ways of delivering nursing services, such as the move to care outside the institutional setting. This revised *Code of Ethics for Registered Nurses* provides nurses with direction for ethical decision-making and practice in everyday situations as they are influenced by current trends and conditions. It applies to nurses in all practice settings, whatever their position and area of responsibility.

Ethical problems and concerns, as well as ethical distress at the individual level, can be the result of decisions made at the institutional, regional, provincial and federal levels. Differing responsibilities, capabilities and ways of working toward change also exist at the client, institutional and societal levels. For all contexts the code offers guidance on providing care that conforms with ethical practice, and on actively influencing and participating in policy development, review and revision.

The complex issues in nursing practice have both legal and ethical dimensions. The laws and ethics of health care overlap, as both are concerned that the conduct of health professionals show respect for the well-being, dignity and liberty of clients. An ideal system of law would be compatible with ethics, in that adherence to the law ought never require the violation of ethics. Still, the domains of law and ethics remain distinct, and the code addresses ethical responsibilities only.

ELEMENTS OF THE CODE

A value is something that is prized or held dear; something that is deeply cared about. This code is organized around seven primary values that are central to ethical nursing practice:

- **Health and well-being**
- **Choice**
- **Dignity**
- **Confidentiality**
- **Fairness**
- **Accountability**
- **Practice environments that are conducive to safe, competent and ethical care.**

Each value is articulated by responsibility statements that clarify its application and provide more direct guidance. Where it is clear that an action or inaction would involve an **ethical violation** (i.e., the neglect of a moral obligation), the level of guidance is prescriptive. The statement is intended to tell the nurse and others what is ethically acceptable and what is not. Where the situation involves an **ethical problem** or dilemma, guidance is advisory. No ready-made answers can be offered and thoughtful consideration is required to increase the quality of decision-making. Where the situation provokes feelings of guilt, concern, or distaste, it is a situation of ethical distress. In instances of **ethical distress** the level of guidance is more limited but there remains a responsibility for the nurse to examine the situation in light of the provisions of the code. Decisions will be influenced by the particular circumstances of the situation. Ethical reflection and judgement are required to determine how a particular value or responsibility applies in a particular nursing context.

There is room within the profession for disagreement among nurses about the relative weight of different ethical values and principles. More than one proposed intervention may be ethical and reflective of good practice. Discussion is extremely helpful in the resolution of ethical issues. As appropriate, clients, colleagues in nursing and other disciplines, professional nurses' associations and other experts are included in discussions about ethical problems. In addition to this code, legislation, and the standards of practice, policies, and guidelines of professional nurses associations may also assist in problem-solving.

The values articulated in this code are grounded in the professional nursing relationship with clients and indicate what nurses care about in that relationship. For example, to identify health and well-being as a value is to say that nurses care for and about the health and well-being of their clients. The nurse-client relationship presupposes a certain measure of trust on the part of the client. Care and trust complement one another in professional nursing relationships. Both hinge on the values identified in the code. By upholding these values in practice, nurses earn and maintain the trust of those in their care. For each of the values, the scope of responsibilities identified extends beyond individuals to include families, communities and society.

HEALTH AND WELL-BEING

Nurses value health and well-being and assist persons to achieve their optimum level of health in situations of normal health, illness, injury, or in the process of dying.

1. Nurses provide care directed first and foremost toward the health and well-being of the client.

2. Nurses recognize that health is more than the absence of disease or infirmity and assist clients to achieve the maximum level of health and well-being possible.

3. Nurses recognize that health status is influenced by a variety of factors. In ways that are consistent with their professional role and responsibilities, nurses are accountable for addressing institutional, social, and political factors influencing health and health care.

4. Nurses support and advocate a full continuum of health services including health promotion and disease prevention initiatives, as well as diagnostic, restorative, rehabilitative and palliative care services.

5. Nurses respect and value the knowledge and skills other health care providers bring to the health care team and actively seek to support and collaborate with others so that maximum benefits to clients can be realized.

6. Nurses foster well-being when life can no longer be sustained, by alleviating suffering and supporting a dignified and peaceful death.

7. Nurses provide the best care circumstances permit even when the need arises in an emergency outside an employment situation.

8. Nurses participate, to the best of their abilities, in research and other activities that contribute to the ongoing development of nursing knowledge. Nurses participating in research observe the nursing profession's guidelines, as well as other guidelines, for ethical research.

CHOICE

Nurses respect and promote the autonomy of clients and help them to express their health needs and values, and to obtain appropriate information and services.

1. Nurses seek to involve clients in health planning and health care decision-making.

2. Nurses provide the information and support required so that clients, to the best of their ability, are able to act on their own behalf in meeting their health and health care needs. Information given is complete, accurate, truthful, and understandable. When they are unable to provide the required information, nurses assist clients in obtaining it from other appropriate sources.

3. Nurses demonstrate sensitivity to the willingness/readiness of clients to receive information about their health condition and care options. Nurses respect the wishes of those who refuse, or are not ready, to receive information about their health condition.

4. Nurses practice within relevant legislation governing consent or choice. Nurses seek to ensure that nursing care is authorized by informed choice, and are guided by this ideal when participating in the consent process in cooperation with other members of the health team.

5. Nurses respect the informed decisions of competent persons to refuse treatment and to choose to live at risk. However, nurses are not obliged to comply with clients' wishes when doing so would require action contrary to the law. If the care requested is contrary to the nurse's moral beliefs, appropriate care is provided until alternative care arrangements are in place to meet the client's needs.

6. Nurses are sensitive to their position of relative power in professional relationships with clients and take care to foster self-determination on the part of their clients. Nurses are sufficiently clear about personal values to recognize and deal appropriately with potential value conflicts.

7. Nurses respect decisions and lawful directives, written or verbal, about present and future health care choices affirmed by a client prior to becoming incompetent.

8. Nurses seek to involve clients of diminished competence in decision-making to the extent that those clients are capable. Nurses continue to value autonomy when illness or other factors reduce the capacity for self-determination, such as by providing opportunities for clients to make choices about aspects of their lives for which they maintain the capacity to make decisions.

9. Nurses seek to obtain consent for nursing care from a substitute decision-maker when clients lack the capacity to make decisions about their care, did not make their wishes known prior to becoming incompetent, or for any reason it is unclear what the client would have wanted in a particular circumstance. When prior wishes of an incompetent client are not known or are unclear, care decisions must be in the best interest of the client and are based on what the client would want, as far as it is known.

DIGNITY

Nurses value and advocate the dignity and self-respect of human beings.

1. Nurses relate to all persons receiving care as persons worthy of respect and endeavor in all their actions to preserve and demonstrate respect for each individual.

2. Nurses exhibit sensitivity to the client's individual needs, values, and choices. Nursing care is designed to accommodate the biological, psychological, social, cultural, and spiritual needs of clients. Nurses do not exploit clients' vulnerabilities for their own interests or gain, whether this be sexual, emotional, social, political, or financial.

3. Nurses respect the privacy of clients when care is given.

4. Nurses treat human life as precious and worthy of respect. Respect includes seeking out and honoring clients' wishes regarding quality of life. Decision-making about life-sustaining treatment carefully balances these considerations.

5. Nurses intervene if others fail to respect the dignity of clients.

6. Nurses advocate the dignity of clients in the use of technology in the health care setting.

7. Nurses advocate health and social conditions that allow persons to live with dignity throughout their lives and in the process of dying. They do so in ways that are consistent with their professional role and responsibilities.

CONFIDENTIALITY

Nurses safeguard the trust of clients that information learned in the context of a professional relationship is shared outside the health care team only with the client's permission or as legally required.

1. Nurses observe practices that protect the confidentiality of each client's health and health care information.

2. Nurses intervene if other participants in the health care delivery system fail to respect client confidentiality.

3. Nurses disclose confidential information only as authorized by the client, unless there is substantial risk of serious harm to the client or other persons, or a legal obligation to disclose. Where disclosure is warranted, both the amount of information disclosed and the number of people informed is restricted to the minimum necessary.

4. Nurses, whenever possible, inform their clients about the boundaries of professional confidentiality at the onset of care, including the circumstances under which confidential information might be disclosed without consent. If feasible, when disclosure becomes necessary, nurses inform clients what information will be disclosed, to whom, and for what reasons.

5. Nurses advocate policies and safeguards to protect and preserve client confidentiality and intervene if the security of confidential information is jeopardized because of a weakness in the provisions of the system, e.g., inadequate safeguarding guidelines and procedures for the use of computer databases.

FAIRNESS

Nurses apply and promote principles of equity and fairness to assist clients in receiving unbiased treatment and a share of health services and resources proportionate to their needs.

1. Nurses provide care in response to need regardless of such factors as race, ethnicity, culture, spiritual beliefs, social or marital status, gender, sexual orientation, age, health status, lifestyle or the physical attributes of the client.

2. Nurses are justified in using reasonable means to protect against violence when they anticipate acts of violence toward themselves, others or property with good reason.

3. Nurses strive to be fair in making decisions about the allocation of services and goods that they provide, when the distribution of these is within their control.

4. Nurses put forward, and advocate, the interests of all persons in their care. This includes helping individuals and groups gain access to appropriate health care that is of their choosing.

5. Nurses promote appropriate and ethical care at the institutional/agency and community levels by participating, to the extent possible, in the development, implementation, and ongoing review of policies and procedures designed to make the best use of available resources and of current knowledge and research.

6. Nurses advocate, in ways that are consistent with their role and responsibilities, health policies and decision-making procedures that are fair and comprehensive, and that promote fairness and inclusiveness in health resource allocation.

ACCOUNTABILITY

Nurses act in a manner consistent with their professional responsibilities and standards of practice.

1. Nurses comply with the values and responsibilities in this *Code of Ethics for Registered Nurses* as well as with the professional standards and laws pertaining to their practice.

2. Nurses conduct themselves with honesty and integrity.

3. Nurses, whether they are engaged in clinical, administrative, research or educational endeavors, have professional responsibilities and accountabilities toward safeguarding the quality of nursing care clients receive. These responsibilities vary but are all oriented to the expected outcome of safe, competent and ethical nursing practice.

4. Nurses, individually or in partnership with others, take preventive as well as corrective action to protect clients from unsafe, incompetent or unethical care.

5. Nurses base their practice on relevant knowledge, and acquire new skills and knowledge in their area of practice on a continuing basis, as necessary for the provision of safe, competent and ethical nursing care.

6. Nurses, whether engaged in clinical practice, administration, research or education, provide timely and accurate feedback to other nurses about their practice, so as to support safe and competent care and contribute to ongoing learning. By so doing, they also acknowledge excellence in practice.

7. Nurses practice within their own level of competence. They seek additional information or knowledge; seek the help, and/or supervision and help, of a competent practitioner; and/or request a different work assignment, when aspects of the care required are beyond their level of competence. In the meantime, nurses provide care within the level of their skill and experience.

8. Nurses give primary considerations to the welfare of clients and any possibility of harm in future care situations when they suspect unethical conduct or incompetent or unsafe care. When nurses have reasonable grounds for concern about the behavior of colleagues in this regard, or about the safety of conditions in the care setting, they carefully review the situation and take steps, individually or in partnership with others, to resolve the problem.

9. Nurses support other nurses who act in good faith to protect clients from incompetent, unethical or unsafe care, and advocate work environments in which nurses are treated with respect when they intervene.

10. Nurses speaking on nursing and health-related matters in a public forum or a court provide accurate and relevant information.

PRACTICE ENVIRONMENTS CONDUCIVE TO SAFE, COMPETENT AND ETHICAL CARE

Nurses advocate practice environments that have the organizational and human support systems, and the resource allocations necessary for safe, competent and ethical nursing care.

1. Nurses collaborate with nursing colleagues and other members of the health team to advocate health care environments that are conducive to ethical practice and to the health and well-being of clients and others in the setting. They do this in ways that are consistent with their professional role and responsibilities.

2. Nurses share their nursing knowledge with other members of the health team for the benefit of clients. To the best of their abilities, nurses provide mentorship and guidance for the professional development of students of nursing and other nurses.

3. Nurses seeking professional employment accurately state their area(s) of competence and seek reasonable assurance that employment conditions will permit care consistent with the values and responsibilities of the code, as well as with their personal ethical beliefs.

4. Nurses practice ethically by striving for the best care achievable in the circumstances. They also make the effort, individually or in partnership with others, to improve practice environments by advocating on behalf of their clients as possible.

5. Nurses planning to participate in job action, or who practice in environments where job action occurs, take steps to safeguard the health and safety of clients during the course of the action.

APPENDIX D

Code for Nurses–
Ethical Concepts
Applied to Nursing
International Council of Nurses

Reproduced with permission from the International Council of National Representatives in 1973 and reaffirmed in 1989. ICN Code for Nurses: Ethical Concepts Applied to Nursing. Geneva

The fundamental responsibility of the nurse is fourfold: to promote health, to prevent illness, to restore health and to alleviate suffering.

The need for nursing is universal. Inherent in nursing is respect for life, dignity and rights of man. It is unrestricted by considerations of nationality, race, creed, colour, age, sex, politics or social status.

Nurses render health services to the individual, the family and the community and coordinate their services with those of related groups.

NURSES AND PEOPLE

The nurse's primary responsibility is to those people who require nursing care.

The nurse, in providing care, promotes an environment in which the values, customs and spiritual beliefs of the individual are respected.

The nurse holds in confidence personal information and uses judgment in sharing this information.

NURSES AND PRACTICE

The nurse carries personal responsibility for nursing practice and for maintaining competence by continual learning.

The nurse maintains the highest standards of nursing care possible within the reality of a specific situation.

The nurse uses judgment in relation to individual competence when accepting and delegating responsibilities.

The nurse when acting in a professional capacity should at all times maintain standards of personal conduct which reflect credit upon the profession.

NURSES AND SOCIETY

The nurse shares with other citizens the responsibility for initiating and supporting action to meet the health and social needs of the public.

NURSES AND CO-WORKERS

The nurse sustains a cooperative relationship with co-workers in nursing and other fields.

The nurse takes appropriate action to safeguard the individual when his care is endangered by a co-worker or any other person.

NURSES AND THE PROFESSION

The nurse plays the major role in determining and implementing desirable standards of nursing practice and nursing education.

The nurse is active in developing a core of professional knowledge.

The nurse, acting through the professional organization, participates in establishing and maintaining equitable social and economic working conditions in nursing.

Glossary

Accountability   The state of being answerable to someone for something one has done.

Active voluntary euthanasia   An act in which the physician both provides the means of death for a patient, such as a lethal dose of medication, and administers it.

Activism   A passionate approach to everyday activities that is committed to seeking a more just social order through critical analysis, provocation, transformation, and rebalancing of power.

Act-utilitarianism   A basic type of utilitarianism that suggests people choose actions that will, in any given circumstance, increase the overall good.

Administrative law   The branch of law that consists mainly of the legal powers granted to administrative agencies by the legislature and the rules that the agencies make to carry out their powers.

Advance directives   Instructions that indicate which health care interventions to initiate or withhold, or which designate someone who will act as a surrogate in making such decisions, in the event that a person loses decision making capacity.

Allocative policies   Policies designed to provide net benefits to some distinct group or class of individuals or organizations, at the expense of others, in order to ensure that public objectives are met.

Anonymity   A situation in which even the researcher cannot link information with a particular participant in a study.

Appeals to conscience   Personal and subjective beliefs, founded on a prior judgment of rightness or wrongness, that are motivated by personal sanction rather than external authority.

Assault   The unjustifiable attempt or threat to touch a person without consent that results in fear of immediately harmful or threatening contact.

Assisted suicide   A situation in which patients receive the means of death from someone such as a physician, but activate the process themselves.

Authority   The state of having legitimate power and sovereignty.

Autonomy   An ethical principle that literally means self-governing. It denotes having the freedom to make independent choices.

Axiology   The branch of philosophy that studies the nature and types of values.

Battery   The unlawful touching of another or the carrying out of threatened physical harm including every willful, angry, and violent or negligent touching of another's person, clothes, or anything attached to his or her person or held by him or her.

Belmont Report   Policies developed by the United States National Commission for the Protection of Human Subjects of Biomedical and Behavioral Research (1978) regarding ethical principles for research with human subjects.

Beneficence   The ethical principle that requires one to act in ways that benefit another. *In research*, this implies the protection from harm and discomfort, including a balance between the benefits and risks of a study.

Cartesian philosophy   A widespread belief during the Renaissance related to Descartes's proposal that the universe is a physical thing and all therein is analogous to machines that can be analyzed and understood, and that the mind and body are separate entities.

Categorical imperative   The Kantian maxim stating that no action can be judged as right which cannot reasonably become a law by which every person should always abide.

Character ethics   Theories of ethics, sometimes called virtue ethics, that are related to the concept of innate moral virtue.

Cheating   Dishonesty and deception regarding examinations, projects, or papers.

Civil law   (Also called private law) The law that determines a person's legal rights and obligations in many kinds of activities involving other people.

Codes of nursing ethics   Explicit declarations of the primary goals and values of the profession that indicate the profession's acceptance of the responsibility and trust with which it has been invested by society.

Coercion   Actual or implied threat of harm or penalty for not participating in a research project, or offering excessive rewards for participation in the project.

Common law   A system of law, also known as case law, based largely on previous court decisions. In this system, decisions are based upon earlier court rulings in similar cases, or precedents. Over time these precedents take on the force of law.

Communitarian theories   Theories of justice that place the community, rather than the individual, the state, the nation, or any other entity, at the center of the value system; that emphasize the value of public goods; and that conceive of values as rooted in communal practices.

Compassion   A focal virtue combining an attitude of active regard for another's welfare with an imaginative awareness and emotional response of deep sympathy, tenderness, and discomfort at the other person's misfortune or suffering.

Competence   A person's ability to make meaningful life decisions. A declaration of incompetence involves legal action with a ruling by a judge that the person is unable to make such life decisions.

Complementary therapies   Therapeutic interventions that derive from traditions other than conventional Western medicine which are used by patients with or without the knowledge of conventional medical practitioners.

Confidentiality   The ethical principle that requires nondisclosure of private or secret information with which one is entrusted. *In research*, confidentiality refers to the researcher's assurance to participants that information provided will not be made public or available to anyone other than those involved in the research process without the participant's consent.

Consequentialism   A theory of ethics, sometimes called utilitarianism.

Constitutional law   A formal set of rules and principles that describe the powers of a government and the rights of the people.

Contract   An agreement between two or more people that can be enforced by law.

Contract law   A type of law that deals with the rights and obligations of people who make contracts.

Cosmology   A branch of philosophy that describes the structure, origin, and processes of the universe.

Covert values   Expectations that are not in writing which are often identified only through participation in or controversies within an organization or institution.

Criminal law   A type of law that deals with crimes, or actions considered harmful to society.

Cultural awareness   Knowledge about values, beliefs, behaviors, and the like of cultures other than one's own.

Cultural competence   Skill in dealing with transcultural issues which is demonstrated through cultural awareness and cultural sensitivity.

Cultural sensitivity   The ability to incorporate a patient's cultural perspective into nursing assessments and to modify nursing care in order to be as congruent as possible with the patient's cultural perspective.

Culture   The total lifeways of a group of interacting individuals, consisting of *learned* patterns of values, beliefs, behaviors, and customs shared by that group.

Decision making capacity   The ability of a person to understand all information about a health condition, to communicate understanding and choices, and to reason and deliberate; and, the possession of personal values and goals that guide the decision.

Declaration of Helsinki   Principles issued by the World Medical Assembly to guide clinical research in 1964 and revised in 1975.

Defamation   Harm that occurs to a person's reputation and good name, diminishes others' value or esteem, or arouses negative feelings toward the person by the communication of false, malicious, unprivileged, or harmful words.

Deontology   Related to the term *duty*, deontology is a group of ethical theories based upon the rationalist view that the rightness or wrongness of an act depends upon the nature of the act, rather than the consequences that occur as a result of it.

Discernment   A focal virtue of sensitive insight, acute judgment, and understanding that eventuates in decisive action.

Disease   The biomedical explanation of sickness.

Distributive justice   Application of the ethical principle of justice that relates to fair, equitable, and appropriate distribution in society determined by justified norms that structure the terms of social cooperation. Its scope includes policies that allot diverse benefits and burdens such as property, resources, taxation, privileges, and opportunities.

Diversity The experience within nursing of differences among colleagues and patients in areas such as gender, age, socioeconomic position, sexual orientation, health status, ethnicity, race, or culture.

Do not resuscitate (DNR) orders Written directives placed in a patient's medical chart indicating that cardiopulmonary resuscitation is to be avoided.

Durable power of attorney Allows a competent person to designate another as a surrogate or proxy to act on her or his behalf in making health care decisions in the event of the loss of decision making capacity.

Egalitarian theories Theories of justice that promote ideals of equal distribution of social benefits and burdens and recognize the social obligation to eliminate or reduce barriers that prevent fair equality of opportunity.

Empirical Knowledge gained through the processes of observation and experience.

Empowerment A helping process and partnership, enacted in the context of love and respect for self and others, through which individuals and groups are enabled to change situations, and are given skills, resources, opportunities and authority to do so. It involves creating a vision, taking risks, making choices, and behaving in authentic ways.

Ethical dilemma Occurs when there are conflicting moral claims.

Ethical principles Basic and obvious moral truths that guide deliberation and action. Major ethical principles include autonomy, beneficence, nonmaleficence, veracity, confidentiality, justice, fidelity, and others.

Ethical treatment of data Implies integrity of research protocols and honesty in reporting findings.

Ethic of care An approach to ethical decision making grounded in relationship and mutual responsibility in which choices are contextually bound and strategies are focused on maintaining connections and not hurting anyone.

Ethic of justice An approach to ethical decision making based on objective rules and principles in which choices are made from a stance of separateness.

Ethics A formal process for making logical and consistent decisions based upon moral beliefs.

Ethnocentrism Judging behaviors of someone from another culture by the standards of one's own culture.

Euthanasia Causing the painless death of a person in order to end or prevent suffering.

Expertise The characteristic of having a high level of specialized skill and knowledge.

External locus of control The belief that forces outside of oneself direct or rule one's life, whether these be generalized forces such as fate or other persons who are perceived as more powerful.

External standards of nursing practice Guides for nursing care that are developed by non-nurses, legislation, or institutions.

Faith A generic feature of the human struggle to find and maintain meaning flowing from an integration of ways of knowing and valuing.

False imprisonment The unlawful, unjustifiable detention of a person within fixed boundaries, or an act intended to result in such confinement.

Felonies Serious crimes that carry significant fines and jail sentences. Examples of felonies include first and second degree murder, arson, burglary, extortion, kidnaping, rape, and robbery.

Fidelity An ethical principle related to the concept of faithfulness and the practice of promise-keeping.

Forgery Includes fraud or intentional misrepresentation.

Formalism A term often used to refer to deontology.

Fraud A deliberate deception for the purpose of securing an unfair or unlawful gain.

Full disclosure Indicates that a research participant must be fully informed of the nature of a study, anticipated risks and benefits, time commitment, expectations of the participant and the researcher, and the right to refuse to participate.

Genetic diagnosis A process of biopsy of embryos to determine the presence of genetic flaws and gender prior to implantation.

Genetic engineering The ability to genetically alter organisms for a variety of purposes, particularly to promote their health and strength.

Genetic screening A process for determining whether persons are predisposed to certain diseases and whether couples have the possibility of giving birth to a genetically impaired infant.

Grassroots lobbying Lobbying efforts that involve mobilizing a committed constituency to influence the opinions of policy makers.

Guardian *ad litem* A court appointed guardian for a particular action or proceeding; such a guardian may not oversee all of the person's affairs.

Health policies Authoritative decisions focusing on health that are made in the legislative, executive, or judicial branches of government and are intended to direct or influence the actions, behaviors, or decisions of others; their lifestyles and personal behaviors; and improvements in the availability, accessibility, and quality of their health care services.

Illness A personal response to disease flowing from how one's culture teaches one to be sick.

Informed consent A process by which patients are informed of the possible outcomes, alternatives, and risks of treatments and required to freely give their consent. This implies legal protection of a patient's right to personal autonomy by providing the opportunity to choose a course of action regarding plans for health care, including the right to refuse medical recommendations and to choose from available therapeutic alternatives. *In research*, this refers to consent to participate in a research study after the research purpose, expected commitment, risks and benefits, any invasion of privacy, and ways that anonymity and confidentiality will be addressed have been explained.

Integrity   Refers to adherence to moral norms that is sustained over time. Implicit in integrity is trustworthiness and a consistency of convictions, actions, and emotions.

Intentional torts   Willful or intentional acts that violate another person's rights or property.

Internal locus of control   The belief that one is able to influence or control things that happen in one's life.

Internal standards of nursing practice   Standards of nursing practice that are developed within the profession of nursing.

Invasion of privacy   Includes intrusion on the patient's physical and mental solitude or seclusion, public disclosure of private facts, publicity that places the patient in a false light in the public eye, or appropriation for the defendant's benefit or advantage of the patient's name or likeness.

Journals   Personal written records kept on a periodic or regular basis containing factual material and subjective interpretations of events, thoughts, feelings, and plans.

Judicial decisions   Authoritative court decisions that direct or influence the actions, behaviors, or decisions of others.

Justice   An ethical principle that relates to fair, equitable, and appropriate treatment in light of what is due or owed to persons, recognizing that giving to some will deny receipt to others who might otherwise have received these things. *In research*, justice implies the rights of fair treatment and privacy, including anonymity and confidentiality.

Kantianism   A deontological theory of ethics based upon the writings of the philosopher Immanuel Kant.

Law   The system of enforceable principles and processes that governs the behavior of people in respect to relationships with others and with the government.

Libel   Printed defamation by written words and images that injure a person's reputation or cause others to avoid, ridicule, or view the person with contempt.

Libertarian theories   Theories of distributive justice that propose that the just society protects the rights of property and liberty of each person, allowing citizens to improve their circumstances by their own effort.

Living wills   Legal documents developed voluntarily by persons giving directions to health care providers related to withholding or withdrawing life support if certain conditions exist.

Lobbying   The art of persuasion—attempting to convince a legislator, a government official, the head of an agency, or a state official to comply with a request—whether it is convincing them to support a position on an issue or to follow a particular course of action.

Locus of control   Beliefs about the ability to control events in one's life.

Loyalty   Showing sympathy, care, and reciprocity to those with whom we appropriately identify; working closely with others toward shared goals; keeping promises; making mutual concerns a priority; sacrificing personal interests to the relationship; and giving attention to these over a substantial period of time.

Malpractice   The form of negligence in which any professional misconduct, unreasonable lack of professional skill, or nonadherence to the accepted standard of care causes injury to a patient or client.

Managed care   An integrated form of health care delivery and financing that represents attempts to control costs by modifying the behavior of providers and patients.

Material rules   Rules by which distributive justice decisions regarding entitlement are made.

Medical futility   Situations in which medical interventions are judged to have no medical benefit, or in which the chance for success is low.

Misdemeanor   A criminal offense of a less serious nature than a felony, usually punishable by a fine or short jail sentence, or both.

Moral development   A product of the sociocultural environment in which one lives and develops that reflects the intellectual and emotional process through which one learns and incorporates values regarding right and wrong.

Moral distress   The reaction to a situation in which there are moral problems that seem to have clear solutions, yet one is unable to follow one's moral beliefs because of external restraints. This may be evidenced in anger, frustration, dissatisfaction, and poor performance in the work setting.

Moral integrity   A focal virtue that relates to soundness, reliability, wholeness, an integration of character, and fidelity in adherence to moral norms sustained over time.

Moral philosophy   The philosophical discussion of what is considered to be good or bad, right or wrong.

Moral thought   Individuals' cognitive examination of right and wrong, good and bad.

Moral values   Preferences or dispositions reflective of right or wrong, should or should not, in human behavior.

Naturalism   A view of moral judgment that regards ethics as dependent upon human nature and psychology.

Negligence   The omission to do something that a reasonable person, guided by those ordinary considerations that ordinarily regulate human affairs, would do, or doing something that a reasonable and prudent person would not do.

Noncompliance   Denoting an unwillingness on the part of the patient to participate in health care activities that have been recommended by health care providers.

Nonmaleficence   An ethical principle related to beneficence that requires one to act in such a manner as to avoid causing harm to another, including deliberate harm, risk of harm, and harm that occurs during the performance of beneficial acts.

Nuremberg Code A set of principles for the ethical conduct of research against which the experiments in the Nazi concentration camps could be judged.

Nurse practice acts Legislative statutes within each state that define nursing, describe boundaries of practice, establish standards for nurses, and protect the domain of nursing.

Nursing process A model commonly used for decision making in nursing.

Nursism A form of sexism that maligns the caring role in society and leads to discrimination in nursing by virtue of the role undertaken, regardless of gender.

Obligation Being required to do something by virtue of a moral rule, a duty, or some other binding demand such as a particular role or relationship.

Overt values Values of individuals, groups, institutions, and organized systems that are explicitly communicated through philosophy and policy statements.

Parentalism A nongender term that parallels the meaning of paternalism while avoiding gender bias.

Partisan Adherence to the ideology of a particular political party.

Paternalism A gender biased term that literally means acting in a "fatherly" manner, the traditional view of which implies well intended actions of benevolent decision making, leadership, protection, and discipline, which, in the health care arena, manifest in the making of decisions on behalf of patients without their full consent or knowledge.

Patient Self-Determination Act A federal law requiring institutions such as hospitals, nursing homes, health maintenance organizations, and home care agencies receiving Medicare or Medicaid funds to provide written information to adult patients regarding their rights to make health care decisions.

Philosophy The intense and critical examination of beliefs and assumptions.

Plagiarism Taking another's ideas or work and presenting them as one's own.

Plaintiff The term used for the complaining or injured party in a lawsuit.

Policy formulation A phase of the policy making process that includes such actions as agenda setting and the subsequent development of legislation.

Policy implementation A phase of the policy making process that follows enactment of legislation and includes taking actions and making additional decisions necessary to implement legislation such as rule making and policy operation.

Policy modification A phase of the policy making process that exists to improve or perfect legislation previously enacted.

Political Relates to the complex process of policy making within the government.

Political issues Those issues that are regulated or influenced by decisions within either the executive, judicial, or legislative branches of government.

Political parties Organized groups with distinct ideology that seek to control government.

Power The ability to do or act; the capability of doing or accomplishing something.

Practical dilemma   A situation in which moral claims compete with nonmoral claims.

Practical imperative   The Kantian maxim requiring that one treat others always as ends and never as a means.

Precedents   Court rulings upon which subsequent rulings in similar cases are based. Over time these precedents take on the force of law.

Principles   Basic and obvious truths that guide deliberation and action.

Private law   (Also called civil law) The law that determines a person's legal rights and obligations in many kinds of activities involving other people.

Profession   A complex, organized occupation preceded by a long training program geared toward the acquisition of exclusive knowledge necessary to provide a service that is essential or desired by society, leading to a monopoly that provides autonomy, public recognition, prestige, power, and authority for the practitioner.

Public law   Law that defines a person's rights and obligations in relation to government and describes the various divisions of government and their powers.

Quality of life   A subjective appraisal of factors that make life worth living and contribute to a positive experience of living.

Racism   The assumption that members of one race are superior to those of another.

Rationalism   A view of moral judgment that regards truth as necessary, universal, and superior to the information received from the senses—having an origin in the nature of the universe or in the nature of a higher being.

Regulatory policies   Policies that are designed to influence the actions, behaviors, and decisions of others through directive techniques.

Religion   The codification of beliefs and practices concerning the Divine and one's relationship with the Divine that are shared by a group of people.

Religiosity   Beliefs and practices that are the expressive aspects of religion.

Respect for human dignity   Implies the rights of patients to full disclosure and self-determination regarding participation in research and in making health care choices.

Respect for persons   An attitude by which one considers others to be worthy of high regard.

Right to fair treatment   Assures equitable treatment of participants in the research selection process, during the study, and after the completion of the study.

Right to privacy   The right to be left alone or to be free from unwanted publicity. *In research*, this is the right of research participants to determine when, where, and what kind of information is shared, with an assurance that information and observations are treated with respect and kept in strict confidence.

Rules or **regulations**   Policies that are established to guide the implementation of laws and programs.

Rule-utilitarianism   A type of utilitarianism that suggests people choose rules that, when followed consistently, will maximize the overall good.

Self-awareness   Conscious awareness of one's thoughts, feelings, physical and emotional responses, and insights in various situations.

Sexism   The assumption that members of one sex are superior to those of the other.

Sexual harassment   All unwelcome sexual advances, request for sexual favors, and other conduct of a sexual nature.

Slander   Defamation that occurs when one speaks unprivileged or false words about another.

Spectrum of urgency   A spectrum depicting the degree of urgency in health care decision making, ranging from minor and nonurgent to severe and very urgent.

Spirituality   The animating force, life principle, or essence of being that permeates life and is expressed and experienced in multifaceted connections with self, others, nature, and God or Life Force.

Standards of nursing practice   Written documents outlining minimum expectations for nursing care.

Statutes or **laws**   Legislation that has been enacted by legislative bodies and approved by the executive branch of government.

Statutory (legislative) law   Formal laws written and enacted by federal, state, or local legislatures.

Stereotyping   Expecting all persons from a particular group to behave, think, or respond in a certain way based on preconceived ideas.

Sympathy   Sharing, in imagination, of others' feelings.

Theory   A proposed explanation for a class of phenomena.

Tort   A wrong or injury that a person suffers because of someone else's action, either intentional or unintentional. The action may cause bodily harm; damage a person's property, business, or reputation; or make unauthorized use of a person's property.

Trustworthiness   A focal virtue that results in recognition by others of one's consistency and predictability in following moral norms.

Unintentional torts   Torts that occur when an act or omission causes unintended injury or harm to another person.

Utilitarianism   A moral theory which holds that an action is judged as good or bad in relation to the consequence, outcome, or end result derived from it.

Utility   The property of usefulness in any object, whereby it tends to produce benefit, advantage, pleasure, good, or happiness or prevent mischief, pain, evil, or unhappiness.

Values   Ideals, beliefs, customs, modes of conduct, qualities, or goals that are highly prized or preferred by individuals, groups, or society.

Values clarification   Refers to the process of becoming more conscious of and naming what one values or considers worthy.

Values conflict   Internal or interpersonal conflict that occurs in circumstances in which personal values are at odds with those of patients, colleagues, or the institution.

Veracity Truth-telling.

Victim blaming Holding the people burdened by social conditions accountable for their own situations and responsible for needed solutions.

Virtue ethics Theories of ethics, usually attributed to Aristotle, which represent the idea that an individual's actions are based upon innate moral virtue.

Index

Italicized page numbers indicate illustrations

A

Abortion, 211–212
Academic honesty, 219–220
Accountability, 141–145
Achterberg, Jeanne, 6–7, 9–12, 15, 236, 302–303
Active voluntary euthanasia, 212
Activism, 264
Act-utilitarianism, 29
Adams, K., 84
Administrative law, 112
Advance directives, 186, 205–206
Africa, 246
African-American nurse, 304
African-Americans, 293, 297
Agency for Health Care Policy and Research, 262
AIDS, 55, 213–214, 246
Alexander the Great, 236
Allanach, E.J., 89
Allocative policies, 257
Altruism, 158
American Assembly for Men in Nursing, 306
American Journal of Nursing, 135
American Medical Association (AMA), 139, 241
American Nurses Association (ANA), 141, 144, 221, 302
    guidelines for human rights protection, *222–223*
Americans with Disabilities Act (1990), 167
Amott, T., 303–304
Ancient cultures, 6–7
Anonymity, 224
Appeals to conscience, 153
Aristotle, 33–34
Aroskar, M.A., 337
Artificial sources of nutrition, 185–186
Asia, 246
Assault, 120–121
Assisted suicide, 212
Attitudes, 191
Authority, 145–146
Autonomy, 40–47, 127, 138–141, 197–199, 295
    defined, 40–41
    four elements of, 41
    informed consent, 44
    noncompliance, 46–47
    paternalism, 45–46
    violations of in patients, 42–44
Axiology, 81
Aydelotte, M., 146

B

Baldwin, C., 84
Baldwin, D., 303
Bandman, B., 274–275
Bandman, E.L., 274–275
Barstow, A.L., 14–15
Batra, C., 262
Battery, 120–121
Beauchamp, T., 34–35, 64, 260–261, 273, 277
Begany, T., 306
Beletz, E., 137, 147
Belmont Report, 222
Beneficence, 47–48, 175, 222–223, 294–295
Benjamin, M., 163
Benokraitis, N.V., 310
Bentham, Jeremy, 28–29
Bethiaume v. Pratt, 119–120
Big Town Nursing Home, Inc. v. Newman, 121
Bill of Rights, 111
Bixler, Genevieve, 135–136, 145
Bixler, Roy, 135–136, 145
Blackman for Blackman v. Rifkin, 121
Blue Cross, 242
Bok, S., 52
Brody, H., 183
Brown, L.S., 293
Buber, Martin, 23, 50
Buddha, 23
Bullough, V., 307
Burg, M.A., 288
Burns, 118–119
Butler, S.S., 289

C

Califano, A.A., Jr., 279
California, 305
Callahan, S., 68–69
Campbell, D.W., 297
Campbell-Heider, N., 310
Canada, 245
Cardiopulmonary resuscitation (CPR), 183–185
Caring, 192–193, 306–307
Cartesian philosophy, 10
Categorical imperative, 31
Certificate of Need programs, 279
Character ethics, 33
Charnock, A., 311
Cheating, 219
Childress, J., 34–35, 64, 153, 260–261, 273, 277
China, 246–247

Chinn, P.L., 306
Christian era, early, 7–8, 12
Christianity, 237
Christian sects, 329
Christrooms, 7
Civil law, 114–122
Civil Rights Act (1964), 166, 304
Civil Rights Act (1991), 168
Claims-made policies, 128
Clinton, Bill, 280
Cobb, A.K., 353
Code for Nurses (International Council of Nurses), 382–383
Code for Nurses with Interpretive Statements (ANA), 357–369
Code of Ethics (AMA), 52
Code of Ethics for Registered Nurses (Canadian Nurses Association), 374–381
Code of Federal Regulations, 225–226
Codes of nursing ethics, 142
Coercion, 224
Cognitive development, stages of (Piaget), 96
Common law, 112
Communication, 126, 191–192, 326
    and gender, 308–310
Communitarianism, 277–278
Compassion, 35
Complementary therapies, 210, 325–326
Confidentiality, 53–56, 214, 224
Confucius, 23
Connelly, L.M., 353
Conscientious practice, 126–127
Consequentialism, 28
Constitutional law, 111
Contract, 114
Contract law, 114
Cosmology, 6
Counterculture, 329
Covert values, 87
Creighton, H., 115–117, 121
Criminal law, 112–113
Crusades, 9, 12–13
Cuba, 244
Cultural awareness, 318
Cultural competence, 318
Cultural sensitivity, 318
Culture, 319
Curtin, Leah, 162, 165, 186, 343, 345–346
Curtis, J., 163

D

Dark Period of Nursing, 10

Davidhizar, R.E., 322
Davis, A.J., 192
Death and dying, 176–179, 324
DeBlois, Jean, 272, 280
Declaration of Helsinki, 222
Defamation, 121–122
Demi, A.S., 297
Deontology, 31–32, 110
Descartes, Rene, 10
Desmond, S.M., 295
Diagnostic Related Grouping, 243, 279
Discernment, 35
Discrimination, 165–169
Disease, 320
Disparate impact, 166
Disparate treatment, 166
Distributive justice, 57, 57, 273
    distribution of resources, 276
    entitlement, 273–276
    fair distribution, 276
    theories of, 277–278
Diversity, 318, 344
Dock, Lavinia Lloyd, 16, 262
Doctor-nurse game, 308–309
Dolan, J.A., 7–8
Domestic violence, 289–290
Donabedian, A., 141, 145–146
Donahue, M.P., 10
Do not resuscitate (DNR) order, 181, 183–185
Dowell, M., 166
Doyle, E.I., 91
Durable power of attorney, 205–206

E

Economic issues, 271–273
    distributive justice, 273–278
    recent trends in, 278–282
Egalitarianism, 278
Ehrenreich, B., 15
Eisler, R., 289
Elderly, 291–292
Eldridge, N.S., 297
Ellin, Joseph, 52
Emotional distress, intentional infliction of, 117
Emotions, 68–69
Empirical, 8
Employer-sponsored coverage, 128
Employment negotiated insurance plans, 279
Empowerment, 127
    for nurses
        compared with power, 340–341
        personal, 341–343
        professional, 343–344
    for patients, 350–354
English, D., 15
Entitlement, 273–276
Eoff, T.A., 295
Epicurus, 28

Equal Employment Opportunity Commission (EEOC), 166, 307
Erb, G., 109
Esposito, C.N., 290
Ethical decision making
    and emotions, 68–69
    and nursing process, 67
    process of, 69–72, 72–73
        applying, 73–75
    and scientific process, 67–68
Ethical dilemma, 64–65
Ethical principles
    autonomy, 40–47
    beneficence, 47–48
    confidentiality, 53–56
    defined, 40
    fidelity, 58
    justice, 57–58
    nonmaleficence, 48–49
    veracity, 50–53
Ethic of caring, 98
Ethic of justice, 98
Ethics
    defined, 24
    and law, 109–110
    in managed care, 281–282
    and nursing, 22–23
    in policy making, 260–261
    and social issues, 294–295
    theories of, 26–27
        deontology, 31–32
        philosophical basis for, 25–26
        utilitarianism, 28–30
        virtue ethics, 33–36
Ethnocentrism, 319
Euthanasia, 179–180, 212
Ewing, W.A., 296
Expertise, 137
Expert witnesses, 128–129
External locus of control, 352
External standards of nursing practice, 143

F

Fair distribution, 276
Fair treatment, right to, 224
Faith, 99
    development, stages of (Fowler), 99–100
Falls, 116
False imprisonment, 121
Farquhar, M., 174
Feagin, J.R., 310
Fee-for-service, 272
Feelings, 342
Feist-Price, S., 307
Felony, 113
Fidelity, 58
Fiesta, J., 116, 120, 123, 280–281
Fishman, D., 129
Flaherty, M., 162
Flexner, Abraham, 135–136
Floating, 155
Focal virtues, 34–35

Folk healers, 13
Foolchand, M., 304
Foot, Phillipa, 34
Foreseeability, 56
Forgery, 219
Formalism, 31
Fowler, B.A., 293
Fowler, J.W., 95–96, 99–100, 102, 136
France, 244
Fraud, 119
Friedman, J., 168
Full disclosure, 224
Furrow, B.R., 117

G

Gadow, S., 153
Gallop, R., 306
Gays, 311–312
Gender issues
    communication, 308–310
    historical perspectives on, 302–303
    and race, 303–304
    sex discrimination in nursing, 304–307
    sexism, 310–311
    sexual harassment in nursing, 307–308
    sexual orientation, 311–312
Genetic diagnosis, 189
Genetic engineering, 189
Genetic screening, 189
Germany, 244
Gibson, C.H., 340, 350–351
Gibson, J., 67
Giger, J.N., 322
Gilligan, C., 96, 98–100
Gilloran, A., 305
Gingerich, B.S., 88
Glossary, 385–395
Golden, B.M., 89
Golden mean, 34
Goodman, L.A., 293
Gossip, 310
Grassroots lobbying, 264
Great Britain, 245
Great Depression, 242
Greeks, 236
Grigsby, K., 306
Group, T.M., 16
Group coverage, 128
Group practices, 241
Gruending, D.L., 134
Guardian *ad litem,* 187
Guido, G.W., 128
Gurka, A.M., 340

H

Hadley, E., 263
Hagerdorn, S., 264
Harassment, 165–169
Hardwig, J., 199

Harm principle, 55–56
Hart, C., 310
Hartman Value Profile, 88
Healer, 6
Health care delivery, 235
　　alternative traditions in, 246–247
　　and culture, 324
　　global concerns, 243–245
　　history of
　　　　early eras of, 236–237
　　　　Middle Ages and Reformation, 237
　　　　in United States, 238–243, *239–240*
　　for rural and urban populations, 247–248
Health care financing, 272
Health care reform, 280
Health insurance, 242–243
Health policy
　　defined, 257
　　ethics in, 260–261
　　formulation of, 258–259
　　implementation of, 259–260
　　modification of, 260
　　and nursing, 262–263
　　regulatory policies, 257–258
　　research data in, 261–262
Henderson, Virginia, 45
Heterosexism, 311
Hill-Burton Act (1946), 242
Hippocratic Oath, 52–53, 134
Hispanics, 293
HIV, 213–214
Homelessness, 288
Homophobia, 311
Hooker, Worthington, 30
The Hospital Hotel, 302–303
Hospitals, 238
Hostile work environment, 168
Howell, T., 309
Hufford, D.J., 325
Husted, G.L., 219
Husted, J.H., 219

I

Illness, 320
Incident reports, 160
India, 246
Individual coverage, 128
Industrial Revolution, 237
Informed consent, 44, 200
　　decision making capacity, 200–202, *201*
　　information component, 202, *202*
　　meaning of, 202–203
　　nursing role in, 204–205
　　and research subjects, 225–226
Integrity, 35, 83
Internal locus of control, 352
Internal standards of nursing practice, 142–143
Invasion of privacy, 119–120

J

Jameton, A., 3, 50–51, 66, 137–139, 147, 158, 160, 344
Japan, 244
Jecker, N.S., 176
Jehovah's Witness, 329
Jennings, C., 264
Jesus, 12
Johnson, S.H., 117
Joint Commission on Accreditation of Healthcare Organizations, 143
Jost, T.S., 117
Journaling, 84, *85*
Judeo-Christian values, 324
Judicial branch, 254
Judicial decisions, 257
Justice, 57–58, 199, 224, 273, 294. *See also* Distributive justice

K

Kant, Immanuel, 31–32, 50
Kantianism, 31
Kavanagh, K., 303
Keele, B.S., 353
Kelly, N., 169
King, Martin Luther, Jr., 110
Klein, Cathy A., 124
Kleinbeck, S.V.M., 353
Kohlberg, L., 96–98, 100–101
Korea, 246
Kozier, B., 109

L

Laing, M., 310
Language of violence, 296
Lantos, J.D., 182
Law
　　administrative, 112
　　common, 112
　　constitutional, 111
　　defined, 109
　　and ethics, 110
　　functions of, 109
　　private, 114–122
　　public, 112–114
　　statutory/legislative, 111–112, 257
　　and technology, 186–187
　　trends in, 122–124
Leininger, M., 95, 320
Lesbians, 311–312
Lewenson, 302–304
Liability insurance, 127–128
Libel, 121–122
Libertarian theories, 277
Licensure, 146
Limandri, B.J., 295
Lipkin, M., 51–52
Listening skills, 126, 351
Living wills, 205
Lo, B., 180, 183, 213
Lobbying
　　defined, 264
　　letter writing campaign, 265

methods of, 264–265
　　personal visits, 266
　　political campaigns, 267
Lockwood, M., 53
Locus of control, 352
Longest, B.B., Jr., 257, 259
Low birth weight infants, 176
Loyalty, 160–161, 339
Lyon, B., 140

M

Mahowald, M.B., 212
Malleus Maleficarum (Kramer & Sprenger), 14
Malpractice, *115,* 115–119, 279
　　claims against nurses, 123–124
　　policies, 128
　　reducing risk of litigation, *125,* 125–128
Managed care
　　ethics in, 281–282
　　legal trends involving, 122–123
　　move toward, 280–281
Markus, A., 53
Material rules, 273
Matthaei, J., 303–304
Medical futility, 180–182
Medicare, 242–243
Medication errors, 116
Megel, M., 306
Men in nursing, 305–306
Mental impairment, 167
Mentally ill, 9
Middle Ages, 8–9, 12–15, 237
Midwest Bioethics Center, 281–282
Midwives, 237
Mill, John Stuart, 29, 50
Mind sets, 337–338
Misdemeanor, 113
Monasticism, 8
Mondragon, D., 288, 293
Montessori, Maria, 165
Moral development, 95
　　theory of (Kohlberg), 97–98
Moral distress, 65–66, 88
Moral philosophy, 24
Moral thought, 3, 81
Moral values, 81
Mosaic health code, 7
A Multicultural Economic History of Women in the United States, 303–304
Munhall, P.L., 225, 229
Murphy, J.D., 144

N

National Association of Colored Graduate Nurses (NACGN), 304
National Council of State Boards of Nursing, Inc., 144
National health insurance, 245
National Organization for Women (NOW), 308

Native Americans, 293, 324
Naturalism, 25–26
Negligence, 114–115
Nietzsche, Friedrich, 58
Nightingale, Florence, 10–11, 16, 137, 168, 237, 307
Nightingale Pledge, 53, 134
Noncompliance, 43, 46–47, 208–210
Nonmaleficence, 48–49, 175, 294
Norris, P., 272
Nuremberg Code, 222
Nurse practice acts, 144–145
Nurses
    criminalization of professional negligence, 124
    empowerment for, 337–346
    as expert witnesses, 128–129
    malpractice claims against, 123–124
    and patient empowerment, 350–352
    and political issues, 255, *255–256*
    as professionals, 136–137
    relationships
        with institutions, 157–160
        with other nurses, 160–161
        with physicians, 162–164
        with subordinates, 164–165
    role in informed consent, 204–205
Nursing, 3
    and ethics, 22–23
    history of, 6–11
    men in, 305–306
    metaphors of, 338–339
    perception of by others, 339–340
    policy goals for, 263
    political strengths and weaknesses of, 263
    re-visioning, 344–346
    and role of women in society, 11–17
    sex discrimination in, 304–307
    sexual harassment in, 307–308
    and technology, 190–193
    and values development, 101–102
Nursing: A Social Policy Statement (ANA), 5
Nursing process, 67
Nursing's Agenda for Health Care Reform (ANA), 258–259
Nursing's Social Policy Statement (ANA), 5, 144
Nursism, 302
Nutrition, artificial sources of, 185–186

O

Obligations, 153–154
Occurence-based policies, 128
Old thinking, 342
Omery, A., 81

Omnibus Budget Reconciliation Act (1989), 262
Ondeck, D.A., 88
Organ transplantation, 189–190
O'Rourke, K., 272
Orthodox Muslims, 329
Oswald v. LeGrand, 117
Overt values, 87

P

Partisan, 253
Paternalism, 45–46, 197–199, 302
Patient
    belongings, loss or damage of, 116
    empowerment of, 350–354
    self-determination
        autonomy and paternalism, 197–199
        informed consent, 200–207, *201–202*
        life and health choices, 207–214
A Patient's Bill of Rights (AHA), 370–373
Patient Self-Determination Act, 206–207
Pay gap, 304
Pearlin, L.J., 292
Peer Review Organizations, 279
Pender, N.J., 90–91, 261
Peter, E., 306
Philosophy, 23–24
Physical impairment, 167
Physicians, 13, 238
Piaget, J., 96
Plagiarism, 219
Plaintiff, 114
Political, 253
Political campaigns, 267
Political issues, 253–255, *255–256*
    health policy, 257–263
    lobbying, 264–267
Political parties, 253
Position Statement on Cultural Diversity in Nursing Practice (ANA), 319
Position Statement on Nursing and the Patient Self-Determination Act (ANA), 206
Poverty, 286–287
Power, 340–341
Practical dilemma, 65
Practical imperative, 31
Precedents, 112
President's Commission for the Study of Ethical Problems, 274
Price, J.H., 295
Privacy, right of, 119, 224
Private law, 114–122
Problem solving, 152–157
Profession, 134
Professional liability insurance, 128
Professional practice standard, 202

Professional Standards Review Organizations, 279
Professional status, 134–137
Progoff, I., 84
Psychological development of women, study of (Gilligan), 98–99
Public law, 112–114

Q

Quality of life, 174
Quid pro quo sexual harassment, 168

R

Racial discrimination, 166
Racism, 293–294, 304
Rand, Ayn, 24, 158
Raphael, D.D., 24, 26, 32
Rationalism, 26
Rawls, John, 278
Reasonable person standard, 202
Reformation, 10–11, 16–17, 237
Registered Care Technician, 139
Regulations, 257
Regulatory policies, 257–258
Religion, 329
Religiosity, 330
Renaissance, 10–11, 16–17
Reproductive technology, 188
Research, 221. *See also* Scholarship issues
    characteristics of beyond human rights protection, 227–228
    ethical issues, 222–225
    informed consent, 225–226
    vulnerable populations, 227
Research data, 229–230, 261–262
Resources, distribution of, 276
Respect for human dignity, 40, 222–224
Reverby, S., 306
Risk management, *125,* 125–128
Risner, P.B., 293
Roberts, J.I., 16
Robertson v. Provident House, 120
Rodwell, C.M., 340–341
Roman Catholic Church, 9
Roman Empire, 236–237
Roosevelt, Theodore, 241
Rules, 257
Rule-utilitarianism, 29–30
Rural populations, 247–248
Russia, 243–244

S

Saint Jerome, 12
Saint Louise De Marillac, 8
Saint Thomas Aquinas, 12
Schessler v. Keck, 122
Schneider, J.K., 353
Scholarship issues
    academic honesty, 219–220
    data treatment, 229–230

research ethics, 221–228
and social concerns, 296–297
Schoof, 88
Schwartz, R.L., 117
Scofield, G.R., 185
Self-awareness, 82–83
enhancing, 83–85
Sexism, 310–311
Sexual discrimination, 304–307
Sexual harassment, 168–169,
307–308
Sexual orientation, 311–312
Shoemaker, M., 169
Sines, D., 295
Slander, 121
Slonaker, W., 165–166
Smelko v. Brinton, 119
Social issues
domestic violence, 289–290
elderly, 291–292
ethical principles applied to,
294–295
homelessness, 288
impediments to intervening with
vulnerable groups, 295–296
poverty, 286–287
racism, 293–294
and scholarship, 296–297
Social need, 3–6
Socrates, 23
South Africa, 244
Spectrum of urgency, 163
Spigner, C., 297
Spirituality, 327
assessment of, 328
defined, 327
nurturing, 331
and religion, 329–330
Sponge counts, 117
Squires, T., 305–306
Standards of nursing practice,
142–143
Standards of Nursing Practice
(ANA), 142
Stark, P.L., 291
*Statement on a Patient's Bill of
Rights* (AHA), 51
State of Louisiana v. Brenner, 113
Statutory law, 111–112, 257
Steele, T., 169
Stein, L., 309
Stereotyping, 319
Strickland, O., 129
Stromberg, A., 303
Subjective standard, 202
Sumerians, 236
Supreme Court, U.S., 254
Swart, J., 165–166
Sympathy, 26

T

Tail, 128
Tannen, D., 309
Tarsoff case, 55–56

Technology, 173
artificial sources of nutrition,
185–186
benefits and challenges of,
173–175
death and dying, 176–179
do not resuscitate orders, 181,
183–185
genetic diagnosis, engineering,
screening, 189
legal issues related to, 186–187
medically futile care, 179–182
and nursing practice, 190–193
organ/tissue transplantation,
189–190
reproductive technology, 188
withholding care, 175–176
Thailand, 246
Theory, 96
Thompson, F.J., 260
Tilden, V.P., 295
Time, 311
Tissue transplantation, 189–190
Tomlinson, T., 183
Tort law, 114–122
Torts, 114
intentional, *119,* 119–122
unintentional, 114–119
Transcultural issues, 318
complementary therapies,
325–326
cultural values and beliefs,
320–322, 320–323
culture and the health care
system, 324
legal considerations, 326
understanding culture, 319
Tripp-Reimer, T., 95
Truhitte v. French Hospital, 117
Trustworthiness, 35

U

Uganda, 246
Undue hardship, 167
United States
health care finances, 244
history of health care in,
238–243, *239–240*
United States Constitution, 111
Unity, 146–147
Universal Declaration of Human
Rights, 274
Urban populations, 247–248
Utilitarianism, 28–30, 110
Utilitarian theories, 277

V

Valentine, P., 309
Values, 81, 191
acquiring, 81–82
Values clarification
defined, 83
enhancing self-awareness, 83–85

impact of institutional values,
87–88
with patients, 89–91
in professional situations, 85–87
Values conflict, 85–87
Values development
Fowler's stages of faith
development, 99–100
Gilligan's study of the
psychological development of
women, 98–99
Kohlberg's theory of moral
development, 97–98
nursing considerations, 101–102
Piaget's stages of cognitive
development, 96
transcultural considerations in, 95
Van Ooijen, E., 311
Vasquez, M.J.T., 297
Veracity, 50–53
Victim, 343
Victim blaming, 295
Virtue ethics, 33–36
Vulnerability principle, 56
Vulnerable populations, 227,
295–296

W

Wakefield, M., 267
Warren, N.A., 297
*Washington Hospital Center v.
Butler,* 116
Watts, D., 309
Weatherley, R.A., 289
Welfare economics, 271
Wendt, A., 165–166
Western biomedical model, 324
Williams, Christine, 305–306
Wilson, H.S., 227–228
Winslow, G.R., 338
Winston, M.E., 55
Witch hunts, 14–15
Woman as Healer (Achterberg), 302
Women. *See also* Sexism
psychological development of
(Gilligan), 98–99
role of in society, 11–17
Workers' compensation, 241
World Health Organization (WHO),
246
World War I, 241
World War II, 241–242

Z

Zurlinden, J., 311